GET
THROUGH

MRCPsych CASC

GET THROUGH

MRCPsych CASC

Edited by

Melvyn W.B. Zhang, MBBS, DCP, MRCPsych,
National HealthCare Group, Singapore

Cyrus S.H. Ho, MBBS, DCP, MRCPsych,
National University of Singapore

Roger C.M. Ho, MBBS, DPM, DCP,
Gdip Psychotherapy, MMed (Psych), MRCPsych, FRCPC,
National University of Singapore

Basant K. Puri, MA, PhD, MB, BChir, BSc (Hons) MathSci,
DipStat, PG Dip Maths, MMath, FRCPsych, FRSB,
Hammersmith Hospital and Imperial College London, UK

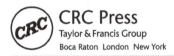

CRC Press
Taylor & Francis Group
Boca Raton London New York

CRC Press is an imprint of the
Taylor & Francis Group, an **informa** business

CRC Press
Taylor & Francis Group
6000 Broken Sound Parkway NW, Suite 300
Boca Raton, FL 33487-2742

© 2017 by Taylor & Francis Group, LLC
CRC Press is an imprint of Taylor & Francis Group, an Informa business

No claim to original U.S. Government works

Printed on acid-free paper
Version Date: 20160128

International Standard Book Number-13: 978-1-4987-0789-3 (Paperback)

Library of Congress Cataloging-in-Publication Data

Names: Zhang, Melvyn W. B., author. | Ho, Cyrus S. H., author. | Ho, Roger, author. | Puri, Basant K., author.
Title: Get through MRCPsych CASC / Melvyn W.B. Zhang, Cyrus S.H. Ho, Roger C.M. Ho, Basant K. Puri.
Other titles: Get through.
Description: Boca Raton : CRC Press/Taylor & Francis, 2016. | Series: Get through! | Includes bibliographical references and index.
Identifiers: LCCN 2016003181 (print) | LCCN 2016003998 (ebook) | ISBN 9781498707893 (pbk. : alk. paper) | ISBN 9781498707909 (e-book)
Subjects: | MESH: Psychiatry | Mental Disorders | Examination Questions
Classification: LCC RC457 (print) | LCC RC457 (ebook) | NLM WM 18.2 | DDC 616.890076--dc23
LC record available at http://lccn.loc.gov/2016003181

Visit the Taylor & Francis Web site at
http://www.taylorandfrancis.com

and the CRC Press Web site at
http://www.crcpress.com

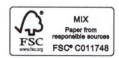

CONTENTS

PREFACE

This book consists of 152 practice stations for the Royal College of Psychiatrists Clinical Assessment of Skills and Competencies (CASC) examination. The stations have been designed to reflect the style and the types of stations commonly encountered in the MRCPsych examination at the time of this writing.

The first 135 stations modelled against the core themes have been tested in the recent MRCPsych CASC examination. While conventional CASC revision materials provide trainees with only a description of the task required in each station and the core points to cover, this book differentiates itself from other revision materials. In each of the stations covered, we provide trainees with additional information such as an outline of the station and a CASC grid with questions commonly asked in each station. The CASC grid aims to help both junior and senior trainees remember what to ask in each station. In addition, we have provided a brief synopsis of relevant conceptual information that trainees need to meet the requirements and obtain a passing grade for each station. References are provided to which the reader can refer if they are in doubt about any of the theoretical concepts.

In addition, the authors have conceptualized 15 new stations. In the MRCPsych CASC examination, it is not uncommon for entirely new stations to appear. The authors hope that including these new stations will help trainees prepare for any unexpected stations in the membership examination. The new stations have been conceptualized based on the clinical experiences of the authors as well as the latest updates on mental health information issued by the Royal College of Psychiatrists.

Trainees who are preparing for the MRCPsych examination are still encouraged to keep themselves up to date with the latest regulations and guidance issued by the Royal College of Psychiatrists.

We welcome any feedback from our readers. Please also let us know further types of questions you would like to see in the next edition of this book.

We wish to again thank all the authors who have contributed to this revision guidebook.

Melvyn W.B. Zhang, Cyrus S.H. Ho, Roger C.M. Ho, Basant K. Puri
Singapore, Cambridge and London
2015

AUTHORS

Melvyn W.B. Zhang, MBBS, DCP, MRCPsych, is a specialist registrar/senior resident at the National Healthcare Group, Singapore. He graduated from the National University of Singapore and received postgraduate training at the Institute of Mental Health, Singapore. He has a special interest in the application of web-based and smartphone technologies for education and research and has published extensively in this field. He is a member of the editorial board of the *Journal of Internet Medical Research* (Mental Health).

Cyrus S.H. Ho, MBBS, DCP, MRCPsych, is an associate consultant psychiatrist and clinical lecturer from the National University Hospital, Singapore. He graduated from the National University of Singapore, Yong Loo Lin School of Medicine, and subsequently obtained a Diploma of Clinical Psychiatry from Ireland and membership in the Royal College of Psychiatrists from the United Kingdom. As a certified acupuncturist with a graduate diploma in acupuncture conferred by the Singapore College of Traditional Chinese Medicine, he hopes to integrate both Western and Chinese medicine for holistic psychiatric care. He is actively involved in education and research work. His clinical and research interests include mood disorders, neuropsychiatry, pain studies and medical acupuncture.

Roger C.M. Ho, MBBS, DPM, DCP, GDip Psychotherapy, MMed (Psych), MRCPsych, FRCPC, is an assistant professor and consultant psychiatrist at the Department of Psychological Medicine, National University of Singapore. He graduated from the University of Hong Kong and received training in psychiatry from the National University of Singapore. He is a general adult psychiatrist and runs the Mood Disorder Clinic, National University Hospital, Singapore. He is a member of the editorial board of *Advances of Psychiatric Treatment*, an academic journal published by the Royal College of Psychiatrists. His research focuses on mood disorders, psychoneuroimmunology and liaison psychiatry.

Basant K. Puri, MA, PhD, MB, BChir, BSc (Hons) MathSci, DipStat, PG Dip Maths, MMath, FRCPsych, FSB, is based at Hammersmith Hospital and Imperial College London, United Kingdom. He reads medicine at St John's College, University of Cambridge. He also trained in molecular genetics at the MRC MNU, Laboratory of Molecular Biology, Cambridge. He has authored or co-authored more than 40 books, including *Drugs in Psychiatry* (second edition: Oxford University Press, 2013), *Textbook of Psychiatry* (third edition, with Ian Treasaden: Churchill Livingston, 2011) and *Clinical Neuropsychiatry and Neuroscience Fundamentals* (third edition, with David Moore: Taylor & Francis, 2012).

AUTHORS

STATION I: ANXIETY DISORDERS

Information to candidates

Name of patient: Sarah Green

A 35-year-old housewife has been referred by her general practitioner (GP) to your service for further assessment. She has given birth to her son, Jordan, 6 weeks ago. She has been increasingly troubled by fears that Jordan might be infected with the new variant of the H1N1 influenza virus. Owing to her distressing worries, she has been finding it increasingly difficult to care for her young baby.

Task

Take a history to arrive at a potential diagnosis.

Outline of station

The purpose of providing an outline of the station is to allow candidates to be familiar with the structure of the station. This outline could also be helpful when candidates practice for the MRCPsych, joining with their colleagues to act out the station.

Please note that the outlines provided are based on the experiences of the authors. There may be variations in the actual examination.

You are Sarah Green and have just delivered your son, Jordan, 6 weeks ago. This is your first pregnancy. You used to have obsessive–compulsive disorder (OCD), which was first diagnosed by your GP when you were age 25. You have been treated with clomipramine previously, but this medication was stopped because of excessive sedation you had from the medication. You were switched over to sertraline and have been on a stable dose. This medication was stopped around 1 year ago, when your symptoms markedly improved after a combination treatment with medication (sertraline) and psychotherapy (exposure and response prevention). After the birth of your child, those symptoms reappeared. You are troubled by recurrent ruminations pertaining to fears of contamination. This has resulted in you having to sterilize the milk bottles of your infant a fixed number of times (eight times). In addition, you have begun to have obsessional doubts and realize that you need to check things (such as switches) eight times. Your mood has been affected by your symptoms, but you still struggle to get by each day. Your family has been largely supportive, and your husband has taken over much of the care of Jordan, as you have been finding it increasingly difficult to care for your child and to ensure that he is getting his feeds on time. You start off the station telling the candidate that your mood has not been good recently after the birth of the baby. Do not be too forthcoming about your personal psychiatric history unless the candidate demonstrates empathy towards your condition.

CASC construct table

The CASC construct table is formatted such that candidates will be able to cover adequately both the range and the depth of the assessment required in this station.

Approach:
Starting off: 'Hello, I am Dr Melvyn. I have received some information from your GP regarding the difficulties that you have been having. Would you mind telling me more?'
Establishment of rapport and demonstration of empathy: 'It must have been a difficult time for you'.

Core OCD symptoms	Origin of thoughts	Nature of thoughts	Exploration of other obsessional thoughts	Exploration of compulsions	Exploration of other compulsions
a. Assessment of obsessions and compulsions – elicit origin, recurrence rate and nature of unpleasant obsessions. Elicit other obsessions. Elicit current compulsions and other associated compulsions (obsessions include fear of contamination, doubts, fear of illness and germs, symmetry and sexual or aggressive thoughts; compulsions include checking, washing and counting).	Can you tell me more about the worries that you have been having? Do the thoughts come from within your mind or are they imposed by outside persons or influences?	Are the thoughts that you have repetitive in nature? Are they bothering you consistently even though you do not wish to have them?	Are you also concerned about needing to arrange things in a special way? Do you also have thoughts, images or doubts that keep coming to your mind? *Please also ask about obsessions involving aggression, guilt, religion, sexual, etc.*	Tell me more about how you have been dealing with those obsessional thoughts. How do you feel after performing the rituals?	As a result of your obsessions, do you find yourself needing to check things very frequently? Do you find yourself needing to perform other rituals to prevent something bad from happening? Is there a particular number ritual which you need to follow? Do you have a magical number in mind?

(Continued)

Current functioning b. *Assessment of impact of illness of current functioning*	Impact of illness Can you tell me how these rituals have impacted on your life?	Have they affected other areas of your life, such as your relationships/work, etc.?	Progression of symptoms Have these symptoms worsened?		
Risk assessment c. *Assessment of risk to son, herself and others*	Risk assessment to son I am sorry to learn of the difficulties that you have been having. Are you so distressed by your circumstances that you have had thoughts of harming Jordan?	Risk assessment to patient Are you so distressed about your current circum-stances that you have thoughts of harming yourself?	Parenting abilities Are you still able to manage your son? • Attending to his daily needs • Any abuse/ neglect? Do you currently need anyone else to help you with the care of your son?		
Other symptoms d. *Exploration of comorbid mood and anxiety symptoms*	Assessment for depressive symptoms How has your mood been? Are you still interested in things you used to enjoy?	Assessment for depressive symptoms How have you been sleeping? How has your appetite been?	Assessment for depressive symptoms Have these mood symptoms come on before or after your OCD symptoms?	Assessment for depressive symptoms Are there other worries that you have been having?	Assessment for depressive symptoms Any psychotic symptoms (auditory/ visual, etc.)?
Coping mechanisms e. *Elicit coping mechanisms*	It has been a difficult time for you. Have you used alcohol to help you get through this difficult time?	Have you used any recreational substances to help you cope with this difficult time?	Any friends/ family to talk to about your problems?		

It is important to ask about the circumstances that led to onset of symptoms, previous psychiatric history and previous compliance to medications. It would also be pertinent to ask about the support given by family, possible stressors the patient faced and circumstances of pregnancy (planned/unplanned, support of husband, any problems with pregnancy).

Common pitfalls

a. Failure to demonstrate empathy towards the patient's current difficulties hence leading to failure in eliciting core symptomatology
b. Failure to cover the range and depth of the OCD symptoms – need to elicit the inherent characteristics of 'obsession' and 'compulsion'
c. Failure to perform a comprehensive risk assessment

Quick recall: OCD*

Epidemiology:

Lifetime prevalence of around 1.9%–3.0%.
Affects males and females equally.
Usual onset either between the age of 12 and 14 years or between the age of 20 and 22 years.

Diagnostic criteria (adapted from *International Statistical Classification of Diseases and Related Health Problems*, 10th revision [*ICD-10*])

a. The symptoms have to be present for at least 2 weeks in duration.
b. Obsessional symptoms are recognized as one's own.
c. There must be at least one act or thought that cannot be resisted.
d. Thoughts of carrying out the compulsion are not pleasurable.
e. Thoughts, images and impulses are experienced as being unpleasant in nature.
f. There must be interference in existing functioning.

Most common obsessions (in descending order):

a. Fear of contamination
b. Doubting
c. Fear of illness, germs or bodily symptoms
d. Symmetry
e. Sexual or aggressive thoughts

Most common compulsions (in descending order):

a. Checking
b. Washing
c. Counting

Suggested References: NICE Guidelines for OCD and BDD: http://guidance.nice.org.uk/CG26; J.L. Kolada, R.C. Bland and S.C. Newman (1994). Obsessive-Compulsive disorder. *Acta Psychiatr. Scand.* (Suppl. 376): 24–35.

---

* Adapted from B.K. Puri, A. Hall and R. Ho (2014). *Revision Notes in Psychiatry.* London, UK: CRC Press, pp. 418–420.

STATION 2: PSYCHOSIS

Information to candidates

Name of patient: John Smith

John Smith has been brought in to the hospital for an assessment today, as he went to the police and told them that he was surrendering for a terrible crime that he had committed. The medics have done basic blood and radiological investigations, and their findings indicated his physical health was normal. They have called you, the psychiatric trainee on call, to assess him.

Task

Perform a mental state examination (MSE), looking in particular for any delusional beliefs and any other psychopathology that he has.

Outline of station

You are John Smith, a 45-year-old postman. You surrendered yourself to the police today, as you firmly believe that you are totally responsible for the war that has occurred between Russia and Ukraine. You are extremely guilty for causing the war, as you feel that it is all because of a silly mistake which you made 3 months ago whilst sorting out the mails in the Royal Mail headquarters. It troubles you greatly when you see or hear of the death toll from the war. You decide to surrender yourself today as the police have been commenting and telling you that you should. Your mood is terrible, and you have been having poor sleep as the police keep speaking to you. You are extremely afraid whenever you see a white car, as you believe that it might be the police who are monitoring your every move. You have had passive suicidal ideations but have not made any suicide plans. On seeing the doctor, you demand that he give you an injection immediately, as you feel you might be better off dead than to feel guilty constantly. You will appear distracted and preoccupied at times. When asked, you tell the candidate that the police are around and speaking directly to you.

CASC construct table

The CASC construct table is formatted such that candidates will be able to cover adequately both the range and the depth of the assessment required in this station.

Approach: Be prepared for a patient who might be unforthcoming and irritable or demand an injection to end his life.
Starting off: 'Hello, I am Dr Melvyn, one of the psychiatrists from the mental health unit. I understand that the police brought you here today. Can you tell me more?'
If the patient is difficult: 'It seems to me that you are quite distressed at the moment. I'm here to help you. Can you tell me more about why you're here today?'

(Continued)

Core delusion a. Eliciting delusional beliefs and challenging beliefs	Can you tell me more as to why you feel this way?	Do you feel that you are guilty and responsible for all that has happened? Assess degree of conviction: How convinced are you: totally or partially? How did you arrive at this conclusion?	Could there be any other alternative explanations for this? Could it be because there are long-standing political tensions between the two countries?	
Other delusions b. Eliciting other delusions, such as delusional perception	Do you feel that other people are trying to harm you in any way?	Do you feel that other people are talking about you?	Do you feel that you have some special powers or abilities?	Do you feel that certain things have special meaning for you?
Hallucinations c. Eliciting hallucinations in all other modalities	Auditory hallucinations Do you hear sounds or voices that others do not hear? How many voices can you hear? Are they as clear as our current conversation? What do they say?	Second person auditory hallucinations Do they speak directly to you? Can you give me some examples of what they have been saying to you?	Third person auditory hallucinations Do they refer to you as 'he' or 'she', in the third person? Do they comment on your actions? Do they give you orders or commands as to what to do?	How do you feel when you hear them? Could there be any alternative explanation for these experiences that you have been having? Assess for other modalities of hallucination: visual, gustatory, olfactory, tactile.
Thought disorders d. Elicit thought disorders	Thought interference Do you feel that your thoughts are being interfered with? Who do you think is doing this?	Thought insertion Do you have thoughts in your head you feel are not your own? Where do you think these thoughts come from?	Thought broadcasting Do you feel that your thoughts are being broadcasted, such that others would know what you are thinking?	Thought withdrawal Do you feel that your thoughts are being taken away from your head by some external force?
e. Elicit passivity experiences	Do you feel in control of your own actions and emotions?	Do you feel that someone or something is trying to control you? Who or what do you think this would be?		
f. Impact on mood, risk assessment and coping	Has this affected your mood in any way? Are you still interested in things you used to enjoy?	Are you feeling so troubled that you have entertained thoughts of ending your life? What plans have you made?	I understand that this must be a difficult time for you. How have you been coping?	Have you made use of any substances, such as alcohol, to help you cope? What about street drugs?

Common pitfalls

a. Failure to take control of the interview/inadequate knowledge on how to handle a difficult patient
b. Failure to challenge the core delusion adequately
c. Failure to elicit other delusional beliefs and cover the range and depth of other perceptual abnormalities
d. Failure to perform a risk assessment

Quick recall*

A delusion is a false belief based on an incorrect inference about external reality that is firmly sustained despite what almost everyone else believes and despite what constitutes incontrovertible and obvious proof or evidence to the contrary. The belief is not ordinarily accepted by members of the person's culture or subculture.

It is important to differentiate between the following delusional beliefs:

a. Mood-congruent delusion: The content of the delusion is appropriate to the mood of the person.
b. Mood-incongruent delusion: The content of the delusion is not appropriate to the mood of the person.
c. Primary delusion: This refers to a delusion that arises fully formed without any discernible connection with previous events. It may be preceded by a delusional mood in which the person is aware of something strange and threatening happening.
d. Bizarre delusion: A delusion involving a phenomenon that the person's culture would regard as totally implausible.

Suggested Reference: NICE. NICE guidelines for schizophrenia: http://guidance.nice .org.uk/CG82 (accessed 1 June 2014).

STATION 3: OUTPATIENT MSE REVIEW

Information to candidates

Name of patient: Brian
Brian has been known to the mental health service since the age of 20 years. He has been previously diagnosed with schizophrenia and has had multiple previous admissions. He is here today for his routine outpatient review.

Task
Perform an MSE.

---

* Adapted from B.K. Puri, A. Hall and R. Ho (2014). *Revision Notes in Psychiatry*. London, UK: CRC Press, p. 6.

Outline of station

You are Brian and have had schizophrenia since you were 20 years old. You used to have multiple admissions to the mental health service, mostly under section. Your relapses were common due to your non-concordance to medications. In the past 2 years, you have been more regular with your medications, as you now have a community psychiatric nurse supervising you and your medications. You have been concordant to your medications since. You are here today for your routine review and will report to the psychiatrist that you have been feeling increasingly anxious recently. You do not have all the symptoms typical of an anxiety disorder. Later in the interview, you disclose to the psychiatrist that you have been feeling increasingly anxious, as you can hear the neighbours making demeaning remarks about you having schizophrenia. You hear them commenting loudly near the wall next to their house. You do not have any other first-rank symptoms. You do not use any alcohol or other recreational substances.

CASC construct table

The CASC construct table is formatted such that candidates will be able to cover adequately both the range and the depth of the assessment required in this station.

Approach: Be prepared for a patient who might be minimizing all the psychotic symptoms. Demonstration of empathy is crucial towards eliciting symptomatology.				
Starting off: 'Hello, I am Dr Melvyn, one of the psychiatrists from the mental health unit. I understand that you are here today for your routine appointment'. 'How have you been?'				
Eliciting auditory hallucinations	Auditory hallucinations Do you hear sounds or voices that others do not hear? How many voices can you hear? Are they as clear as our current conversation? What do they say?	Second person auditory hallucinations Do they speak directly to you? Can you give me some examples of what they have been saying to you?	Third person auditory hallucinations Do they refer to you as 'he' or 'she', in the third person? Do they comment on your actions? Do they give you orders or commands as to what to do?	How do you feel when you hear them? Could there be any alternative explanation for these experiences that you have been having?
Eliciting hallucinations in all other modalities	Olfactory Recently, has there been anything wrong with your sense of smell? Can you tell me more about it?	Gustatory Have you noticed that food or drink seemed to have a different taste recently?	Somatic Have you had any strange feelings in your body?	Visual Have you been able to see things that other people cannot see? What kind of things can you see? Can you give me an example? How long has this been occurring?

(Continued)

Elicit thought disorders	Thought interference	Thought insertion	Thought broadcasting	Thought withdrawal
	Do you feel that your thoughts are being interfered with? Who do you think is doing this?	Do you have thoughts in your head which you feel are not your own? Where do you think these thoughts come from?	Do you feel that your thoughts are being broadcasted, such that others would know what you are thinking?	Do you feel that your thoughts are being taken away from your head by some external force?
Elicit passivity experiences	Do you feel in control of your own actions and emotions?	Do you feel that someone or something is trying to control you? Who or what do you think this would be?		
Impact of symptoms on mood and coping mechanisms	I understand that this must be a difficult time for you. How have you been coping?	Has this affected your mood in any way? Are you still interested in the things you used to enjoy? Are there any difficulties with your sleep or appetite?	Have you made use of any substances, such as alcohol, to help you cope? What about recreational substances?	
Risk assessment – risk to self and others	Are you feeling so troubled that you have entertained thoughts of ending your life? Have you made any plans for how you are going to end your life?	Have you made any plans to confront your neighbours?		

Common pitfalls

a. Failure to cover range and depth of information
b. Failure to engage the patient (who is minimizing his symptoms to avoid being sectioned) and eliciting the core information
c. Poor time management
d. Failure to perform a risk assessment

Quick recall: Psychosis/schizophrenia*

Diagnostic criteria adapted from *ICD-10*

- At least one of the following: thought disturbances, passivity, auditory hallucinations and persistent delusional beliefs; *or*
- Two or more of the following: other persistent hallucinations, formal thought disorder, catatonic behaviour and negative symptoms

These symptoms need to be present for at least 1 month for schizophrenia.

Specifically for this station, the patient might either be still psychotic or might have residual symptoms on presentation to the outpatient clinic. The patient might also develop post-schizophrenic depression. These might be a future variation to this station.

Residual/chronic schizophrenia: This is characterized by predominantly negative symptoms. There has been past evidence of at least one schizophrenic episode and a period of at least 1 year in which the frequency of positive symptoms has been minimal, and negative schizophrenic syndrome has been present. There is absence of depression, institutionalization or dementia or other brain disorders.

Post-schizophrenic depression: This is a depressive episode arising after a schizophrenic illness. Schizophrenic illness must have occurred within the last 12 months, some symptoms still being present. Depressive symptoms fulfil at least the criteria for a depressive episode and are present for at least 2 weeks. There is an increased risk of suicide.

Diagnostic criteria Adapted from *Diagnostic and Statistical Manual of Mental Disorders*, 5th edition (*DSM-5*):

- At least two of the following: delusions, hallucinations, disorganized speech, grossly disorganized or catatonic behaviour and negative symptoms.
- Out of the two symptoms, at least one should be delusions, hallucinations or disorganized speech.
- The minimum duration of symptoms is at least 1 month.

Suggested Reference: NICE. NICE guidelines for schizophrenia: http://guidance.nice.org.uk/CG82 (accessed 1 June 2014).

STATION 4: MANIA WITH PSYCHOTIC SYMPTOMS

Information to candidates

Name of patient: Sandra Green

Miss Sandra Green has been brought in to the hospital for an assessment today. She was caught speeding down the M1 motorway at more than 90 miles per hour.

---

* Adapted from B.K. Puri, A. Hall and R. Ho (2014). *Revision Notes in Psychiatry*. London, UK: CRC Press, p. 353.

When the police arrested her, her mood was noted to be irritable. The medical doctor has seen her and done the routine lab work, in which nothing abnormal was found. The medical doctor has given her oral lorazepam to calm her down. She is slightly less irritable now and is more willing to speak to the psychiatrist.

Task
Perform an MSE, looking in particular for any abnormal psychopathology that may be suggestive of mania with psychotic symptoms.

Outline of station
You are Miss Sandra Green, a 29-year-old female. You have been arrested by the police for speeding down the M1 Motorway at more than 90 miles per hour. Your mood has been high for the past week or so. You believe that you have been granted special rights and powers by the royal family and hence you are confident that you will not get into any legal problem if you speed. You are irritated that the police have brought you into the hospital for an assessment for no reason. You share with the doctor that you are the royal family's 'chosen one'. You are convinced about this. You have special rights and abilities that others do not have. You have not been sleeping well due to the increasing number of thoughts that you have. At times, you feel that you can hear the royal family speaking directly to you. Also, you have donated 3000 pounds over the past week to the local charity.

CASC construct table

The CASC construct table is formatted such that candidates will be able to cover adequately both the range and the depth of the assessment required in this station.

Approach: Be prepared to expect a patient with florid manic symptoms, who might be difficult to engage. Be prepared that the patient might be disinhibited – setting of boundaries is crucial and be prepared to call for a chaperone.				
Starting off: 'Hello, I am Dr Melvyn, one of the psychiatrists from the mental health unit. I understand that the police brought you here today. Can you tell me more?'				
Eliciting core manic symptoms	How has your mood been? If I were to ask you to rate your mood on a scale from 1 to 10, what score would you give to your mood now? Have others commented that you have been more irritable recently?	How has your energy level been? How has your sleep been? Are you still as energetic as ever despite the decreased amount of sleep? How has your appetite been?	Are you able to think clearly? Do you feel that there are many thoughts racing through your mind at any moment?	How long have you been feeling this way?

(Continued)

Eliciting grandiose delusional beliefs and challenging beliefs	It seems to me that you feel that you are specially chosen. Can you tell me more?	Are there any special powers or abilities that you have that others do not have? Can you tell me more about it? How convinced are you that this is true?	Could there be any other explanations for why you are having all these symptoms/all these special abilities? Could it be because you have been unwell?	Do you feel increasingly more confident about yourself recently?
Eliciting hallucinations in all other modalities, elicit thought disorders, elicit passivity experiences	Auditory hallucinations Do you hear sounds or voices that others do not hear? How many voices can you hear? Are they as clear as our current conversation? What do they say?	Second person auditory hallucinations Do they speak directly to you? Can you give me some examples of what they have been saying to you?	Third person auditory hallucinations Do they refer to you as 'he' or 'she', in the third person? Do they comment on your actions? Do they give you orders or commands as to what to do?	How do you feel when you hear them? Could there be any alternative explanation for these experiences that you have been having? Do you feel that your thoughts are being interfered with by an external force? Do you feel in control of your own actions and emotions?
Risk assessment – risk of excessive spending, intimacy, self-harm, violence	Have you engaged in any activities recently that might be dangerous? By that, I mean have you been involved with the police recently?	Have you been spending more money than usual? Gambling? Use of alcohol/ recreational substances?	Have you been thinking about sex more often recently? Any engagement in promiscuous, unprotected sexual activity? Is this your usual behaviour?	Have you been so troubled by all these things that you have entertained thoughts of ending your life? Have you got into fights with others around you?
Impact and coping mechanisms	How have you been coping with all these things?	Have you made use of any substances, such as alcohol, to help you cope?	What about street drugs?	

It would be helpful to use reflective interview techniques in this case to demonstrate symptoms portrayed by the patient. For example, 'I can see that you are talking very fast now . . . I'm wondering if your thoughts are racing just as fast?'; 'You are talking really fast and seem to have a lot of energy. Am I right? I'm wondering, how has your sleep been?' In these two illustrations, one can also link up and cluster symptoms together to make the flow of interview more seamless and logical.

Common pitfalls

a. Failure to take control of the station
b. Failure to set boundaries with patient
c. Failure to elicit core manic symptoms from patient/failure to cover the range and depth of the station
d. Failure to perform a complete risk assessment

Quick recall*

ICD-10 criteria for manic episode (F30 manic episode)
The fundamental disturbance is an elevation of mood to elation, with concomitant increase in activity level. Three degrees of manic episode are specified, all used for a single manic episode only.

a. Hypomania: There is persistent elevated mood, increased energy and activity, feelings of well-being and reduced need for sleep. Irritability may replace elation. Work is considerably disrupted. There are no hallucinations or delusions.
b. Mania without psychotic symptoms: Mood is elated, with almost uncontrollable excitement. There is over-activity, pressured speech; distractible, inflated self-esteem and grandiose thoughts. Perceptual heightening may occur. The person may spend excessively and become aggressive.
c. Mania with psychotic symptoms: The symptoms are as mentioned earlier but with delusions and hallucinations, usually grandiose. There may be sustained physical activity, aggression and self-neglect.

It is recommended to remember the *DSM-5* criteria for bipolar I disorder:

Duration: 1 week
To fulfil the diagnosis of bipolar I disorder, there must be at least one manic episode.

Manic episode: at least three of the following symptoms or four or more if only irritability is present:

a. Inflated self-esteem or grandiosity
b. Decreased need for sleep
c. More talkative than usual or pressure to keep talking
d. Flight of ideas or subjective experience that thoughts are racing
e. Distractibility
f. Increase in goal-directed activity or psychomotor agitation
g. Excessive involvement in activities that have a high potential for painful consequences (such as over-spending, sexual indiscretions or foolhardy investments)

There must be functional impairment and exclusion of other causes.

---

* Adapted from B.K. Puri, A. Hall and R. Ho (2014). *Revision Notes in Psychiatry*. London, UK: CRC Press, p. 375.

Suggested Reference: NICE. NICE guidelines for schizophrenia: http://guidance.nice .org.uk/CG38 (accessed 1 June 2014).

STATION 5: HYPOMANIA

Information to candidates

Name of patient: Chris Brown

Mr Chris Brown has been referred by his GP to the psychiatry for an assessment today. He has gone to the GP today, seeking to have a look at his hospital records. He has been refusing to tell his GP he wishes to have access to his hospital records. You have been asked to speak to him, to perform an MSE.

Task

Perform an MSE, looking in particular for any abnormal psychopathologies that may be suggestive of hypomania.

Outline of station

You are Mr Chris Brown, a 30-year-old male. You have approached your GP today as you wish to have access to your hospital records. You are upset that your GP cannot treat you, but you are sure that the psychiatrist you will be seeing will be able to help. You are slightly disinhibited at the start of the interview and refuse to let go of the doctor's handshake. You make inappropriate comments about the doctor and his or her dress.

The reason you wish to have access to your hospital records is that you wish to change the diagnosis that you have been previously labelled with. You also wish to document some plans on the hospital records. You have this massive plan to help the NHS reduce the waiting time for elderly patients seeking treatment. You believe that if you document this, this plan will eventually be implemented, when the hospital conducts their routine audit.

Your mood has been higher than normal over the past 4 days, and you have been requiring much less sleep than usual. At times, you feel that your thoughts are racing. You have been coping well with work thus far, as you feel more productive at work because you have more energy than usual. You have not been having any abnormal perceptions, such as auditory hallucinations. You donated around 1000 pounds to the local charity just 2 days ago. You have not done any other adventurous things recently. You have not been involved with the police. You have not used any alcohol or substance to help you cope.

CASC construct table

The CASC construct table is formatted such that candidates will be able to cover adequately both the range and the depth of the assessment required in this station.

Approach: Be prepared that the patient might be disinhibited – setting of boundaries is crucial, and be prepared to call for a chaperone.

Starting off: 'Hello, I am Dr Melvyn, one of the psychiatrists from the mental health unit. I understand that your local GP has referred you here today. Can you tell me more?'

Eliciting core hypomanic symptoms	How has your mood been? If I were to ask you to rate your mood on a scale from 1 to 10, what score would you give your mood now? Have others commented that you have been more irritable recently?	How has your energy level been? How has your sleep been? Are you still as energetic as ever despite the decreased amount of sleep? How has your appetite been?	Are you able to think clearly? Do you feel that there are many thoughts racing through your mind at any given moment?	How long have you been feeling this way?
Eliciting delusional beliefs and challenging beliefs (to explore and challenge more about the delusional ideations pertaining to his plans of accessing his records)	It seems to me that you have some specific plans in mind. Can you tell me more?	Does that mean that you have special powers or abilities that others do not have? Can you tell me more about it?	Can you tell me how it is possible that others would come to know of your plan?	Could there be any other explanations for why you are having all these symptoms/all these special abilities? Could it be because you have been unwell?
Eliciting hallucinations in all other modalities, eliciting thought disorders, eliciting passivity experiences	Auditory hallucinations Do you hear sounds or voices that others do not hear? How many voices can you hear? Are they as clear as our current conversation? What do they say?	Second person auditory hallucinations Do they speak directly to you? Can you give me some examples of what they have been saying to you?	Third person auditory hallucinations Do they refer to you as 'he' or 'she', in the a third person? Do they comment on your actions? Do they give you orders or commands as to what to do?	How do you feel when you hear them? Could there be any alternative explanation for these experiences that you have been having? Do you feel that your thoughts are being interfered with by an external force? Do you feel in control of your own actions and emotions?

(Continued)

Risk assessment – risk of excessive spending, intimacy, self-harm, violence	Have you engaged in any activities recently that might be dangerous? By that, I mean have you been involved with the police recently?	Have you been spending more money than usual?	Have you been recently involved in any intimate relationships with others?	Have you been so troubled by all these that you have entertained thoughts of ending your life? Have you gotten into trouble with others around you?
Impact and coping mechanisms	How have you been coping with all these?	Have you made use of any substances, such as alcohol, to help you cope?	What about street drugs?	

Common pitfalls

a. Failure to take control of the station
b. Failure to set boundaries with patient
c. Failure to elicit core hypomanic symptoms from patient/failure to cover the range and depth of the station
d. Failure to adequately challenge his or her delusional beliefs
e. Failure to perform a complete risk assessment

Quick recall*

ICD-10 criteria for manic episode (F30 manic episode)
The fundamental disturbance is an elevation of mood to elation, with concomitant increase in activity level. Three degrees of manic episode are specified, all used for a single manic episode only.

a. Hypomania: There is persistent elevated mood, increased energy and activity, feelings of well-being and reduced need for sleep. Irritability may replace elation. Work is considerably disrupted. There are no hallucinations or delusions.
b. Mania without psychotic symptoms: Mood is elated, with almost uncontrollable excitement. There is over-activity, pressured speech; distractible, inflated self-esteem and grandiose thoughts. Perceptual heightening may occur. The person may spend excessively and become aggressive.
c. Mania with psychotic symptoms: The symptoms are as mentioned earlier but with delusions and hallucinations, usually grandiose. There may be sustained physical activity, aggression and self-neglect.

---

* Adapted from B.K. Puri, A. Hall and R. Ho (2014). *Revision Notes in Psychiatry*. London, UK: CRC Press, p. 375.

It is recommended to remember the *DSM-5* criteria for bipolar II disorder:

1. The duration of the symptoms must be at least 4 days.
2. There must be one previous major depressive episode and at least one hypomanic episode.
3. Hypomanic episode has the same requirement of the number of symptoms as manic episode.
4. The only difference is that patients should have no impairments in their functioning.

Suggested Reference: NICE. NICE guidelines for schizophrenia: http://guidance.nice .org.uk/CG38 (accessed 1 June 2014).

STATION 6: DELIRIUM TREMENS

Information to candidates

Name of patient: Thomas Smith

Mr Thomas Smith, a 65-year-old man, has just been admitted to the orthopaedic ward after sustaining a fracture of his hip, when he slipped and fell whilst bathing. He had his hip operation 2 days ago and is currently being nursed in the Surgery High Dependency unit. He has been complaining to the nurses that he has been seeing Spanish guerrillas around. He has been aggressive and agitated most of the time, as he believes that these Spanish guerrillas might harm him.

Task

Please assess him for his psychopathology and perform a risk assessment.

Outline of station

You are Thomas Smith, a 65-year-old man who has just been admitted to the orthopaedic ward. You have just recently undergone a hip replacement operation and are currently still in some pain. Things have not been the same for you, as you have been seeing Spanish guerrillas whilst you are on the ward. You appear to be very frightened and distressed by what you are seeing.

You start the station by telling the doctor, 'There is no point for us having a chat . . . Look, they are coming to get me, I think we better escape from this war-zone right now'.

You will then share (only if the doctor is able to take control of the interview and is empathetic) further information. You will share more about your visual and auditory hallucinations. You will then share some information about your alcohol history, stating that your last drink was around 3 days ago, and that you have been a chronic drinker since your teenage years. With regard to risk, you will tell the doctor that you might think of absconding from the inpatient unit as this is too troubling for you. There might be a chance you will consider ending your life.

CASC construct table

The CASC construct table is formatted such that candidates will be able to cover adequately both the range and depth of the assessment required in this station.

Approach: Be prepared that the patient may be difficult and reluctant to engage in an interview – take control by reassuring the patient, inviting him to have sit down. If he refuses, sit down and start the station.				
Starting off: 'Hello, I am Dr Melvyn, one of the psychiatrists from the mental health unit. I received some information about you from my medical colleagues. Can you tell me more about what happened that led to your current admission?'				
Alternatively, for a difficult patient:				
'It seems to me that you are feeling very bothered at the moment. Please let me reassure you that this is the hospital and I'm one of the doctors. Can we have a chat?'				
Eliciting core visual hallucinations	I can see that you seemed to be quite distressed at the moment. Are you able to tell me more about what you can see?	Do these people appear to be much smaller than usual? How long have you been troubled by these experiences? Have you had such experience before?	How do you feel when you see them? I understand that this must be a highly distressing situation for you. Do you feel that they are real? Is there any possibility of stopping them?	Why do you think they are troubling you? Do you have an explanation for these experiences? Could it be due to the fact that you are not well at the moment?
Eliciting hallucinations in all other modalities, elicit thought disorders and elicit passivity experiences	Auditory hallucinations Do you hear sounds or voices that others do not hear? How many voices can you hear? Are they as clear as our current conversation? What do they say?	Second person auditory hallucinations Do they speak directly to you? Can you give me some examples of what they have been saying to you?	Third person auditory hallucinations Do they refer to you as 'he' or 'she', in the third person? Do they comment on your actions? Do they give you orders or commands as to what to do?	How do you feel when you hear them? Could there be any alternative explanation for these experiences that you have been having?
	Has there been anything wrong with your sense of smell recently?	Have you noticed that food or drink seemed to have a different taste recently?	Do you have any strange feelings in your body?	Do you feel in control of your thoughts, emotions and actions?
Check for orientation to time, place and person	Do you know where you are at the moment?	Do you know roughly what time it is right now?	Do you know who I am?	

(Continued)

Elicit alcohol history if possible	I understand that you have used alcohol before you came into the hospital. How often do you drink?	When did you first start to drink? Have you been increasing your alcohol intake recently?	Do you remember when you had your last drink?	Have you tried to quit using alcohol previously? What was the outcome when you tried?
Risk assessment	With all these troubling experiences, have you thought of ending your life?	Have you thought of taking revenge on the people you think are troubling you?		

Common pitfalls

a. Failure to take control of the station/failure to reassure the patient
b. Failure to cover the range and depth of the station
c. Conducting the clinical interview standing throughout the entire 7 minutes as the patient refuses to sit
d. Failure to ascertain that the patient was disoriented

Quick recall*

The peak onset is usually within 2 days of abstinence, and usually the entire episode will last for around 5 days. In chronic heavy drinkers, this is due to a fall in the blood alcohol concentration that leads to withdrawal symptoms.

There might be a prodromal period with the following clinical symptoms: anxiety, insomnia, tachycardia, tremor and sweating.

The onset of delirium is characterized by the following:

a. Disorientation
b. Rapidly changing level of consciousness
c. Intensely fearful affect
d. Hallucinations
e. Misperceptions
f. Tremor
g. Restlessness
h. Autonomic overactivity

The hallucinations are usually visual and are commonly Lilliputian in nature. Auditory and tactile hallucinations, and secondary delusions, may also be present. There is an estimated morality rate of around 5%, usually associated with cardiovascular collapse or infection.

---

* Adapted from B.K. Puri, A. Hall and R. Ho (2014). *Revision Notes in Psychiatry*. London, UK: CRC Press, p. 516.

With regard to the treatment, it is usually supportive with fluid and electrolytes replacement and high-potency vitamins (especially thiamine to prevent an unrecognized Wernicke's encephalopathy progressing onto Karsakov's psychosis).

Summarization of the National Institute for Health and Care Excellence (NICE) guidance on the management of delirium tremens or seizures

a. Oral lorazepam should be considered to be used as the first-line treatment for delirium tremens or seizures.
b. If the symptoms persist, or if it is tough for the patient to tolerate oral lorazepam, parental route of administration should be considered. Parental haloperidol and parental olanzapine could also be given. The medications suggested do not have UK marketing authorization for treating delirium tremens or seizures. Hence, informed consent should be obtained and documented whenever possible.
c. Phenytoin should not be considered for usage in the treatment of alcohol withdrawal seizures.

Suggested Reference: NICE. NICE guidelines for drug misuse: http://guidance.nice .org.uk/CG51 and 52 (accessed 2 June 2014).

STATION 7: ANXIETY DISORDERS (PANIC DISORDER WITH AGORAPHOBIA)

Information to candidates

Name of patient: Janice Thomas

Ms Janice Thomas is a 35-year-old housewife. Her husband has brought her to the GP as she has been having increasing anxiety about heading out from her house. Her GP has referred her over to the local mental health service for an assessment and potentially for psychological treatments.

Task

Please take a history.

Outline of station

You are Janice Thomas, a 35-year-old housewife. You have been having increasing anxieties about leaving home, and this first started around 6 months ago. Six months ago, you were travelling in the tube when something nasty happened. The tube broke down, and you were trapped there with all the other passengers. There was not much ventilation, and you felt dizzy and nearly collapsed. That episode lasted for around 30 minutes before you recovered and managed to leave the tube. Ever since that episode, you have been having increasing anxiety about leaving home. Even if you are with your husband, you worry that something similar might happen. Recently, you went out to shop for household items and the same physical and psychological symptoms returned to trouble you. You recall that during the last episode, you had palpitations, shortness of breath, giddiness and fear of losing control and dying. Since then, you have not been able to leave the house. You have resorted to purchasing items online and have also rejected all social invitations. Your mood has been affected. You have not been using alcohol or any other substances to cope. You desperately want help. Begin the station by telling the doctor, 'I think I have a serious problem. I don't think you can help me'.

CASC construct table

The CASC construct table is formatted such that candidates will be able to cover adequately both the range and the depth of the assessment required in this station.

Approach: Be prepared that the patient may be difficult to engage at the start of the interview, as she has been feeling quite helpless about her situation. She might be quite anxious about coming to the doctor's appointment, and hence, if open questioning does not work, the candidate should consider closed-ended questioning to elicit the core symptoms.				
Starting off: 'Hello, I am Dr Melvyn, one of the psychiatrists from the mental health unit. I understand that you have been referred by your GP for anxiety symptoms. Can you tell me more?'				
History and eliciting core anxiety symptoms (physical and psychological)	Can you tell me how long this has been troubling you for? Do you remember when this first started? Can you tell me more about your experiences during the first episode? Do you remember how long the episode lasted for?	Physical symptoms Can you tell me more about the bodily symptoms that you have during those episodes? • Palpitation • Sweating • Trembling • Dry mouth • Difficulty breathing • Chest pain • Nausea or stomach churning	Psychological symptoms When you have those bodily symptoms, what runs through your mind? Are you worried about losing control? Are you worried about dying or going crazy? Are you also afraid that something awful might happen?	How have you been in between those episodes? How frequently do these episodes occur now? Do you feel restless, and keyed up, always on the edge? Have you ever had exaggerated responses to minor surprises? Do you worry much about when the next attack might occur? Are there specific situations in which these symptoms come on? For example, in situations which you cannot leave easily? Do you tend to avoid these situations?

(Continued)

Rule out other anxiety symptomatology and comorbid	Do you worry a lot about everyday little things? Do you tend to get anxious when you have to make conversations with people or give a presentation? Are there specific things that you are afraid of?	Do you have excessive checking or any washing behaviour? Do you have nightmares or flashbacks related to previous traumatic experiences?	I know this has been a difficult time for you. With all this going on, how has your mood been? Are you still able to keep up with your interests? What about your sleep and appetite?	
Impact and coping	How have these symptoms affected your life? Are you able to cope?	Have you used any alcohol to help you cope with your symptoms?	Have you used any other drugs to help you with all your symptoms?	Have you sought medical help previously?
Personal history	Is this the first time that you are seeing a psychiatrist? Does anyone in your family have any mental health problems?	How were things when you were a child? Were there any difficulties?	Can I know whether you have any chronic medical condition? For the conditions that you have mentioned, are you on long-term medications?	How would you describe yourself in terms of your personality before all this came on?

Common pitfalls

a. Failure to engage the patient as she might be overtly anxious
b. Failure to recognize the need to switch to closed-ended questioning if the patient does not answer open-ended questions
c. Failure to cover the range and the depth of the station/failure to rule out other anxiety conditions and assess mood

Quick recall*

For this station, it is essential to recognize the common epidemiology of panic disorders: Women aged 25–44 years, with a family history of panic disorder, divorced or separated are at the highest risk.

To elicit history from the patient, candidates need to know either the *ICD-10* or the *DSM-5* diagnostic criteria:

---

* Adapted from B.K. Puri, A. Hall and R. Ho (2014). *Revision Notes in Psychiatry.* London, UK: CRC Press, p. 413.

ICD-10	DSM-5
• Episodic paroxysmal anxiety not confined to predictable situations. • Several attacks occur within I month. • Discrete episode of intense fear or discomfort, abrupt onset, reaches a maximum within a few minutes; autonomic arousal symptoms with freedom from anxiety symptoms between attacks. • Symptoms involve the chest and abdomen. • Symptoms involve the mental state.	• Recurrent unexpected panic attacks with symptoms similar to the *ICD-10* criteria. • At least one of the attacks has been followed by at least I month of persistent concern or worry about additional panic attack and maladaptive change in behaviour related to the attacks. Common symptoms: Palpitations, sweating, trembling, dry mouth, difficulty breathing, choking sensation, chest pain, nausea or stomach churning, giddiness, fainting, derealization, depersonalization, fear of losing control, fear of dying or 'going crazy', feeling afraid as if something awful may happen, hot flushes, numbness, tingling, restlessness, keyed up, trouble relaxing

Comorbidity

One-third develop secondary depression following the onset of panic disorder. If depression does occur, the course is shorter. Agoraphobia usually occurs with panic disorder but can also occur separately. There is estimated to be an increased lifetime prevalence (54%) of alcohol abuse and dependence and an increased lifetime prevalence (43%) of drug abuse and dependence. Some use substances as a complication of their panic disorder; others develop panic disorder as a result of the withdrawal from substances.

Suggested Reference: NICE. NICE guidelines for anxiety: http://guidance.nice.org .uk/CG22 (accessed 2 June 2014).

STATION 8: ANXIETY DISORDERS (SOCIAL PHOBIA)

Information to candidates

Name of patient: Mr Lewis

Mr Lewis is a 30-year-old man who has been referred to your clinic by his GP. He has recently visited his GP as he has been increasingly concerned about his upcoming marriage. He is reluctant to share further details with his GP. He has been insistent on getting medications to help him with his condition from the GP.

Task

Please take a history to come to a diagnosis. In addition, please elicit a history about possible aetiological factors.

Outline of station

You are Mr Lewis and have been referred by your GP to see the psychiatrist. You are not very keen to see the psychiatrist, as you do not want to be perceived to be having any mental health problems, given that a major life event (your marriage) is coming up soon in 2 weeks. All you want from the GP are some medications that might calm you down during the event. Since you were young, you have been having difficulties in various social situations. You are not able to give a presentation in front of others, and you dislike social gatherings, avoiding them at all cost. There are symptoms that previously manifested during those social situations that are particularly troubling for you. These include the sensation of blushing, dryness of mouth, palpitations and the sensation of butterflies in your stomach. Because of your difficulties since graduation, you have been forced to settle for a job as a chemist in the local lab. You always wanted to do finance and business management, but with your ongoing symptoms you have to give up that career option. You met your fiancé 2 years ago and your relationship with her is good. She understands your problem, but she is insisting on having a church wedding (with approximately 200 guests), to which you have disagreed. All you want is a small event. What is more troubling for you is that you need to give a speech during the wedding in front of others. You cannot perceive yourself doing that.

Your mood has been much affected by this. You still have retained interest and are still able to function at your workplace. You do not have any other anxiety symptoms such as panic attacks or fear of going out. You do have a positive family history of mental health disorders: neither of your parents have anxiety disorder. You have not used any substances to cope with your current difficulties.

You are expecting to be anxious throughout the interview, avoiding and hesitating to answer questions about your condition. A good candidate will be able to engage you after trying close-ended questioning later in the interview.

CASC construct table

The CASC construct table is formatted such that candidates will be able to cover adequately both the range and the depth of the assessment required in this station.

Approach: Be prepared that the patient may be difficult to engage at the start of the interview, as he has been feeling quite helpless about her situation. He might be quite anxious about coming to the doctor's appointment, and hence, if open questioning does not work, the candidate should consider closed-ended questioning to elicit the core symptoms.				
Starting off: 'Hello, I am Dr Melvyn, one of the psychiatrists from the mental health unit. I understand that you have been referred by your GP for anxiety symptoms. Can you tell me more?'				
History and core anxiety symptoms	How long has this been troubling you? Can you explain to me in what context or situations you feel this way?	Can you tell me more about your symptoms? What are the symptoms that you have in those situations? • Blushing • Dryness of mouth • Palpitations	How do you respond when you feel this way?	

(Continued)

		• Shaking • Urgency • Fear of micturition/ defecation		
Psycho-social impact of anxiety symptoms	Do you tend to avoid certain situations?	Do you have any difficulties with your daily work?	Does this have any impact on your current relationships?	Is it true that because of your current symptoms, you have resorted to avoiding certain situations, choosing to work in occupations that do not need much social interaction?
Rule out comorbidities	Do you worry a lot about everyday little things? Have you had panic attacks before? Do you have difficulties going out of the house? Are there specific things that you are afraid of?	Do you have excessive checking or any washing behaviour? Do you have nightmares or flashbacks related to previous traumatic experiences?	I know this has been a difficult time for you. With all this going on, how has your mood been? Are you still able to keep up with your interests? What about your sleep and appetite?	Have you used any alcohol or substances to help you cope with your current situation?
Personal history/ aetiology	Is this the first time that you are seeing a psychiatrist? Does anyone in your family have any mental health problems?	How were things when you were a child? Were there any difficulties?	Can I know whether you have any chronic medical conditions? For the conditions that you have mentioned, are you on long-term medications?	How would you describe yourself in terms of your personality before all these came on? Are you someone who always worries a lot?

Common pitfalls

a. Failure to engage the patient as he might be overtly anxious
b. Failure to recognize the need to switch to closed-ended questioning if the patient does not answer open-ended questions
c. Failure to cover the range and depth of the station/failure to rule out other anxiety conditions and assess mood
d. Failure to elicit the aetiologies: the precipitating, the perpetuating and the protective factors

Quick recall*

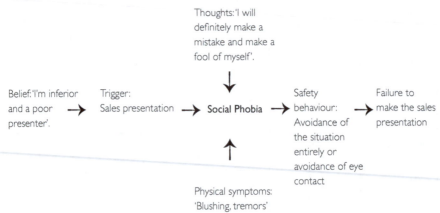

Cognitive model (adapted) of an individual with social anxiety

ICD-10 diagnostic criteria	DSM-5 diagnostic criteria
Symptoms are manifestations of anxiety and not secondary to other symptoms. Anxiety is largely restricted to or predominates in particular social situations. The phobic situation is avoided whenever possible. There is marked fear of being the focus of attention and marked avoidance of being the focus of attention. At least two symptoms must be present: Blushing or shaking, fear of vomiting and urgency or fear of micturition or defecation.	Based on the DSM-5 diagnostic criteria, it is characterized by marked fear or anxiety about one or more social situations in which the individual is exposed to possible scrutiny or being negatively evaluated by others. The fear is out of proportion and lasts for 6 months or longer.

The treatment of social phobia is similar to panic disorder, but beta-blockers can be used to reduce autonomic arousal. Beta-blockers are used to help reduce the amount of performance anxiety.

Suggested Reference: NICE. NICE guidelines for anxiety: http://guidance.nice.org.uk/CG22 (accessed 2 June 2014).

---

* Adapted from B.K. Puri, A. Hall and R. Ho (2014). *Revision Notes in Psychiatry*. London, UK: CRC Press, p. 408.

STATION 9: MSE FOR PATIENT GOING ON LEAVE

Information to candidates

Name of patient: Mr Gordon

Mr Gordon is a 20-year-old gentleman who has been sectioned to the mental health unit, after attempting to jump into the river 3 weeks ago. He shared with the team of doctors that he has been experiencing auditory hallucinations, command hallucinations and delusional ideations for the past 4 months. The team doctors have diagnosed him with first episode psychosis and have since started treatment for him. He is due to go for his home leave this weekend. The ward manager has requested for you to come and assess his mental state and his risk prior to him going for the planned home leave.

Task

Please perform an MSE and a relevant risk assessment.

Outline of station

You have been sectioned for admission to the mental health unit 3 weeks ago, after attempting to jump into the Thames River. You wanted to end your life at that time as you have been increasingly troubled by auditory hallucinations and used to hear multiple voices that were making demeaning remarks and at times also commenting on your actions. The voices did sound as clear as any conversation you have had with others. The voices commanded you to jump into the river previously. You have also been increasingly troubled and have been feeling that there are spy cameras that are monitoring your actions. Your mood has been much affected by these experiences. You have been more settled whilst you are inpatient and since the commencement of medications.

You have been exercising quite a lot in the ward throughout your admission. Some residual voices are telling you to do so, as they tell you that the closer you get to the core of the earth, the chances of you becoming well again are higher. You have plans to head out for your scheduled home leave with your sister, as you are keen to find another river that is deeper than the previous one, so that you can immerse yourself deep within and get rid of these experiences that have been troubling you. You do not think that this is dangerous.

CASC construct table

The CASC construct table is formatted such that candidates will be able to cover adequately both the range and the depth of the assessment required in this station.

Approach: Be prepared for a patient who might be minimizing his symptoms to go on home leave.				
Starting off: 'Hello, I am Dr Melvyn, one of the psychiatrists from the mental health unit. I understand that you are scheduled to go on your home leave. Can we have a chat as to how you have been?'				
Eliciting auditory hallucinations	**Auditory hallucinations** I understand the circumstances that led to your current admission. How have things changed? Do you still hear sounds or voices that others do not hear? How many voices can you hear? Are they as clear as our current conversation? What do they say?	**Second person auditory hallucinations** Do they speak directly to you? Can you give me some examples of what they have been saying to you?	**Third person auditory hallucinations** Do they refer to you as 'he' or 'she', in the third person? Do they comment on your actions? Do they give you orders or commands as to what to do?	How do you feel when you hear them? Could there be any alternative explanation for these experiences that you have been having?
Eliciting delusions	I understand from the team that you have been exercising a lot in the ward. Can you tell me more about this?	How is it possible that by exercising you could have more strength to deal with your experiences?	Are there any other alternative explanations for why you are thinking this way?	Could it be that you have not yet been well?
Elicit thought disorders	**Thought interference** Do you feel that your thoughts are being interfered with? Who do you think is doing this?	**Thought insertion** Do you have thoughts in your head that you feel are not your own? Where do you think these thoughts come from?	**Thought broadcasting** Do you feel that your thoughts are being broadcasted, such that others would know what you are thinking?	**Thought withdrawal** Do you feel that your thoughts are being taken away from your head by some external force?
Elicit passivity experiences	Do you feel in control of your own actions and emotions?	Do you feel that someone or something is trying to control you? Who or what do you think this would be?		

(Continued)

Impact of symptoms on mood and insight	I understand that this must be a difficult time for you. How have you been coping?	Since admission till now, how has your mood been? Are you still interested in things you used to enjoy?	I understand that the team doctors have started you on some medications. Did they share with you what might be wrong with you? Do you believe them? Do you feel safe in the ward?	Do you know why you need the medications?
Risk assessment – risk to self and others	I understand that you are due for a home leave today. What plans do you have in mind? *Need to probe and get patient to elaborate*	Do you have plans to repeat what you did 3 weeks ago? Have you felt that life is no longer worth living? Do you have any thoughts of ending your life? What plans do you have?	Do you think you will return back to the ward for continued treatment after your home leave? *Assess history of suicide/self-harm attempts. Does the patient have any access to weapons or items that can cause harm (drugs, etc.)?*	(If patient vocalizes paranoid ideations) Do you have any intentions to do anything nasty to the people who are troubling you?

Common pitfalls

a. Failure to engage with a patient who might be minimizing his symptoms
b. Failure to cover the range and depth of the station
c. Failure to perform an adequate risk assessment – need to take into consideration risk of harm to self, others and also risk of absconding and not returning to the ward
d. Failure to assess history of suicide/self-harm episodes and their severity/lethality

Quick recall: Psychosis/schizophrenia and suicide/violence risk*

The relevant information pertaining to the diagnostic criteria for schizophrenia and psychosis can be found in the earlier stations. As this station essentially involves a risk assessment, further information about schizophrenia and its association with suicide and violence will be covered.

Suicide: It has been estimated that approximately 10% of patients with schizophrenia commit suicide; this usually happens early in the course of their illness. Suicide is more likely in the following cases: male gender, younger

---

* Adapted from B.K. Puri, A. Hall and R. Ho (2014). *Revision Notes in Psychiatry*. London, UK: CRC Press, p. 370.

patients, unemployment, having chronic illness with relapses, having a higher educational status prior to the onset of the illness, akathisia, abrupt stoppage of the psychotropic medication and recent discharge from inpatient care.

Patients with paranoid schizophrenia have been estimated to have an increased incidence of three times compared with non-paranoid patients.

Violence: The prevalence of aggressive behaviour amongst patients with schizophrenia in the outpatient has been estimated to be 5%. The most common type of violence is verbal aggression, followed by physical violence towards objects, violence towards others and then self-directed violence. Family members are usually the victims. Chances of a family member being attacked are as high as 50%, compared with the general population, in which the chances are only 20%.

Suggested Reference: NICE. NICE guidelines for schizophrenia: http://guidance.nice .org.uk/CG82 (accessed 1 June 2014).

STATION 10: DEPRESSION WITH PSYCHOTIC FEATURES

Information to candidates

Name of patient: Ms Brown

You are the core trainee 3 on call. Your medical colleagues from the emergency services have asked you to help assess a 70-year-old female who has just been transferred to their service via the ambulance. You have been informed that she tried to burn herself alive in her backyard, but her neighbours noticed it and called the police. You have been told that she has been vocalizing to the medical doctors that she thinks she is already dead and does not want them to do anything for her. Your medical colleagues have done the necessary blood investigations and have deemed her to be medically stable.

Task

Please find out more about the abnormal beliefs the patient has and also perform an appropriate risk assessment.

Outline of station

You are Ms Brown, and you regret that your attempt to burn yourself in your backyard has not been successful. You feel that your neighbours are troublemakers and that they should not have contacted the police and the ambulance. You are convinced that you are already dead, and your plan today was to get rid of your physical body as you know that it is rotting away already. You are convinced, as around 1 month ago, when you awoke and saw the angel at the foot of your bed, and that was a clear sign for you that you were dead. You will begin the station telling the candidate 'I am dead' and 'You are talking to my soul' and repeat it no matter what the candidate asks or says. Only if the candidate asks, 'What happened before you realized you were dead?' and appears to be empathetic would you be willing to engage more. You will have absolutely no eye contact with the candidate, and your mood is very low.

You will share with the candidate that you have been feeling low in your spirits since a few months ago, when you were made redundant at your workplace and when your youngest son passed on from a silent heart attack. Since then, your mood has been pervasively low. Your sleep and appetite are affected and you have active ideations of doing something similar again, on discharge, as you cannot envision living on.

CASC construct table

The CASC construct table is formatted such that candidates will be able to cover adequately both the range and the depth of the assessment required in this station.

Approach: Be prepared for a patient who is very depressed and delusional and not willing to engage. Demonstrate empathy and if the patient keeps insisting that she is dead, please ask her, 'What happened before you died?' to attempt to elicit the range and depth of information required in the station.				
Starting off: 'Hello, I am Dr Melvyn, one of the psychiatrists from the mental health unit. Can you tell me more about what has happened?'				
Eliciting nihilistic delusions and challenging delusions	It does sound like things have been difficult for you. How long have you been feeling this way?	What does it mean when you say you are dead? Do you feel that particular parts of your body are rotting? Was that the reason that led you to do what you did today? How convinced are you that you are dead?	How do you know that you are dead? Did anything happen that led you to believe so?	How is it possible for us to be having a conversation now if you are already dead? Could there be an alternative explanation to all these?
Eliciting depressive symptoms	Key question: Can you tell me more about how things have been for you before you died?	With all this going on, how is your mood? Are you able to enjoy things you used to enjoy?	How has your sleep been? Have there been any problems with your appetite? How are your energy levels?	Have you had thoughts that life was not worth living? What are your plans for the future?
Eliciting psychotic symptoms?	Have there been times when you were alone and were bothered by unusual experiences? Do you hear voices when no one is around?	Do you feel that your thoughts are being interfered with?	Do you feel in control of your own emotions?	Do you feel in control of your own actions?

(Continued)

Risk assessment	This must be an extremely difficult time for you.	What were your intentions when you tried to burn yourself today? How did you do it? Was anyone hurt or properties damaged?	Do you still have thoughts of ending your life right now? What plans do you have in mind?	Is there anything that would prevent you from doing so?

Common pitfalls

a. Failure to engage with a patient who is supposed to be extremely depressed in this station
b. Failure to cover the range and depth of the station (failure to elicit both the depressive and the psychotic symptoms and adequately challenge the delusional beliefs)
c. Failure to perform an adequate risk assessment – includes harm to self, others and damage to properties

Quick recall: Depression in the elderly*

There are noted similarities and differences in terms of depressive symptomatology between the young and the old.

The following are more common for depressed elderly individuals:

a. Behavioural disturbances such as food refusal
b. Complaints about loneliness
c. Complaints of pain of unknown origin
d. Depressive pseudo-dementia (poor concentration and memory)
e. Hypochondriacal preoccupations
f. Irritability or anger
g. Loss of interest often replaces the depressed mood in the elderly
h. Denial or minimization of low mood
i. Neuro-vegetative symptoms
j. Neurotic symptoms
k. Psychomotor retardation or agitation
l. Paranoid and delusional ideation

With regard to treatment, it should be noted that newer antidepressants such as selective serotonin reuptake inhibitors (SSRIs) and serotonin norepinephrine reuptake inhibitors (SNRIs) are better tolerated than tricyclic antidepressants (TCAs) because SSRIs have low anticholingeric activity.

Deluded depressed patients would require the addition of an antipsychotic.

With regard to prognosis and risks, 70% of the elderly depressive patients would recover within a year, but 20% will relapse. Only 10%–15% are considered to suffer

---

* Adapted from B.K. Puri, A. Hall and R. Ho (2014). *Revision Notes in Psychiatry*. London, UK: CRC Press, p. 710.

from treatment-resistant depression. The death rate is higher for late life depressives than for non-depressed patients. Hence, risk assessment is important and crucial.

STATION 11: DEPRESSION WITH PSYCHOTIC FEATURES

Information to candidates

Name of patient: Ms White

You are the core trainee 3 on call. You have been asked to assess a 55-year-old female who has been brought into the emergency services by the police. You received information that she has attempted to surrender herself today to the police as she is convinced that she has committed a terrible crime many years ago. The medics have performed the basic blood works for her and have cleared her medically.

Task

Please question the patient to find out more about the abnormal beliefs she has and also perform an appropriate risk assessment.

Outline of station

You are Ms White, a 55-year-old female. You have decided to surrender yourself to the police station today, as you strongly believe that you have committed a serious crime and mistake years ago. This came to your realization a month ago, when you were watching a documentary about adoption of children on BBC channel 1. This reminded you that you had intentionally left out the name of your daughter's father on her birth certificate, as you had a conflict with your husband back then and decided not to include his name. You know that your daughter's marriage is undergoing a tough time and believe that this is all because of you intentionally leaving out the name of your husband. You have told your husband about your concerns, but he does not believe you.

Your mood has been low for the past month or so. You cannot enjoy the things you used to enjoy. The house is in a state of mess as you have barely sufficient energy to do the housework. Your sleep is disrupted, and your appetite is poor, as you constantly ruminate over the serious crime that you have committed. Recently, you have not dared to watch the television, as you feel that the people in the television programs might talk about your crime. At times, you hear voices when you are alone which sound like those of your husband, asking you to surrender yourself to the police for the serious mistake you have committed. You do feel that your life is meaningless and have had passive ideations of suicide. You are very afraid that you might do something to end your life as this is troubling you very much.

CASC construct table

The CASC construct table is formatted such that candidates will be able to cover adequately both the range and the depth of the assessment required in this station.

Approach: Be prepared for a patient who might be quite restless, anxious and preoccupied with thoughts that she has indeed committed a major crime. Use empathetic statements to engage the patient.

Starting off: 'Hello, I am Dr Melvyn, one of the psychiatrists from the mental health unit. Can you tell me more about what happened prior to your current admission?'

Eliciting delusional beliefs and challenging beliefs	I can see that you looked very distressed. Can you tell me more about what has been troubling you?	Can you tell me more as to why you are feeling this way? Did anything remind you of what happened previously?	Do you feel that you are guilty and responsible for all that has happened to your daughter's relationship? How convinced are you? Can there be any other alternative explanations for this?	Can it be possible that your daughter already has some marital issues to begin with?
Eliciting depressive symptoms	With all this going on, how is your mood? Are you able to enjoy things you used to enjoy?	How has your sleep been? Have there been any problems with your appetite? How are your energy levels?	Have you had thoughts that life is not worth living? What are your plans for the future?	
Eliciting psychotic symptoms	Have there been times when you are alone and you have been bothered by unusual experiences?	Do you feel that your thoughts are being interfered with?	Do you feel in control of your own emotions?	Do you feel in control of your own actions?
Risk assessment	This must be an extremely difficult time for you.	Have you previously had thoughts of ending your life?	Do you still have thoughts of ending your life right now?	What plans do you have in mind? Is there anything that will prevent you from doing so?

Common pitfalls

a. Failure to engage with the patient.
b. Failure to challenge her delusional beliefs adequately.
c. Failure to cover the range and depth of the station (failure to elicit both the depressive and the psychotic symptoms). There is also a need to establish the onset of mood and psychotic symptoms – which comes first.
d. Failure to perform an adequate risk assessment.

Quick recall: Delusions and management of psychotic depression*

A delusion is a false belief based on an incorrect inference about external reality that is firmly sustained despite what almost everyone else believes and despite what constitutes incontrovertible and obvious proof or evidence to the contrary. The belief is not ordinarily accepted by members of the person's culture or subculture.

It is important to differentiate between the following delusional beliefs:

a. Mood-congruent delusion: The content of the delusion is appropriate to the mood of the person.
b. Mood-incongruent delusion: The content of the delusion is not appropriate to the mood of the person.
c. Primary delusion: This refers to a delusion that arises fully formed without any discernible connection with previous events. It may be preceded by a delusional mood in which the person is aware of something strange and threatening happening.
d. Bizarre delusion: A delusion involving a phenomenon that the person's culture would regard as totally implausible.

In terms of management of psychotic depression, Spiker et al. (1985) have found a superior response when an antidepressant and an antipsychotic were used in combination in delusional depression.

STATION 12: DELUSION OF LOVE/EROTOMANIA

Information to candidates

Name of patient: Mr Jordan

You are the core trainee 3 on call, and you have been informed by the emergency services receptionist to evaluate a man who has turned up unexpectedly and is now demanding to see the nurse who treated him 3 weeks ago.

Task

Please speak to the patient and assess his psychopathology. In addition, please perform an assessment of risk.

Outline of station

You are Mr Jordan, and you have returned to the emergency department today, requesting to see the nurse who attended to you around 3 weeks ago. You are quite insistent on seeing her today as you came believing that she is in love with you and are extremely convinced about this, from the special way that she treated

---

* Adapted from B.K. Puri, A. Hall and R. Ho (2014). *Revision Notes in Psychiatry*. London, UK: CRC Press, pp. 6, 392.

you 3 weeks ago and also from the way she smiles at you. You are keen to meet up with her today and take this relationship further. In addition, you have made some plans of what you wish to do if she is willing to go on a date with you. You want to have a good meal with her and then take it further from that. You desire intimacy and have been thinking of chaining her to the bed and being intimate with her. You have done this before with your previous two girlfriends, who have since left you. There was one occasion in which one of your girlfriends reported you to the police for the acts that you had done against her.

You do not know much about the nurse whom you met 3 weeks ago. All you know is that she works in the hospital, and that her shift is usually around this time. You do not have additional details such as where she stays or her telephone number and have not attempted to stalk her or follow her home.

You are very insistent on meeting the nurse today and are upset that the receptionist could not facilitate this. Now, you think that it is absurd that you have to meet up with a psychiatrist to discuss this with him or her. You have been holding on to a bag, which contains a knife, and you would consider using the knife to deal with anyone who interferes with your plan.

CASC construct table

The CASC construct table is formatted such that candidates will be able to cover adequately both the range and the depth of the assessment required in this station.

Approach: The patient is expected to be very demanding and insisting on meeting up with the nurse. He might be aggressive and hostile as well. Pay attention to non-verbal cues, as he might be holding a bag with a knife within. Make use of the initial few minutes to establish rapport.					
Starting off: 'Hello, I am Dr Melvyn, one of the psychiatrists from the mental health unit. I understand that you have come here today, requesting to see one of my psychiatric nurses. Can you tell me more?' (The nurse's name is assumed to be 'Sarah'.)					
Introduction and establishment of rapport	I understand that you are very keen to see Sarah. However, it has been a surprise that you have come today.	I am here to help you, but firstly, I need to understand a bit more. Can you tell me more?	How do you know Sarah?	Can you tell me more about when you first met her?	
Explore and challenge existing delusions	What is your relationship with Sarah? When did you first feel that Sarah started to love you?	What made you think so? How do you know that she is indeed in love with you?	Has she told you anything? How likely is this feeling?	From my understanding, you only met her once. Can this be possible? How convinced are you?	Could it not be possible that this is how she is, and she treats all patients the same way?

(Continued)

Knowledge about victim	Thanks for sharing with me so patiently. Can you tell me how much you know about Sarah?	Apart from knowing that she works here, do you know where she stays?	Do you know her mobile number? Have you looked her up in the local phone directory?	Have you ever followed her home before? How about social media such as Facebook and Twitter?	Do you know whether she is in a current relationship? What are your thoughts towards her boyfriend?
Explore and assess other psychiatric pathology	How has your mood been thus far? Do you still have interest in what you loved to do? What do you work as and whom do you live with?	Have there been any changes in your sleep or your appetite recently? Are you currently working? If not, why?	Do you feel more self-confident compared with others? Do you feel that you have some special abilities that others do not have?	Have you ever had strange experiences, such as hearing voices when no one is there or seeing things when no one is there?	Have you used substances like alcohol or other street drugs to help you cope with your anxiety previously?
Forensic history and risk assessment	Can you tell me more about what plans you have in mind if you are able to meet Sarah tonight? Do you have plans to get intimate with her?	Is this the first relationship you have had? You mentioned your previous girlfriends; can you tell me more about how those relationships went?	Why were the police involved? Have you been involved with the police for other reasons? Do you have access to any weapons?	What will happen if Sarah decides not to meet you? Do you have thoughts of ending it all? Do you have thoughts of harming yourself, Sarah and her boyfriend?	It has been quite a surprise for us that you turned up today. What if we say that we need more information from Sarah before we allow her to see you?

Common pitfalls

a. Failure to engage with a difficult patient.
b. It is important to stay calm and firm as the patient will keep insisting to see Sarah. Remember to cover all grounds.
c. Failure to challenge the patient's delusional beliefs adequately.
d. Failure to cover the range and depth of the station (failure to elicit more background information from the patient regarding his knowledge about the nurse, failure to elicit and consider other psychiatric diagnosis).
e. Failure to ask question about his previous forensic history.
f. Failure to ask about drugs and substance usage.
g. Failure to perform an adequate risk assessment.

Identification of childhood history to support a previous diagnosis of ADHD	Can you tell me more about when your ADHD was first diagnosed? Do you remember what were the main problems back then?	Did you have any other difficulties when you were younger besides ADHD? Has your academic performance been affected as well?	Can you tell me more about the previous treatments that you have had? Do you remember the reasons why the medication that was previously started for you was stopped?
Consideration of other psychiatric comorbidities	How has your mood been recently? Are you still able to have interest in things that you used to be interested in?	Have you used any substance such as alcohol or drugs to help you cope with your current condition?	Any medical issues, such as heart problems and seizures?
Risk assessment	Have you been involved with the police previously? Can you tell me more?	Have you or people around you noticed that you have been more irritable recently? Have you got into any trouble with others?	Do you find yourself being more impulsive and more reckless when driving?
Address current concerns	I understand that you are concerned about whether you will be eligible for the upcoming international competition.	I could help you with a medical memo, but before that I might need to contact your previous psychiatrist and any other doctors to get more information. Will that be alright?	Do you have any other concerns? I understand that your coach is here to speak to me. Will it be alright for me to speak to him? *(Remember to take consent from the patient in a paired station)*

Common pitfalls

a. Failure to engage with a patient who might be very anxious initially and keeps requesting for help with a medical memo.
b. Failure to elicit current core ADHD symptoms.
c. Failure to assess impact of current core ADHD symptoms on his level of functioning.
d. Failure to elicit comprehensive childhood history of ADHD.
e. Failure to elicit previous medications history and contraindications to specific medications tried previously.
f. Need to adequately assess how the patient is currently doing so far in the area that he is concerned about (in this case doing sports), and whether he really needs stimulants.
g. Failure to adequately address his current concerns. (Some candidates might mention that they will write him a memo immediately, without getting further

collaborative history from his previous clinical notes and previous attending psychiatrists.)
h. Failure to tactfully assess for secondary agenda of getting stimulants in a non-judgemental manner.

Quick recall: Adult ADHD*

Current studies have demonstrated that for adult ADHD, the symptoms of ADHD tend to be focused more upon the inattentive symptoms. Symptoms of hyperactivity usually improve over time.

The following are the common symptoms of adult ADHD:

a. Irritability
b. Impatience
c. Forgetfulness
d. Inattention
e. Impulsivity
f. Disorganization
g. Distractibility
h. Chronic procrastination with many projects underway at the same time and having difficulties with completing them
i. Difficulties with tolerating boredom

NICE guidance for the treatment of ADHD in adults:

Pharmacological treatment: Methylphenidate is the first-line treatment. Dose: 5 mg three times daily (TID) and increase to a maximum of 100 mg/day. Target dosage is usually 1 mg/kg/daily. Consider atomoxetine if drug diversion is a problem. Maintenance dose is 80–100 mg/day.
Interventions: It would be ideal to offer a comprehensive treatment program (group or individual cognitive behavioural therapy [CBT]) addressing psychological, behavioural and occupational needs.

ADHD symptoms do persist at the age of 30 years in one-quarter of the ADHD children. Most patients do not require medications when they get older. However, it is appropriate to consider treatment in adults whose ADHD symptoms remain disabling to them. Although symptoms of hyperactivity often improve as the child grows older, inattention is likely to persist. Predictors for the persistence of ADHD symptoms into adulthood include the following:

a. Having a positive family history of ADHD
b. Psychosocial adversity
c. Comorbid conduct disorder
d. Comorbid depressive disorder
e. Comorbid anxiety disorder

---

* Adapted from B.K. Puri, A. Hall and R. Ho (2014). *Revision Notes in Psychiatry*. London, UK: CRC Press, p. 631.

STATION 14: ADULT ADHD PAIRED STATION

Information to candidates

Name of patient: Mr Thomas Foster

You are a core trainee 3, and you have just seen James Hunt, one of the star players in Mr Thomas Foster's soccer team. Mr Foster is here today to understand more about your assessment, and he wants to clarify some of his concerns.

Task

Please speak to the team manager, Mr Foster, to explain your assessment of his player and also address all his views, concerns and expectations.

Outline of station

You are Mr Thomas Foster and are here today as you have some concerns about your star player, James Hunt. You understand that he is on a stimulant medication for his psychiatric condition. You are very concerned about him being on the stimulant medication, as he is going to represent your team in the upcoming World Cup. You are concerned that with him taking stimulants, your team might be disqualified from the match.

You are keen to listen to the assessment that has just been done by the core trainee. However, you need to disagree that continuation of his current medications is the best management option. You are insistent and request that he be taken off his stimulant medications immediately. You will ask whether there are other medications that are non-stimulant in nature that he could possibly take.

You raised your concerns about him taking a banned drug that would have severe implications on the team's participation in the upcoming competition. You have heard of some herbal remedy and have researched more about it online. You have found at least 10 research articles documenting its clinical efficacy. You inform the core trainee about it and are insistent that he be switched over to this herbal remedy if he still needs some form of medication for his symptoms. If the core trainee is insistent that the player needs to be maintained on the stimulant medication, you will ask him how best to let the authorities know.

CASC construct table

The CASC construct table is formatted such that candidates will be able to cover adequately both the range and the depth of the assessment required in this station.

Approach: In this station, you should be prepared to expect a coach who will disagree with the assessment you have performed and is keen to get his player off the stimulant medications. It is important to acknowledge his concerns, but it is also important to tactfully explain to him the rationale for continuation of the existing medications and tactfully handle all his other concerns.

Starting off: 'Hello, I am Dr Melvyn, one of the psychiatrists from the mental health unit. I understand that you came to see us today as you have some concerns about your player, James Hunt. Can you tell me more?'

Clarify current assessment	I understand that this has been a difficult time for you. Please allow me some time to explain my assessment, after having seen your player.	It does seem to me that he still has persistent symptoms of inattention at the moment. My understanding is that he was diagnosed with ADHD when he was a child and has been started on medications since then.	Do you have any questions pertaining to my current assessment? Have there been any issues with his performance in the team? Have there been times in which you have noticed that he is distracted and not able to focus?
Clarify rationale for continuing on existing medications	Given the current symptoms that he is still having, he might benefit from the medications that he has been on previously. Do you have any concerns about continuing the medications that he has been on previously?	I understand that you are concerned that methylphenidate is a stimulant medication. There are other medications that could be considered. However, he has tried the alternative medications previously, and it has resulted in liver side effects, and hence it might not be appropriate to restart him on his previous medication.	It might be wiser to continue him on his current medications, so that he could function and perform in your team.
Address concerns	Do you have other concerns?	It seems to me that you are very keen for James to be started on this alternative herbal medication. My concern is that it is not recommended in the clinical guidelines.	
Future management plans	I understand that you are distressed about the fact that your team might be banned in view of James being on a stimulant medication.	As James does have residual symptoms and is likely to benefit from the medications, we could help by applying for a medical dispensation. Before applying for a medical dispensation, we might, however, need to obtain further collateral history from the psychiatrists who have treated him previously.	We like to do our best to help James and yourself. There are quite a lot of individuals with ADHD who do quite well in specific sports, so it is essential to see how best we could support them in what they are inclined to do.

Common pitfalls

a. Failure to engage with a patient who might be difficult and challenging. It is important to address his concerns.
b. Being unsure of the clinical guidelines and recommendations for the treatment of adult ADHD.
c. Failure to explain to the concerned coach about future management plans.
d. Failure to recognize that stimulants may be detected present on urine drug screen.

There may be several versions to this station: The coach may be very insistent for the patient to be on stimulants or he may be very against it. Nevertheless, it is still essential to adequately assess the functional status of the patient in the first part of the paired station and make the appropriate recommendation.

STATION 15: PANIC DISORDER (PAIRED – PART 1)

Information to candidates

Name of patient: Thomas Smith

You are a core trainee 3 and are running the outpatient specialist service. You have received a referral from your cardiology colleague, who has referred a 23-year-old man to you. On the referral letter, it states that the gentleman has frequent episodes of chest pain with palpitations, and the cardiologist has done a whole host of investigations, which found all heart functions were normal. The patient, Thomas Smith, remains very concerned about his condition nevertheless and feels that the cardiologist might be missing something.

Task

Please speak to the patient and elicit a detailed history from him to arrive at a diagnosis. Please also elicit the relevant aetiological factors. In addition, please inform the patient that you will be speaking to his mother in the next station.

Outline of station

You are Mr Thomas Smith, a 23-year-old university student. Over the past 3 months or so, you have been troubled by frequent sudden onset of the following symptoms: chest pain, palpitations, shortness of breath. These physical symptoms are associated with worries that you might lose control of yourself and even faint during the episode. These episodes usually come on suddenly, and the peak of the symptoms usually lasts for around 15 minutes. You worry very much about when the next attack might come on. You do not have any medical history of note, but you have since consulted several doctors, and none of them could give you a definitive answer as to why you are having these symptoms.

You worry that this might be a heart condition which the cardiologist has missed. You have an uncle who passed on at the age of 30 years due to sudden cardiac arrest. Since you were young, your family has been very health conscious. In addition, you are someone who worries a lot in terms of your personality. You get the attacks whether you are at home or in crowded spaces. You appeared to be anxious about your current health condition, but you are not depressed. You do not have any specific fears or fears of presenting in front of others. You do not have obsessional thoughts or commit compulsive acts.

CASC construct table

The CASC construct table is formatted such that candidates will be able to cover adequately both the range and the depth of the assessment required in this station.

Approach: Be prepared that the patient may be difficult to engage at the start of the interview, as he might not want to be seen by a psychiatrist. Be empathetic towards the patient, stating that you are involved in his care as part of a collaborative approach to help him with his symptoms.				
Starting off: 'Hello, I am Dr Melvyn, one of the psychiatrists from the mental health unit. I understand that the cardiologist has referred you. Can you tell me more?'				
History and eliciting core anxiety symptoms (physical and psychological)	Can you tell me how long this has been troubling you? Do you remember when this started? Can you tell me more about your experiences during the first episode? Do you remember how long the episode lasted?	Physical symptoms Can you tell me more about the bodily symptoms that you have during those episodes? • Palpitation • Sweating • Trembling • Dry mouth • Difficulty breathing • Chest pain • Nausea or stomach churning	Psychological symptoms When you have those bodily symptoms, what runs through your mind? Are you worried about losing control? Are you worried about dying or going crazy? Are you also afraid that something awful might happen?	How have you been in between those episodes? How frequently do these episodes occur now? Do you feel restless and keyed up, always on the edge? Have you ever had exaggerated responses to minor surprises? Do you worry much about when the next attack might occur? Are there specific situations in which these symptoms come on? For example, in situations in which you cannot leave easily? Do you tend to avoid these situations?

(Continued)

Rule out medical comorbidity and other anxiety symptomatology	I understand that the cardiologist has done a series of tests for you. Are you aware of the tests results? I know that you are very concerned about your current symptoms. Can I find out a bit more so that I can help you?	Apart from what you have shared, do you worry a lot about everyday little things? Do you tend to get anxious when you have to make conversation with people or give a presentation? Are there specific things that you are afraid of?	Do you have excessive checking or any washing behaviour? Do you have nightmares or flashbacks related to previous traumatic experiences?	I know this has been a difficult time for you. With all these going on, how has your mood been? Are you still able to keep up with your interests? What about your sleep and appetite?
Impact and coping	How have these symptoms affected your life? Are you able to cope?	Have you used any alcohol to help you cope with your symptoms?	Have you used any other drugs to help you with all your symptoms?	Have you sought medical help previously?
Personal history	Is this the first time that you are seeing a psychiatrist? Does anyone in your family have any mental health problems?	How were things when you were a child? Were there any difficulties?	Can I know whether you have any chronic medical conditions? For the conditions that you have mentioned, are you on long-term medications? Does anyone in the family have any medical history?	How would you describe yourself in terms of your personality before all these symptoms came on?
Diagnosis	Thanks for sharing with me your concerns.	From the symptoms that you have shared, it seemed to me that you have an anxiety disorder called panic attack. Have you heard about it before?	I understand that your mother is here. Would it be alright for me to speak to her?	

Common pitfalls

a. Failure to engage a patient who might be reluctant to speak to a psychiatrist as he thinks that his symptoms are medical in nature
b. Failure to elicit a full history of the presenting complaint – not eliciting information such as the duration of the symptoms, the onset, etc.
c. Failure to cover the aetiological factors that might contribute to his current illness
d. Inadequate usage and demonstration of empathy to reassure the patient throughout the interview

Quick recall*

To elicit history from the patient, candidates need to know either the *ICD-10* or the *DSM-5* diagnostic criteria:

ICD-10	DSM-5
• Episodic paroxysmal anxiety not confined to predictable situations • Several attacks occur within 1 month • Discrete episode of intense fear or discomfort, abrupt onset, reaches a maximum within a few minutes; autonomic arousal symptoms with freedom from anxiety symptoms between attacks • Symptoms involve the chest and abdomen • Symptoms involve the mental state	• Recurrent unexpected panic attacks with symptoms similar to the *ICD-10* criteria. • At least one of the attacks has been followed by at least 1 month of persistent concern or worry about additional panic attack and maladaptive change in behaviour related to the attacks. Common symptoms: Palpitations, sweating, trembling, dry mouth, difficulty breathing, choking sensation, chest pain, nausea or stomach churning, giddiness, fainting, derealization, depersonalization, fear of losing control, fear of dying or 'going crazy', feeling afraid as if something awful may happen, hot flushes, numbness, tingling, restlessness, keyed up, trouble relaxing

Aetiology of panic disorders

1. Genetic factors: The morbid risk for panic disorder in relatives of probands has been estimated to be around 15%–30%, much higher than that in the general population. Female relatives tend to be at higher risk compared with male relatives.
2. Cognitive theories: classical conditioning and negative catastrophic thoughts during panic attacks.
3. Psychoanalytic theory: Panic attacks arise from unsuccessful attempts to defend against anxiety-provoking techniques.
4. Neurochemistry: Noradrenaline, serotonin, gamma-aminobutyric acid (GABA) and other neurochemicals such as cholecystokinin (CCK) and sodium lactate have been implicated.

---

* Adapted from B.K. Puri, A. Hall and R. Ho (2014). *Revision Notes in Psychiatry.* London: CRC Press, p. 413.

5. There has been sub-sensitivity of the 5-hydroxytryptamine, 5-HT (5HT1A) receptors and exaggerated postsynaptic receptor response.
6. Life events: usually an excess of stressful life events in the year prior to the onset of panic disorder, especially illness or death of a cohabitant or relative.

Differential diagnosis:

a. Respiratory disorders such as chronic obstructive pulmonary disease (COPD), asthma and mitral valve prolapse
b. Endocrine disorders such as diabetes, hypoglycaemia, thyrotoxicosis, hypo-parathyroidism, phaeocheomocytoma and anaemia

Management guidelines (NICE)

1. The NICE guidelines recommend SSRI as the first-line treatment of panic disorder. Examples include citalopram, escitalopram, fluoxetine, fluvoxamine, paroxetine or sertraline. If an SSRI is unsuitable and there is no improvement, there is a need to consider either imipramine or clomipramine but not venlafaxine.
2. The TCAs and SSRIs are efficacious in the treatment of panic disorder. The downregulation of 5HT-2 receptors may be responsible for the therapeutic effects, which take up to 4 weeks to appear. Increased anxiety or panic may occur in the first week of treatment.
3. Benzodiazepines reduce the frequency of panic attacks in the short term. There is a need to maintain treatment in the long term, with the risk of dependency.
4. Psychological treatment: CBT should be offered to generalized anxiety disorder (GAD) and panic disorder in primary care. For panic disorder, CBT should be delivered by trained and supervised therapists, closely adhering to the treatment protocol. CBT should be offered weekly with duration of 1–2 hours and be completed within 4 months. The optimal range is 7–14 hours in total.

Suggested Reference: NICE. NICE guidelines for anxiety: http://guidance.nice.org.uk/CG22 (accessed 02 June 2014).

STATION 16: PANIC DISORDER (PAIRED – PART 2)

Information to candidates

Name of patient: Mrs Smith

You are a core trainee and are running the outpatient specialist service. You have received a referral from your cardiology colleague, who has referred a 23-year-old man to you. In the referral letter, it states that the man has frequent episodes of chest pain with palpitations, and the cardiologist has done a whole host of investigations, which found all heart functions were normal. The man, Thomas Smith, remains very concerned about his condition nevertheless and feels that the cardiologist might be missing something.

Task

You have spoken to the patient previously and have elicited a detailed history from him to arrive at a diagnosis. His mother has come along, and she is very concerned about his condition. She wants to know more about the diagnosis. Please address her concerns and expectations and discuss the likely aetiology and treatment options.

Outline of station

You are Mrs Smith, the mother of Thomas. You have been very concerned about his medical condition. Of late, you understand that he has been experiencing sudden onset of palpitations associated with chest pain. Your brother died of a sudden cardiac attack recently, and you are wondering whether Thomas might have a similar condition. You hope that the cardiologist can do more extensive investigations, but you hear from Thomas that the cardiologist has cleared him medically and told him that he has a psychiatric problem. You are very anxious as to what Thomas might be suffering, as you can't help worrying that the doctors might have missed something of significance.

If there is indeed something wrong psychologically, you want to know what could have precipitated this. You hope you have not contributed to this in any way. You seek to know more about the treatment of the current condition – both medical treatments and talking therapy. You are extremely distressed with the symptoms that Thomas is having at the moment and want the doctor with whom speaking to advise you on what best to do when he is having those panic episodes. You want specific answers to your questions.

CASC construct table

The CASC construct table is formatted such that candidates will be able to cover adequately both the range and the depth of the assessment required in this station.

Approach: Be prepared that the patient's mother might be highly anxious about her son's condition and might be difficult to engage. Establish rapport first and help her to understand how best you are trying to help her son.			
Starting off: 'Hello, I am Dr Melvyn, one of the psychiatrists from the mental health unit. I have recently seen your son, Thomas, and I understand you have some concerns. Can I spend some time with you to address the concerns that you have?'			
Clarification of diagnosis	I understand that it has been a difficult time for both yourself and your son. I have assessed him, and I am keen to share more about my assessment. Would that be alright?	Based on the information Thomas has provided, it seems to me that he has what is known as a panic disorder. Have you heard of panic disorder before? How much do you know about panic disorder?	Thanks for sharing with me your understanding. Perhaps, can I take some of your time to explain in more details what panic disorder is all about? I am sorry to hear about what has happened in the family recently. Given that the medical investigations are largely normal, it is possible that Thomas's symptoms are psychological in nature.

(Continued)

			Mention about fight and flight action, and how stimulation of autonomic system causes the sympathetic overdrive.
Clarification of possible aetiological factors	You seemed to be concerned as to what precipitated this entire episode. From my assessment, there might be several factors that cause Thomas to have these episodes.	The possible factors responsible might include a. Recent stressors b. Presence of family history of psychiatric disorder c. Premorbid anxious personality	
Treatment options	Panic disorder is a relatively common disorder, and I am glad that Thomas has sought help early. There are various treatment options, both medications and talking therapies. Which one do you want me to speak about first?	There are medications that could help. Benzodiazepines or hypnotics are helpful generally for acute attacks and for short-term usage. We hope to start Thomas on an antidepressant medication to help him cope with his anxiety condition.	In addition to medication, it might be advisable for Thomas to consider talking therapy as well. The commonest talking therapy used in such condition is CBT. Have you heard of that before? Perhaps, let me share a bit more about CBT.
Support during episodes	I understand how distressing it must be for you to see your son having those episodes.	Thanks for coming to speak with us today. Your understanding of what your son is experiencing is crucial. I will give you some pamphlets to read about the condition and treatment.	You could offer him more support during those episodes by reassurance and encouraging him to use the techniques he has been taught during his sessions with the psychologists.

Common pitfalls

a. Failure to engage the patient's mother, who is likely to be very anxious about her son's diagnosis.
b. Failure to explain the aetiology of the condition.
c. Discussing only the pharmacological management options and not the psychological treatment options.
d. Failure to elaborate more about the possible support during the episodes rendered by caregiver.
e. Patient may ask how being anxious psychologically causes the physical symptoms – it is important to be able to explain the phenomenon adequately.

Quick recall: Psychological treatment for panic disorder*

Based on the NICE guidelines,

a. CBT should be offered in primary care.
b. For panic disorder, CBT should be delivered by trained and supervised therapists who are closely adhering to the treatment protocols. CBT should be offered weekly with a duration of 1–2 hours and be completed within 4 months.

CBT involves the cognitive restructuring of catastrophic interpretation of bodily experience. Exposure techniques that generate bodily sensations of fear during therapy with the aim of habituating the subject to term are effective as well.

STATION 17: HYPER-PROLACTINAEMIA EXPLANATION

Information to candidates

Name of patient: Ms Catherine Woods

You are a core trainee 3 and are running the outpatient service. You are seeing a 30-year-old female, Catherine Woods, who has a chronic history of schizophrenia, which was first diagnosed at the age of 20 years. She has been on long-term psychotropic medications, which she has been concordant in taking. She is currently on risperidone 5 mg. She came today as she has been increasingly concerned that she has not been having her menses for the last year, and you have organized some blood tests prior to the appointment today. The blood tests revealed that her prolactin levels are currently 880 mIU/L.

Task

Please explain to Ms Woods the results of her blood test. Please consider taking a history if necessary to check for prolactin-related symptoms. Please address all her concerns with regard to the future management of her condition. Please do not perform an MSE.

Outline of station

You are Ms Catherine Woods, and you have been diagnosed with schizophrenia since the age of 20 years. You have been sectioned for inpatient admission on three occasions, and your last relapse was around 3 years ago. You have managed well thus far, as you have been compliant with her psychotropic medication: risperidone 5 mg. However, over the past year, you have noticed that you have not had your menses. This is your main concern. In addition to not having your

---

* Adapted from B.K. Puri, A. Hall and R. Ho (2014). *Revision Notes in Psychiatry*. London, UK: CRC Press, p. 416.

menses, you do have other troubling symptoms, which you will disclose only if the doctor is sensitive and demonstrates empathy. You do have milky discharge from your breast occasionally. You want to know the results of your blood test that the doctor has mentioned he will organize for you, and you want to know whether the symptoms that you are having are related to the medications. You also wish to know the long-term side effects of the medications. You wish to discuss with the doctor how best to manage your condition: Would a switch of medication be ideal, and what are the risks?

CASC construct table

The CASC construct table is formatted such that candidates will be able to cover adequately both the range and the depth of the assessment required in this station.

Approach: Be prepared that the patient might be very anxious about her blood test results. She might be shocked to know that her blood test results are abnormal. It is important to reassure her and to demonstrate adequate empathy and sensitivity when asking her for other prolactin-related clinical symptoms.			
Starting off: 'Hello, I am Dr Melvyn, one of the psychiatrists from the mental health unit. I understand that you are here today to find out more about the blood test which was done?'			
Clarification of blood test results and explanation of likely causes for deranged results	Did you come with anyone today? I'd like to share with you the result of the blood test. I'm afraid that the results are abnormal. Would it be alright if I go on?	Based on the results obtained, it does show that your prolactin levels are outside of the normal range. What this means is that you have a higher than normal amount of this hormone called prolactin.	I understand that you are very concerned about the results. Can I clarify that you are only on risperidone 5 mg for your schizophrenia? Very often, the high prolactin levels might be due to the antipsychotic medication that you are on.
Eliciting clinical features of hyper-prolactinaemia	I understand that your menstrual cycle has been abnormal for the past year. Have there been any other bodily changes?	I'd need to ask you some sensitive personal questions to help you with your condition. Apart from the menstrual changes, have there been occasions in which you have discharges from your breasts? Have you noticed any changes in your intimacy recently?	Have there been any times in which you have had other bodily symptoms, such as headaches, blurred vision, weakness and numbness of your limbs? Any fractures so far?

(Continued)

Clarification of long-term side effects	It does seem like the bodily changes you are experiencing are due to the high levels of prolactin caused by the medication you have been on.	Over the long term, there might be a risk of osteoporosis – by that I mean your bones get weaker.	I'm sorry, but there might be also a possible increase in the risk of breast cancer.
Discussion of management plan	There are several options available to help you with these difficulties.	We could consider a switch to other non-prolactin elevating drug, such as antipsychotics like olanzapine and aripiprazole. Have you heard of them before?	The other option would be to add newer antipsychotics like aripiprazole to your existing treatment regimen.

Common pitfalls

a. Failure to explain the results in a simplistic manner whilst being reassuring to the patient
b. Failure to elicit core symptoms and to rule out possible neurological causes
c. Failure to clarify the long-term side effects of having a raised prolactin level
d. Failure to offer plausible treatment alternatives

Quick recall*

Comparison of risperidone versus other antipsychotics:

a. Higher risk of extra-pyramidal side effects (EPSE) and galactorrhoea compared with other second-generation antipsychotics
b. Low risk of sedation

STATION 18: EXPLAIN CLOZAPINE

Information to candidates

Name of patient: Jonathan

Jonathan was diagnosed with schizophrenia at the age of 20 years. He has been concordant with his medications, but he still has had numerous involuntary admissions for relapse of his underlying condition. He has tried several antipsychotics, both from the typical and the atypical classes. Further collaborative history obtained from the family revealed that his medications are supervised, and he has not had any recent substances and drug usage.

His case has been discussed with the other members of the multi-disciplinary team. The ward consultant has decided to start treating him with clozapine as he seemed to

---

* Adapted from B.K. Puri, A. Hall and R. Ho (2014). *Revision Notes in Psychiatry*. London, UK: CRC Press, p. 367.

have rather resistant schizophrenia. The ward consultant hopes that you can discuss more about clozapine with him, as it is likely to be beneficial for his condition.

Task

Please explain to Jonathan the rationale for the team's decision to commence him on an alternative antipsychotic known as clozapine. Please explore his concerns as well as his expectations.

Outline of station

You are Jonathan, and you were diagnosed with schizophrenia 20 years ago. You have had three previous admissions to the inpatient unit for stabilization following a relapse of your condition. You do not use any illegal substances and have been concordant with the recommended dosages of the medications. You feel helpless as the doctors have tried several antipsychotics, but these have not been very helpful for your condition. You are keen to hear of this new medication that the core trainee will be discussing with you. You have only limited understanding of this medication, as you do know of friends who have been on it. You have your concerns: You wish to know more about the medication, how the medication could help you, the side effects of the medication and the necessary monitoring process that needs to be done when you are on the medication. You are concerned about the side effects of the medication. In addition, you are very concerned about the risk associated with relapse if you happen to miss doses of the medications. You wish to ask the doctor whether you can take alcohol with the medication too.

CASC construct table

The CASC construct table is formatted such that candidates will be able to cover adequately both the range and the depth of the assessment required in this station.

Approach: Be prepared that the patient might be extremely anxious about the commencement of this new medication called clozapine. He might be feeling helpless given that he has tried quite a few typical and atypical antipsychotics previously. Try to engage the patient, and start off by asking his understanding about the new medication.			
Starting off: 'Hello, I am Dr Melvyn, one of the psychiatrists from the mental health unit. The team wants me to discuss with you the option of starting a new medication, called clozapine. Will that be alright?'			
Clarify the rationale for commence-ment of clozapine	Can you tell me more about your understanding of clozapine?	Perhaps let me share more about clozapine. Clozapine is an antipsychotic medication that is commonly used to treat patients with treatment-resistant schizophrenia. Schizophrenia is deemed treatment-resistant when three or more medications have been tried and have not helped with the condition.	In schizophrenia, neurochemicals like dopamine are overactive and in excess. Clozapine would help to block some of the dopamine in the brain and hence it will help you with your symptoms. Studies have shown that approximately every 6 of 10 people do benefit from the commencement of clozapine, and we are hopeful it will help you as well.

(Continued)

Describe the investigations necessary for initiation of clozapine and the rationale	I understand that you're concerned as to when you can start clozapine. Before starting clozapine, we need to do some blood tests for you, as well as register you with the clozapine patient monitoring service.	As clozapine could cause a reduction in the white blood cells (which are the cells necessary to fight off any infections) in around two to three in every hundred people taking it, it is a necessity for us to do a baseline blood count. Thereafter, we will need you to repeat the blood tests every week for the first 18 weeks. If things go well, we will then do the blood tests every 2 weeks for the remainder of the year.	Apart from the baseline blood count (full blood count), we will do other blood tests as well as a baseline heart tracing of your heart rhythm before commencing you on clozapine.
Explain common side effects and highlight dangerous side effects	As with all other medications, clozapine does have its side effects as well. Some of the more common side effects include sedation, lowering of blood pressure and increased salivation. Some patients also complaint of weight gain and also constipation.	Our team will start your clozapine at the lowest dose and increase the medication gradually to minimize these side effects.	Apart from the side effects previously mentioned, some of the rarer side effects include a reduction in the total number of white blood cells in the body, which will affect your body's ability to fight off an infection. Also, there is an increased chance for fits for patients who are on high dose of clozapine. We need your help to seek medical advice immediately if you are feeling unwell or down with an infection.
Clarify other concerns	Clozapine is an antipsychotic medication and is not addictive in nature. You do not have to take more of the same dose to get the same effect over time.	The treatment duration varies for every individual. We will monitor your symptoms and advise you accordingly.	We do not advise you to stop the medications, for your symptoms might return. We understand your concerns about missing a dose. If you have missed a dose within 24 hours, please take the medications as prescribed. Do not double the dose. Should you miss the dose for more than 24 hours, please let us know. It would not be advisable for you to mix alcohol and clozapine, as it might cause increased drowsiness.

Common pitfalls

a. Failure to allay the anxiety of the patient regarding his concerns about the new medications and engage him in the interview.
b. Failure to explain a simplified concept of 'treatment-resistant schizophrenia'.
c. Failure to convince the patient to try clozapine, as there is too much emphasis on the side-effect profile. Remember to mention how effective clozapine has been for patients with treatment-resistant schizophrenia.
d. Failure to mention the need for regular blood checking and dose titration for clozapine.
e. Failure to address all the concerns of the patient. (Please leave some time at the end of the interview to ask the patient whether he has further questions.)

Quick recall*

Based on the NICE Guidelines on atypical antipsychotics, clozapine should be introduced if schizophrenia is inadequately controlled despite the sequential use of two or more antipsychotics (one of which should be an atypical antipsychotic) each for at least 6–8 weeks.

Kane's criteria for treatment-resistant schizophrenia:

a. In the past 5 years, the patient has had no good functioning.
b. In the past 5 years, two different antipsychotics have been tried for 6 weeks with at least 1000 mg chlorpromazine equivalent, but unsatisfactory response has been noted.
c. The score of the Brief Psychiatry Rating Scale is larger than 45.
d. The score of the Clinical Global Index (CGI) is larger than 4.

If the patient has failed to respond to a trial of three neuroleptics of different classes, using an adequate dose for an adequate duration, an atypical agent such as clozapine can be tried. Clozapine can cause agranulocytosis, so regular blood counts are necessary. The incidence is 0.8% at 12 months and 0.9% at 18 months with a peak risk in the third month; it is higher in women and older patients. Kane et al. (1988) showed that clozapine was significantly better than chlorpromazine in the treatment of schizophrenia previously resistant to haloperidol. Improvement has been noted in both the positive and the negative symptoms.

In the United Kingdom, patients receiving clozapine are required to have their full blood count monitored at regular intervals.

Characteristic properties of clozapine:

1. The most common side effect is sedation until the next morning.
2. The second most common side effect is hyper-salivation.
3. Clozapine (like olanzapine) carries the highest risk of weight gain.
4. Clozapine is least likely to cause tardive dyskinesia.

Clozapine patient management system (CPMS) summary

---

* Adapted from B.K. Puri, A. Hall and R. Ho (2014). *Revision Notes in Psychiatry*. London: CRC Press, pp. 366–368.

Time 0	1. Information and advice about swapping to clozapine from another antipsychotic should be sought from the pharmacy.
	2. Decide whether it is inpatient or outpatient treatment. Inpatient initiation is indicated for elderly and adolescents of 16–18 years and for those with concurrent medical problems.
	3. Register patient with CPMS and obtain an initial full blood count (FBC).
	4. Start clozapine at 12.5 mg once a green blood result is issued by CPMS.
	5. For inpatient treatment, physical monitoring is required every hour for 6 hours, and patient needs to be accompanied by a carer.
	6. For outpatient treatment, patient and carer must be provided with emergency contact details for the first 24 hours.
	7. Inform his or her GP on the start date.
	8. Baseline physical examination needs to be done: weight, temperature, pulse and blood pressure ([BP], both lying and standing).
	9. For patients with diabetes, HbA1c at baseline; for patients without diabetes, fasting blood glucose.
	10. Other baselines: liver function test (LFT), renal function tests (RFTs), lipids and electrocardiogram (ECG).
Time 0–18 weeks	1. FBC: at least weekly for the first 18 weeks of clozapine treatment.
	2. Fasting plasma glucose at 1 month and then 4–6 monthly.
	3. LFTs, RFTs, lipids: every 6 months for the first year.
	4. Follow standardized clozapine initiation charts.
	5. A slower dose titration in the inpatient setting is required for older adults (>65).
	6. The usual dose is 200–450 mg daily with a maximum dose of 900 mg daily.
	7. For outpatient treatment, increments should not be done over a weekend or holidays.

STATION 19: EXPLAIN LITHIUM AUGMENTATION

Information to candidates

Name of patient: Megan

Megan is a 35-year-old female and has been suffering from depressive disorder since the age of 22 years. She has tried several antidepressants, but the medications have not been helpful for her. She still suffers from frequent relapses that require inpatient stabilization in view of the risk of self-harm. She is currently on citalopram. The team has discussed her condition, and the team consultant wants to consider augmenting her existing antidepressant with lithium. You are the core trainee on the team, and your team consultant wants you to discuss this with her.

Task

Please explain to Megan the rationale for augmentation of her existing antidepressant and address all her concerns.

Outline of station

You are Megan, and this is your third admission to the inpatient unit this year. You were diagnosed with depressive disorder at age of 22 years. You have tried several medications, but none of the antidepressants seemed to help you much with your condition. You still have frequent relapses, which require you to be admitted as whenever you have a relapse, you will be suicidal. You have been on citalopram 20 mg for the past 6 months and have not improved much on this new medication. Your mood is persistently low, and you are always feeling tired. You cannot keep up with any of your interests at all. You understand that the team's doctor is here to discuss with you more about using another medication to enhance your current antidepressant. You are keen to find out more.

With regard to the new medication, you are especially concerned about its side effects. If you hear that it might cause toxicity to your kidneys, you express deep concern, as your father passed on due to kidney failure. You wish to know when you can start the medications, the monitoring process before starting, and what you need to do if you are taking the medication. You have concerns pertaining to whether the medication is addictive and whether you can use alcohol whilst on the medications. You wonder whether the medication might affect the chance of you getting pregnant.

CASC construct table

The CASC construct table is formatted such that candidates will be able to cover adequately both the range and the depth of the assessment required in this station.

Approach: Be prepared that the patient might be reluctant to try any new medications as she has been on several antidepressants previously but with no success. You need to be clear with regard to the rationale for commencing the medications.			
Starting off: 'Hello, I am Dr Melvyn, one of the psychiatrists from the mental health unit. The team wants me to discuss with you the option of starting a new medication, called lithium. Will that be alright?'			
Clarify the rationale for commencement of lithium	Have you heard about lithium before? What is your understanding about the medication? Can I share with you the reasons as to why the team is suggesting adding on lithium to your current medications?	Lithium is a medication that has been used as a mood stabilizer for patients with bipolar disorder.	It can also be used to help patients with depression. How it works is by enhancing the effects of the antidepressants that you are on currently.

(Continued)

Discuss investigations prior to the commencement of lithium	Before we start lithium, we need you to do some basic blood investigations. These include a thyroid function test as well as an RFT.	In addition, we also would recommend a heart tracing be done. Whilst you are on the medication, it is necessary for us to do routine blood tests to measure the lithium level. This enables us to know how much of the medication is in your blood. The normal ranges are between 0.4 and 1.0.	The blood tests (lithium levels) might be quite frequent initially, but once we have adjusted the medication to the right dose for you, we will repeat the test once every 3 months.
Describe side effects – short term and long term	Like all medications, lithium does have its side effects. The common side effects are that of thirst, passing more urine than usual, bad metallic taste and occasional tremors of the hands.	The long-term side effects might include weight gain. In a small percentage of patients, lithium does cause abnormalities in the renal and thyroid functioning. We will do regular blood tests to monitor this. I understand that you are very concerned about lithium and its effect on the kidneys. I'm sorry to learn of what has happened to your father. There are many other causes for renal disease, but I do hear your concerns and we will make sure we will monitor closely.	Other side effects might come on when the lithium levels are too high in the body. This might happen due to drug interactions and dehydration. If the lithium levels in the blood are high, you could have symptoms such as diarrhoea, vomiting, severe hand tremors and maybe even confusion. Please come back to see us immediately.
Address other concerns	The time for a response varies amongst individuals. We are hopeful that the addition of lithium to your existing antidepressant will help you with your recurrent depressive episodes. It is not wise to stop the medications immediately once you feel that you're better. You should come back to us, and we could discuss more about how best to help you.	Lithium is not an addictive medication, and this means that you do not need to take increasing doses to get the same effect. We like you to inform your other doctors that you are on lithium as there are certain medications you cannot take.	As lithium might cause heart abnormalities in a foetus, please let us know if you have plans to start a family. We would not advise you to take lithium in combination with alcohol. I understand that I have given you quite a lot of information. Can I offer you a brochure to help you understand the medication further?

Common pitfalls

a. Failure to engage the patient and discuss with her the rationale for commencement of lithium as she is feeling quite hopeless about her multiple admissions
b. Failure to acknowledge her concerns about renal failure and reassure her that it is not a common side effect and that there would be routine monitoring done for her (should she be on lithium)
c. Failure to adequately address all her concerns
d. Failure to warn her about contraceptives and needing to inform the team should she have any intentions to start a family

Quick recall*

Given that lithium ions is excreted mainly by the kidneys, renal function must be checked before commencing therapy with lithium. As the therapeutic index of lithium is low, regular lithium level monitoring is thus required. The dose should be adjusted to obtain a lithium level of between 0.4 and 1.0, with a much lower level aimed for in the elderly.

The common side effects of lithium therapy include the following: fatigue, sedation, dryness of mouth, metallic taste, polydipsia, polyuria, nausea, vomiting, weight gain, diarrhoea, fine tremor, muscle weakness and oedema.

Long-term treatment with lithium may give rise to the following: thyroid function abnormalities, memory impairment, nephrotoxicity, cardiovascular changes (T-wave flattening on the ECG, arrhythmias).

Signs of intoxications include the following: mild sedation and sluggishness, which might lead to giddiness and ataxia, lack of coordination, blurred vision, tinnitus, anorexia, dysarthria, vomiting, diarrhoea, coarse tremor and muscle weakness.

If the lithium levels are too high (more than 2), the following effects could occur: hyperreflexia and hyperextension of the limbs, toxic psychosis, convulsions, syncope, oliguria, circulatory failure, coma and death.

STATION 20: EXPLAIN ELECTROCONVULSIVE THERAPY (ECT)

Information to candidates

Name of patient: Mr Thomas

Mr Thomas saw the psychiatrist 4 months ago, and he was initially started on fluoxetine for his depressive symptoms. As he did not response to the medication, the dose of fluoxetine was increased to 40 mg, and another antidepressant was added on. He has been concordant and has been taking his medications. However, collaborative history from the wife indicates that his mood is still much the

---

* Adapted from B.K. Puri, A. Hall and R. Ho (2014). *Revision Notes in Psychiatry*. London, UK: CRC Press, p. 253.

same, and he has not improved since the commencement of pharmacological therapy. The team has discussed his case, and the team consultant has decided that Mr Thomas might benefit from ECT. You are the core trainee and have been tasked to provide Mr Thomas with more information about ECT with the aim of enabling him to come to an informed decision.

Task

Please explain to Mr Thomas the rationale for ECT and address all his beliefs, concerns and expectations.

Outline of station

You are Mr Thomas, and you have started seeing the psychiatrist around 4 months ago, after being made redundant at work for depression. He has initially started you on fluoxetine 10 mg, but it did not seemed to help you much with your mood. Hence, the medication (fluoxetine) was increased to 40 mg after 8 weeks. The increased dose of medications did not do you any good, and your mood remained low. An additional antidepressant was added. Your condition has not improved even with the addition of another alternative antidepressant. Your wife also feels that you haven't improved.

You wonder whether the new treatment, now recommended by the team, would really help you with your condition. If the core trainee is empathetic enough towards your condition, you will ask him to explain more about the procedure. You have heard that the procedure was barbaric in nature based on media reports. You have concerns pertaining to the potential benefits, efficacy and side-effect profile, and you also wish to know more about whether the procedure could be stopped once you have made some improvement.

CASC construct table

The CASC construct table is formatted such that candidates will be able to cover adequately both the range and the depth of the assessment required in this station.

Approach: Be prepared that the patient might be reluctant to try any new medications as he has been on several antidepressants previously but with no success. You need to demonstrate empathy towards the patient and explain the rationale for recommending the current treatment.			
Starting off: 'Hello, I am Dr Melvyn, one of the psychiatrists from the mental health unit. The team wants me to discuss with you the option of starting you on ECT. Is that alright with you?'			
Clarification of the rationale for ECT	Can I check with you whether you have heard anything about ECT before? Thanks for sharing with me your understanding. I'd like to explain to you more about ECT. Is that okay?	ECT refers to electroconvulsive therapy. It is one of the commonly used therapies, recommended by NICE, to help people with severe depression who have not benefitted from antidepressants.	ECT has been used for mania and schizophrenia. In your case, my understanding is that the doctors have tried you on two different antidepressants, and your mood has not improved significantly. Hence, we'd like to help you with your condition by using ECT.

(Continued)

Explanation of ECT procedure	Before listing you for the treatment, we need to do some basic blood works and possibly a tracing of your heart rhythm, to make sure you are medically fit to undergo the procedure.	The treatment is usually given two times in a week. During the procedure, the anaesthetist will give you some medications to help you relax and go to sleep. In addition, he will also give you some oxygen to breathe.	When you are relaxed and asleep, we will administer a small amount of electric current, using electrodes to your brain. This will induce a short period of fit. It is believed that the induced fit will alter the levels of brain chemical that are responsible for regulating your mood, appetite and sleep.
Clarifications of concerns relating to ECT	As I have mentioned before, ECT is a commonly used treatment modality in various psychiatric units. It is not a barbaric form of treatment as being portrayed in the media.	The risk associated with ECT is very low. The risk of death is rare and similar in percentages to that of a normal surgery.	
Explain benefits and potential side effects	The reasons why we are keen for you to consider ECT are that you have tried two previous antidepressants, but they have not worked for you.	As with all modalities of treatment, ECT has known side effects. Immediately after the procedure, some patients do complain of muscular aches and headache. We could help with this by giving you painkillers.	Very rarely are the memory side effects permanent. We usually also start ECT with the lowest energy level to minimize its effect on memory.
	We are hopeful that ECT would work for you and enable you to have a quicker recovery. Switching and adjusting medications for your depressive symptoms might take a longer time. Previous research has shown that ECT is helpful in 60% of individuals.	ECT does have effects on your memories – old memories and formation of new memories. Some patients do experience memory difficulties after ECT, but most of their difficulties usually improve with time.	In addition, we could always consider unilateral ECT if the memory difficulties are very prominent. The number of sessions is usually 6–12, depending on your condition, done three times per week.
Discuss about consent issues and address other concerns	As with all procedures, we are required to ask you to sign a consent form for the procedure. Signing the consent form does not mean that you are mandated to undergo all the sessions you have signed for. You can withdraw your consent at any point in time.	Do you have any other queries pertaining to ECT? I understand that I have given you quite a lot of information. Can I offer you a brochure about ECT?	Please feel free to book an appointment to see us again to discuss further about ECT or the other alternative therapies.

Common pitfalls

a. Failure to reassure the patient that ECT is not a barbaric form of treatment and to build rapport with the patient by continuing to explain more about ECT
b. Overemphasis on explanation of the side effects of ECT, and failure to bring across the point as to why the team wishes the patient to consider ECT
c. Failure to address the patient's concern about side effects of ECT and possible remedies such as using unilateral electrode placement

Quick recall*

The NICE guidelines recommend that ECT be used only to achieve rapid and short-term improvement of severe symptoms after an adequate trial of other treatment options has proven ineffective and/or the condition is considered to be potentially life-threatening in individuals with the following:

- Severe depressive illness: Around 60%–80% remission rates, typically attained after 2–4 weeks; relapse rate without maintenance antidepressant treatment is around 50%–95%.
- Life-threatening depression: refusal to eat.
- Depression with strong suicidal ideation.
- Psychotic depression.
- Stupor.
- Puerperal depressive illness.

Pre-ECT assessment and investigations

- Review psychiatric history, medical history, drug history and previous ECT record.
- Perform physical examination.
- Assess patient's dentation.
- Order full blood count, urea and electrolytes and LFT.
- Consult an anaesthetist for assessment.
- Patient receiving ECT should remain nil by mouth from the previous midnight.

With regard to consent, it is important to tell the patient that he or she will retain his or her right to withdraw consent at any point during the course of the ECT.
    Administration of ECT:

Electrode placement: In bilateral ECT, both the cerebral hemispheres are being stimulated.
In unilateral ECT, the electrodes are placed on the non-dominant cerebral hemisphere.
Seizure threshold increases with age. The age-based dosing method formula is computed by Dose in energy = Age divided by 2.

---

* Adapted from B.K. Puri, A. Hall and R. Ho (2014). *Revision Notes in Psychiatry.* London, UK: CRC Press, p. 321.

Frequency of sessions and the total number of treatment:

The usual frequency is twice a week for a total of 6–12 ECT sessions.
Side effects of ECT:

Main early side effects:	Memory impairments:
Headache Myalgia Nausea Dental damage Muscoskeletal (MSK) injuries Temporary confusion after ECT	• Anterograde and retrograde amnesia may occur after ECT. • Retrograde amnesia of events immediately preceding ECT treatments may be permanent. • Anterograde amnesia is usually transient. Anterograde amnesia usually resolves in 6 months. • A small number of patients do experience long-lasting subjective memory impairment, which is not detected objectively by cognitive assessment.

STATION 21: EXPLAIN SCHIZOPHRENIA

Information to candidates

Name of patient: Mr Johnson

Mr Johnson is a 21-year-old university student who has been admitted to the inpatient mental health unit as he was noted by his hostel mates to have been experiencing auditory hallucinations over the past 2 months. The team has done the necessary blood work as well as the radiological imaging and thus far, they are all normal. The team consultant feels that Mr Johnson has a diagnosis of first-episode psychosis and has started him on olanzapine to help him with his unusual experiences. His mother, Sarah, is very frustrated to learn that he has been diagnosed with first-episode psychosis. She has come down today expecting to know more about the diagnosis as well as the prognosis of his condition.

Task

Please explain to Sarah the diagnosis and discuss with her the prognosis of her son's condition.

Outline of station

You are Johnson, and you have been sectioned for an admission to the local mental health unit, following experiencing 2 months of auditory hallucinations. The team doctors have told you that you have first-episode psychosis, and they have started you on a medication known as olanzapine. You feel better since they have commenced the medication, although you do feel quite sedated on taking it. You are keen to get well as soon as possible and be discharged home soon.

Your mother, Sarah, is here, and she appears to be very agitated about learning from the nurses that you have first-episode psychosis. She has researched much about the condition online and is very concerned that you been diagnosed with this condition. She demands to know the prognosis of your condition and also wants to know whether you can get back to university life.

CASC construct table

The CASC construct table is formatted such that candidates will be able to cover adequately both the range and the depth of the assessment required in this station.

Approach: Be prepared that the mother might be very agitated when approached. She is very upset to have heard from the nurses, and not the team doctors, about her son's diagnosis. It is important to apologize for that, and to attempt to engage her by telling her that you represent the team, and you're here to explain and address all her concerns.			
Starting off: 'Hello, I am Dr Melvyn, one of the psychiatrists from the mental health unit. I understand that you are here today as you have some concerns about your son, Mr Johnson. Can we have a chat about it?'			
Clarification of diagnosis	I must apologize that you have learnt about your son's diagnosis from the nurses. It should have come from the doctors. Please let me speak to the team to ascertain why this has happened. I understand how concerned you are with regard to your son's condition. I'm hoping that we could make use of this interview to address all your questions as we would like to work collaboratively with you to get your son better.	I'm sorry to tell you that the team feels that your son has a condition known as schizophrenia. Have you heard about this before? Schizophrenia is a relatively common mental health condition that affects approximately 1% of the population. Patients usually develop symptoms in their 20s.	The common symptoms of schizophrenia include positive and negative symptoms. By positive symptoms, I am referring to the presence of unusual experiences, such as hearing voices, seeing images or having strange feelings in their body. By negative symptoms, I am referring to symptoms such as low mood, low energy levels as well as lack of interest. Are you following me so far?
Explain aetiological causes	I need to reassure you that you are not to be blamed for your son's current condition.	Research has demonstrated that there are multiple causes for schizophrenia: it might be due to someone having a positive family history; or it might also be due to the usage of street drugs or even stress.	Unfortunately, unlike other medical conditions, there are no specific tests that we can do to diagnose someone with schizophrenia.

(Continued)

Explain management plans	Usually when someone is acutely ill, we might need to treat them in our inpatient unit. There are various ways in which we could help them, using medication and other non-medication methods.	We have started your son on a medication known as an antipsychotic. It will help to regulate his brain chemical and control the symptoms. Like all medications, antipsychotics do have their own side effects. The common side effects include sleepiness, weight gain and at times restlessness and muscle stiffness.	Apart from medications, there are other forms of treatment that are helpful. We could make use of talking therapy like CBT to help him deal with his distressing symptoms. Other forms of therapy might include family therapy.
Address concerns and expectations	Your son would need to take the medications for a period. You could help us by supervising him taking his medications. If he stops the medications, there is a high chance that those symptoms that have been bothering him might reappear again.	Despite what is commonly portrayed in the media, patients with schizophrenia are rarely dangerous.	I am hopeful that with the medications that he is on, and with your assistance in supervising his medications, he should be able to eventually return back to his previous work/studies. I have shared quite a lot of information. Can I offer you a leaflet to bring home?

Common pitfalls

a. Failure to apologize to the mother at the start of the interview.
b. Failure to engage the mother. (It is important to tell the mother that you're here to address all her concerns so that you can work collaboratively with her to get her son better.)
c. Failure to identify and alleviate any guilt that the mother may have and to offer to provide support. (It is important to explain that there are multiple aetiological factors that might predispose an individual towards developing psychosis.)
d. Failure to discuss the psycho-social approaches with regard to the management of the condition.
e. Failure to offer the mother a prognosis of her son's condition.

Quick recall*

Epidemiology:

The point prevalence of schizophrenia is approximately 1%.

---

* Adapted from B.K. Puri, A. Hall and R. Ho (2014). *Revision Notes in Psychiatry*. London, UK: CRC Press, p. 358.

The age of onset is usually between 15 and 45 years and is earlier in men than in women. It is equally common in males and females.

Adapted from Royal College of Psychiatrists *Schizophrenia: Key Facts* leaflet by Dr Philip Timms:

- Schizophrenia is a common disorder that tends to affect about 1 in every 100 individuals.
- It is a condition that affects an individual's thinking, feeling and behaviour and causes them to have unusual experiences.
- There are a couple of causes for schizophrenia. Having a family history of psychosis or schizophrenia might be one of the causative factors. Other factors include issues during pregnancy, childhood abuse as well as the usage of drugs. At times, stress might also precipitate an episode.
- The common symptoms of schizophrenia include both positive and negative symptoms.

The positive symptoms include the following:

a. Hallucinations: hearing, seeing or feeling things that are not present in reality
b. Delusions: having a firm belief that something is true despite the fact that the belief is not in keeping with cultural beliefs
c. Passivity experiences/thought disorders: feeling not in control of own thoughts, actions and emotions

The negative symptoms include the following:

a. Low mood
b. Lack of interest
c. Lack of energy

With regard to treatment, antipsychotics, psychological treatments and social support are crucial.

- Antipsychotic medication helps with the positive symptoms. It helps around 80% of patients with their symptoms. It works by helping to reduce the action of a brain chemical known as dopamine. Like all medications, antipsychotics do have side effects. The side effects include sedation/sleepiness, stiffness and restlessness and weight gain (which in the longer term might cause elevated blood pressure, lipids and diabetes mellitus).
- Apart from medications, psychological treatments are effective as well. CBT could help an individual to cope with the unusual experiences. Family therapy could help the family to cope with the illness.
- Apart from the above, other forms of help include day centres (offering classes, advice about education and employment), work projects, art therapies, supported accommodation and having a key worker supporting the individual with the disorder.

Adapted from B.K. Puri, A. Hall and R. Ho (2014). *Revision Notes in Psychiatry.* London, UK: CRC Press, p. 370.

Prognosis
- It has been estimated that approximately 25% of the cases of schizophrenia do show good clinical and social recovery.
- Factors associated with a good prognosis include the following:
  a. Female gender
  b. Being married
  c. Good premorbid social adjustment
  d. Having a family history of a mood condition
  e. Short duration of the illness prior to the treatment
  f. Absence of abrupt onset of the illness
  g. Late onset of the disorder
  h. Having an affective/mood component to the illness
  i. Paranoid ideations
  j. Absence of negative symptoms
  k. Absence of cognitive impairment
  l. Good initial response to treatment

STATION 22: CHRONIC SCHIZOPHRENIA (PAIRED STATION-I)

Information to candidates

Name of patient: James

James is a patient with a chronic history of schizophrenia. He is currently on follow-up with the outpatient services, but he has had multiple inpatient admissions for relapses. His last inpatient admission was about 1 month ago. He has been tried on several medications previously, but they have not been effective for him. Some of his relapses are also due to him being non-concordant with the medications. Since then, your team's community psychiatric nurse has been following up on his care. You have heard that James's father called in to make a complaint, and he wishes to speak to you about the treatment plans.

Task

Please explain the current situation to Sarah, the community psychiatric nurse who has been following James in the community. Please take a history from Sarah with the aim of helping you to understand James's condition better. You will have to speak to his father in the next station.

Outline of station

You are Sarah, the community psychiatric care nurse who has been following up on James since he was discharged from hospital. You are aware that James has chronic schizophrenia and has been tried on several antipsychotics before. For the last admission, he relapsed as he was non-compliant with his medications. He was floridly psychotic when he was admitted but was stabilized on medications. The team suggested clozapine, but James did not agree to the weekly blood tests, and hence the medication was withheld. He was discharged back home with his oral medications. He has capacity during the last admission, and hence the team was not able to start him either on clozapine or an intramuscular depot. You have attempted to visit James on multiple occasions since his discharge. However, all your visitations were futile, as he was not at home. The neighbours have told you that James spends most of his time at the local pub and has been drinking quite a lot.

CASC construct table

The CASC construct table is formatted such that candidates will be able to cover adequately both the range and the depth of the assessment required in this station.

Approach: Please introduce yourself and allow the community practice nurse (CPN) to address you by your name, as she is part of the multidisciplinary team.			
Starting off: 'Hello, I am Dr Melvyn, one of the psychiatrists from the mental health unit. You can call me Melvyn. I understand that you have been following up on James's condition since his discharge. Can I find out more from you?'			
Clarification about last admission	I understand that James has just been discharged from the hospital. Can you tell me more about the last admission? Do you know what were the circumstances that led to the previous inpatient admission?	Do you know what medications the team has started for him? Were there other alternative medications that the team has considered?	Do you know how James was doing prior to his being discharged from the hospital?
Clarification about psychiatric history	Can you tell me more about his previous psychiatric history? Can you tell me when he was first diagnosed? Also, can I understand how many sectioned admission he has had over the years?	Do you know what led to him being admitted previously? Can you share with me more about the medications that he has tried in the past?	Were there previous admissions that were mandated because James was either violent towards himself or others?
Current mental state	I understand that you have been following up with James since he has been discharged from the hospital. Can you tell me more about how he has been?	How has his mood been? How does he spend his typical day? How have his sleep and appetite been?	Have there been any recurrences of his psychotic symptoms? Can you tell me more?
Risk assessment	Has he vocalized any risk to himself or to others?	Do you know whether he has been using alcohol or any street drugs?	

(Continued)

Current issues and concerns	My understanding is that his father is very concerned about him. Do you know why?	Can you share with me whether he is compliant with his medications? Can you share with me the level of support he needs?	Is there anything else you would like me to know about James before I speak to his father?

Common pitfalls

a. Failure to cover the range and depth of information needed for this station
b. Failure to ask the CPN about risk assessment
c. Failure to identify and exclude factors that might account for treatment resistance

Quick recall*

- With regard to service interactions, assertive outreach teams should be developed for patients who engage poorly with services, are considered to be high users of inpatient care and/or are homeless. Crisis resolution and home treatment teams should be made available for those who are in any form of acute crisis.
- The care program approach helps to ensure that services are managed and integrated.

STATION 23: CHRONIC SCHIZOPHRENIA (PAIRED STATION-2)

Information to candidates

Name of patient: James

James is a patient with a chronic history of schizophrenia. He is currently on follow-up with the outpatient services, but he has had multiple inpatient admissions for relapses. His last inpatient admission was about 1 month ago. He has been tried on several medications previously, but they have not been effective for him. Some of his relapses are also due to him being non-concordant with the medications. Since then, your team's community psychiatric nurse has been following up on his care. You have heard that James's father has called in to make a complaint and wishes to speak to you about the treatment plans.

Task

Please talk to James's father, who has called in to make a complaint. Please address all his concerns and expectations.

---

* Adapted from B.K. Puri, A. Hall and R. Ho (2014). *Revision Notes in Psychiatry*. London, UK: CRC Press, p. 365.

Outline of station

You are James's father, Mr Brown, and you have called in to make a complaint as you are very concerned about your son's deteriorating mental health condition, and you feel that the team has not provided him with the best possible care. You are upset that he has not been admitted for treatment. You are very distressed by the increasing frequency of calls that your son, James, has been making to you. In addition, you are very upset that during the last admission, your son was discharged with the same medications, and the doctors did not seem to have done anything to help with his condition. You are concerned that right now, your son has been drinking more as well, and he has missed his last injection appointment. You worry that he might get himself into trouble again, as he has been involved and charged by the police previously. You demand to know how best he could be managed at the moment.

CASC construct table

The CASC construct table is formatted such that candidates will be able to cover adequately both the range and the depth of the assessment required in this station.

Approach: Be prepared that the father might be very agitated and angry.			
Starting off: 'Hello, I am Dr Melvyn, one of the psychiatrists from the mental health unit. I understand that you are here today as you have some concerns about your son. Can we have a chat?'			
Address his concerns	I see that you're quite distressed about your son's condition. I would like to make use of this opportunity to clarify any doubts you have. I hope you understand that we are concerned too and want to work collaboratively with you to help James.	I have just spoken to the community psychiatric nurse who has been following-up with James. Is there anything you wish to know?	It must be a difficult time for you as well, given that James has been consistently calling you and bothering you in the middle of the night. I am glad that you have shared this with us, as we would like to help you and advise you on how best you can care for your son.
Explain current mental state	I understand from the nurse that there has been deterioration in James's mental state since discharge.	I have spoken to the community psychiatrist nurse who has been following up with him. Would it be alright for me to share more?	There are multiple reasons as to why there has been a change in his mental state. It might be due to him not being compliant with the medications we prescribed, or that the depot that we gave him was not effective for him. It might also be due to him using alcohol or street drugs. Are there any changes at home?

(Continued)

Clarify recent admission and management plans	I do hope I can clarify what happened with regard to the previous admission. When James was admitted a month ago, it was a voluntary admission.	As it was a voluntary admission, he was not legally bound to remain in the hospital to receive continued treatment. Whilst he was in the hospital, we offered him a new medication, but unfortunately, he declined and told us he was only willing to take the previous medications. We did not have an opportunity to make use of the Mental Health Act for James, as he improved whilst he remained in the hospital. Hence, we needed to go with his choice.	However, we understand that James has suffered from relapses quite frequently, and hence the team of doctors decided that the community psychiatric nurse should visit James more frequently to check on his mental state and ensure his compliance with medications.
Explain proposed management	I understand how difficult things have been for you. We hope we can work collaboratively to help your son, James. For now, we will ask our community psychiatric nurse to visit James more regularly to check on his mental state. Should there be further deterioration, we might need to invoke the Mental Health Act for him to be admitted.	If he is to be admitted, the team might want to consider him on an alternative medication, known as clozapine. This medication is usually reserved for patients with schizophrenia that has not responded to adequate doses of previous antipsychotics. If we are thinking about starting clozapine, we will need to register him with the CPMS, and we will start him with the lowest dose.	I understand that you are very concerned that James might not agree to an inpatient admission. We will make sure that we do frequent visitations, and we will try to explain to him the reasons for him needing an inpatient stay. If he strongly declines an inpatient admission, we might need to admit him under the Mental Health Act. Unfortunately, even though you are his caregiver, the Act does not allow you to give consent for an involuntary admission.
		Clozapine, like other medications, does have its side effects. The common side effects include sedation, decreased blood pressure and hyper-salivation.	Thanks for sharing with us his drinking issues. It is important for him not to drink if he is started on the new medications. If he is admitted, we will assess his drinking issue in further details and help James with it. Do you have any other concerns that I could address?

Common pitfalls

a. Failure to deal with an angry parent
b. Failure to address all his concerns and expectations (lack of range and depth of information covered in the station)

Quick recall*

NICE Guidelines

a. Clozapine should be introduced if schizophrenia is inadequately controlled despite the sequential use of two or more antipsychotics (one of which should be an atypical antipsychotic) each for at least 6–8 weeks.

For the above station, it is important to also check why the patient has not been adherent to his or her medications. The NICE guidelines recommend the following interventions to enhance adherence:

a. Improve communication with the patient.
b. Increase the patient's involvement – helping the patient to analyse the risks and the benefits to come to a decision.
c. Understanding the patient's perspectives: Does the patient have general or specific concerns with regard to the adverse effects or is the patient worried about dependence?
d. Determine the type of non-adherence: intentional is usually due to beliefs and concerns; unintentional might be due to practical difficulties and cost.
e. Provide information to the patient.
f. Monitor adherence in a non-judgemental way.
g. Additional interventions: psychiatrist could suggest to the patient to record his or her taking medicine with the multi-compartment medicine system.

If the patient is indeed treatment resistant, clozapine should be considered.

Kane's criteria states that clozapine can be considered if a patient has failed to respond to a trial of three neuroleptics of different classes, using an adequate dose for an adequate duration. If the patient is to be commenced on clozapine, the following needs to be done:

Initiation	Register the patient with the CPMS and obtain an initial FBC.
	Start clozapine at the lowest dose of 12.5 mg once a green blood result is issued by CPMS.
	For inpatient treatment, physical monitoring is required every hour for 6 hours, and the patient needs to be accompanied by a carer.
	For outpatient treatment, the patient and carer must be provided with emergency contact details for the first 24 hours.
	Baseline physical examination needs to be done.
	Baseline labs need to be done.

(Continued)

---

* Adapted from B.K. Puri, A. Hall and R. Ho (2014). *Revision Notes in Psychiatry.* London, UK: CRC Press, p. 366.

0–18 weeks	FBC: This needs to be done weekly for at least the first 18 weeks of treatment. LFT, RFT, lipids: every 6 months for the first year. It is crucial to follow standardized clozapine initiation charts. The usual dose is 200–450 mg with a maximum dose of 900 mg daily.
18–52 weeks	FBC: at least 2 weekly from week 18 to week 52 of clozapine treatment. Fasting glucose at 1 month and then 4–6 monthly. LFT, RFT, lipids: every 6 months for the first year.

STATION 24: EXPLAIN BIPOLAR AFFECTIVE DISORDER

Information to candidates

Name of patient: Eunice

Eunice is a 26-year-old administrator who was diagnosed with depression 1 year ago and has been on an antidepressant, citalopram, for the past year. She has been admitted informally to the mental health unit, as her family members realize that she has had a massive change in her mood state. She was noted to be very irritated and at times very elated and was spending huge amounts of money on investments and even harboured unusual ideations that she was the royal family's chosen one. She has since been admitted to the inpatient mental health unit and has been there for 2 weeks. Eunice is aware that the team stopped her antidepressants and then started to treat her with both an antipsychotic and a mood stabilizer, known as sodium valproate. She has been told that she has bipolar affective disorder.

Eunice is very concerned about her diagnosis, as she is afraid of future relapses. She is keen to know more about her condition as well as the medications she has been started on.

Task

Please speak to Eunice with the aim of explaining her diagnosis, clarifying her doubts about her medications and address all her concerns and expectations pertaining to her condition. You do not need to perform an MSE.

Outline of station

Much of the history is in the introductory notes for this station. You are Eunice, and this is the first time you have had a manic episode, after having been treated for what seemed to be depression, 1 year ago. You understand from the team that you have been diagnosed with bipolar affective disorder, but you have limited understanding about it and wish to know more. You are keen to know the reasons why you are predisposed to having it. You are concerned about the medication (sodium valproate) that has been prescribed. You want to know the common side effects. You wish to know more about the prognosis of your condition as it would affect your chances of getting back to work.

CASC construct table

The CASC construct table is formatted such that candidates will be able to cover adequately both the range and the depth of the assessment required in this station.

Starting off: 'Hello, I am Dr Melvyn, one of the psychiatrists from the mental health unit. I understand from the team that you have some concerns. Can we have a chat?'			
Explain bipolar affective disorder	I understand that the team informed you that you have bipolar affective disorder. Have you heard about this before?	Bipolar affective disorder is a common mental health disorder that affects, on average, every 1 in 100 persons. It is called bipolar disorder, as there are two poles in this disorder: mania and depression. When an individual is in the manic phase, he or she feels very elated in mood and full of energy despite not getting much rest. He or she might be spending more money than usual and might be less inhibited in their social activities. They tend to speak very rapidly and might have a lot of plans.	In contrast, when a patient is in the depressive phase, he or she has a low mood with a reduction in interest. There might also be difficulties with sleep and appetite. At the extremes, some people do have suicidal ideations, and some might act on their ideations.
Clarify causes	Bipolar affective disorder usually starts prior to the age of 30 years.	I hear that you are concerned as to what causes you to have this disorder. The exact cause is not known, and research has demonstrated that there might be several factors that might predispose someone to have this disorder.	If you have a family history of a psychiatric disorder, there is a higher chance for you to acquire it. Chemical imbalances and environmental stressors might also be contributing factors.
Explain mood stabilizer (valproate)	Since the time that you were admitted, the team decided to stop your antidepressant as it might worsen your condition. They have started you on a mood stabilizer called sodium valproate. Have you heard about this before?	Sodium valproate is commonly used for those individuals with fits or epilepsy. However, it can also be used as a mood stabilizer for patients who are in the manic phase. It works on a chemical in the brain called GABA.	Other mood stabilizers that could be considered for usage include lithium and carbamazepine.

(Continued)

Explain side effects	Like all medications, sodium valproate does have its side effects.	The common side effects include sleepiness and weight gain, due to increased appetite, in some individuals. Some individuals also experience nausea and hair loss.	A small minority of individuals on the medication might have abnormal LFT, and some females do experience other side effects relating to their menstrual cycle.
Address concerns	I am hopeful that if you are compliant with the medications, you should be able to go back to work.	It is also important to be regular with your appointments.	Before we end this interview, I am hoping I could also provide you with some leaflets about bipolar disorder and how to help yourself. The leaflets can tell you how to cope with your condition, as well as how to recognize the early relapse signs.

It is important not to keep loading the patient with medical information and result in a 'monologue'. Remember to ask about what the patient has experienced in terms of her symptoms and relate them to the characteristics of the condition (this can help to make the discussion more relevant and easy to absorb for the patient). Furthermore, do pause intermittently and check for understanding.

Quick recall*

ICD-10 classification

a. Hypomania: There is persistent elevated mood, increased energy and activity, feelings of well-being and reduced need for sleep. Irritability may replace elation. Work is considerably disrupted. There are no hallucinations or delusions.

b. Mania without psychotic symptoms: Mood is elevated, with almost uncontrollable excitement. There is overactivity, pressured speech, reduced sleep, distractibility, inflated self-esteem and grandiose thoughts. Perceptual heightening may occur. The person may spend excessively and become aggressive, amorous or facetious.

---

* Adapted from B.K. Puri, A. Hall and R. Ho (2014). *Revision Notes in Psychiatry*. London, UK: CRC Press, p. 377.

c. Mania with psychotic symptoms: The symptoms are as mentioned earlier but with delusions and hallucinations, usually grandiose. There may be sustained physical activity, aggression and neglect.

Adapted from Royal College of Psychiatrists *Bipolar Disorder: Key Facts* leaflet by Dr Philip Timms.

Explanation of bipolar disorder and treatment options

- Bipolar disorder is commonly known as a condition in which an individual's mood can swing from being very high or very low, lasting for weeks to months.
- It used to be called manic depression.
- It is a common mental health disorder that affects about 1 individual in every 100.
- There are multiple factors that might cause bipolar disorder. Genetics might be a factor. Stress in itself can also trigger episodes.
- When an individual is undergoing a depressive phase, he or she would experience persistent unhappiness that does not go away. This might be associated with loss of self-confidence, feelings of uselessness, inadequate and hopelessness. They might even entertain thoughts of suicide.
- When an individual is undergoing a manic phase, he or she could be very happy and excited. They are full of new and exciting ideas and tend to move quickly from one idea to another. They are quite disinhibited and might be more interested in sexual activities. They might get irritable with other people and might spend more money than usual.
- With regard to treatment, for a manic episode, lithium, antipsychotics and sodium valproate are medications that have been commonly used. For a depressive episode, antidepressants should be used carefully as they could make people go high. Psychological treatments could be helpful – it is important to educate patients about their conditions and encourage them to do regular mood monitoring.

Adapted from D. Taylor, C. Paton, S. Kapur (2009). *The Maudsley Prescribing Guidelines* (10th edition). London, UK: Informa Healthcare, p. 155.

- Valproate can cause gastric irritation, lethargy and confusion. It can also cause dose-related tremors.
- Hair loss with curly regrowth and peripheral oedema might occur, as can thrombocytopaenia, leucopaenia and red cell hypoplasia and pancreatitis. Valproate could also cause hyperandrogenism in women, and this has been linked with the development of polycystic ovaries.
- In addition, valproate is a major human teratogen. The NICE guidelines recommend that valproate should not be routinely used to treat women who are of child-bearing age.

STATION 25: LITHIUM USAGE DURING PREGNANCY

Information to candidates

Name of patient: Sarah

Sarah is a 28-year-old female who was diagnosed with bipolar affective disorder at the age of 25 years. She has been sectioned for an admission to the inpatient unit on three occasions following manic relapses. The team has since decided to start her on a mood stabilizer, known as lithium carbonate. She has been taking lithium carbonate 400 mg for the last year and has not had a relapse since. She has just gotten married and is keen to start a family. She has been on a contraceptive as advised by the team consultant who saw her previously.

Task

Please speak to Sarah with the aim of addressing all her concerns and expectations. It is not necessary to take a history or to perform an MSE.

Outline of station

Much of the history is in the introductory notes for this station. You are Sarah, and you were diagnosed with bipolar affective disorder at the age of 25 years. You used to suffer from frequent manic relapses, and it was only recently that the team decided to start you on this mood stabilizer, known as lithium carbonate. You have been compliant with the medication and have been on lithium carbonate 400 mg on night. Your serum lithium levels are in the therapeutic range. It might be that the team's decision to keep you on lithium has kept you off a relapse for the past year. The team consultant has previously advised you to use contraceptives in view of the fact that you are on lithium. You have just gotten married and are now keen to start a family with your husband. You wish to discuss more about the usage of lithium in pregnancy. You do not wish the lithium to be stopped abruptly, as you have witnessed its efficacy over the past year. You hope that the doctor will be able to address all your questions and concerns and deal with all your expectations.

CASC construct table

The CASC construct table is formatted such that candidates will be able to cover adequately both the range and the depth of the assessment required in this station.

Approach: Be gentle when exploring the benefits and risks of being on lithium in pregnancy. The patient might be quite reluctant to be off her mood stabilizer, as it has kept her well for the past year.

Starting off: 'Hello, I am Dr Melvyn, one of the psychiatrists from the mental health unit. I understand that you are here today because you have some concerns about your medications. Can we have a chat?'

Clarifications about mood stabilizer	I understand that you have some concerns pertaining to the lithium carbonate that you have been on. Can you tell me more?	Thanks for sharing, and congratulations on getting married. From what you have shared, it seems that lithium carbonate has kept you well over the past year, such that you have had no relapse.	I understand that you are keen to start a family. Has anyone told you about the issues pertaining to the usage of lithium in pregnancy?
Explain risk of lithium in pregnancy	I'm sorry but I have to inform you that mood stabilizers like lithium are contraindicated in pregnancy. If you are on lithium for stabilization of your mood, we will generally recommend you stop the medication. There are other alternatives to keep you well during the pregnancy.	However, given that you have been stable on lithium previously, an abrupt stoppage of the medication might cause a relapse.	Also, I do understand that pregnancy in itself is very stressful. The stress you face during pregnancy might in itself precipitate a relapse. Hence, it is important we have this discussion today for us to work out how best we can help you plan ahead.
Explain risk after pregnancy	Some individuals who are without their usual mood stabilizers do have relapses.	For a minority of individuals who relapse when they are not on their usual medications, they might find themselves having difficulties with caring for their infant.	
Explain risk to infant	In addition, we need to stress that lithium is contraindicated in pregnancy, as it has been known to cause heart defects, known as 'Ebsteins anomaly' in the foetus.	As you have a history of bipolar affective disorder, there is also a heightened chance that your infant might acquire the disorder.	For mothers who do have a relapse during pregnancy, the well-being and the development of their children might be affected.

(Continued)

| Advice on alternative management options | I understand that you are very concerned about the withdrawal of lithium prior to you planning for a pregnancy, and I am aware that you are also concerned about having a relapse. | I would like to suggest that I could try to adjust your lithium and stop it gradually, before we advise you to stop your contraception.
I will keep you free from lithium during the pregnancy.
However, given that you have a history of multiple relapses, we could make use of alternative medications, like older generation antipsychotics (such as haloperidol) to keep your mood stable during pregnancy. | Once you have delivered, I would recommend that you recommence taking lithium as soon as possible.
However, as you have been recommenced on lithium, it is not advisable for you to breastfeed. I will recommend that you give your infant bottle feeds instead.
I know that we have discussed a lot today. Please allow me to give you a leaflet on lithium in pregnancy.
Perhaps we can arrange for another meeting to talk about your decision after you have talked with your family. |

Common pitfalls

a. Failure to cover the range and depth of the station adequately. (You need to explore the risk of withdrawing lithium for the mother during pregnancy and consider the risk after pregnancy as well as the risk to the infant.)
b. Failure to discuss alternative medications during pregnancy to avoid a relapse of her underlying bipolar affective disorder.
c. Failure to highlight that breastfeeding is contraindicated if the mother is on lithium.

It is important not to appear paternalistic about treatment options and insist on stopping lithium or not breastfeeding, etc. It would be better if you can provide a balanced opinion about all possible medical options and let the patient decide, after having some time for consideration.

Quick recall*

It is always best to avoid drug usage during pregnancy if possible. Stable patients may often be withdrawn from medication prior to conception. For those with great risk of relapse, a judgement needs to be made about the relative risk of relapse against the relative risk of taking the medication.

---

* Adapted from B.K. Puri, A. Hall and R. Ho (2014). *Revision Notes in Psychiatry*. London, UK: CRC Press, p. 560.

If there is indeed a need to take a psychotropic medication, the dose should be maintained at the minimum dose during the first and the second trimesters. The dose needs to be increased in the third trimester as a result of the expansion of the blood volume.

Bipolar disorder and pregnancy

The NICE and the Maudsley's guidelines have recommended the following:

- Treat with an antipsychotic if the patient has acute mania or if she is stable.
- Consider ECT or mood stabilizer only if the patient does not respond to an antipsychotic.
- If lithium is used, the women should undergo level 2 ultrasound of the foetus at 6 and 18 weeks of gestation.
- If carbamazepine is used, prophylactic vitamin K should be given to the mother and neonate after delivery.
- The treatment of bipolar depression follows the recommended treatment of depression

Drug choices for bipolar disorder in pregnancy

- Effect on mother and foetus: The risk of relapse is high if medication is stopped abruptly.
- For lithium, the incidence of the Ebstein's anomaly is between 0.05% and 0.1% after maternal exposure to lithium in the first trimester. For valproate, the incidence of foetal birth defect (mainly neural tube defect) is 1 in 100. For carbamazepine, the incidence of foetal birth defect is 3 in 100.
- For mania, the recommended medications are mood-stabilizing antipsychotics such as haloperidol and olanzapine.
- For bipolar depression, CBT is indicated for moderate bipolar depression. Fluoxetine has the most data on safety and is indicated for severe bipolar depression, especially for those patients with very few previous manic episodes.
- Not recommended: Valproate is the most teratogenic mood stabilizer and should not be combined with other mood stabilizers. Lamotrigine requires further evaluation because it is not usually used in pregnancy. It could cause oral cleft (9 in 1000) and Stevens–Johnson syndrome in infants.

STATION 26: TREATMENT-RESISTANT DEPRESSION

Information to candidates

Name of patient: Joseph

Joseph is a 30-year-old male who was first diagnosed with depression in 2011. He was initially treated with fluvoxamine 50 mg in 2011, and his symptoms remitted after 1 year of treatment. The antidepressant was thus stopped. Recently, he was told to leave his workplace, and over the past 3 months, he has what seemed to be a relapse, as he has been having persistent low mood associated with marked loss of interest. He came back to the mental health service, and his original antidepressant was restarted. However, his symptoms did not improve, and hence the dose was further increased. After 6 weeks on the increased dose of the previous antidepressant, the psychiatrist feels that Joseph has not responded to the treatment and has switched him over to venlafaxine 150 mg for now.

Task

Please speak to Joseph and discuss with him the treatment options available, as he is keen to recover as soon as possible. Please do not take a history or perform an MSE.

Outline of station

Much of the history is in the introductory notes for this station. You are Joseph, and you have been diagnosed with depression since 2011. You were started on fluvoxamine 50 mg previously and recovered from that episode. However, 3 months ago, you were told to leave your job as a teacher. Since then, you have been experiencing low mood associated with marked loss of interest. Your psychiatrist has tried to adjust the dose of the antidepressant you had been on previously, but you have not noted much changes after 6 weeks on the higher dose of the medication. Your psychiatrist thus decided to switch you over to venlafaxine 150 mg, hoping that it would do you good. Unfortunately, nothing much has improved. You are keen to get well soon and are keen to hear from the doctor what are the alternatives available that could help you get better soon.

CASC construct table

The CASC construct table is formatted such that candidates will be able to cover adequately both the range and the depth of the assessment required in this station.

Starting off: 'Hello, I am Dr Melvyn, one of the psychiatrists from the mental health unit. I understand that you are here today because you have some concerns about your condition. Can we have a chat?'			
Explore reasons leading to poor response	Can I understand from you more about your condition? When were you diagnosed with depression? Can I check with you whether you have other medical conditions? Are you on any long-term medications for your other medical conditions?	I know that it has been a difficult time for you. How have you been coping? Have you used any alcohol or drugs to help you cope?	Are you taking the antidepressant on a daily basis? Have there been any side effects with the medication? Apart from the stressor you shared, have there been any other problems, such as finances or in your relationships?

(Continued)

Discuss potential alternatives and explore alternatives for his current condition	Can you tell me more about the medications you have tried thus far?	I understand how difficult it must have been for you. What we could do now is increase the dose of the venlafaxine that you have been on and observe your mood. Prior to us increasing the dose of the venlafaxine, can I check with you whether you have any family history of any medical problems? We might need to also perform some basic investigations prior to increasing the dosage.	At times, a combination of medications may be helpful – augmenting with another antidepressant or use of mood stabilizer or antipsychotic medication. Combining medication treatment with talking therapy might also be helpful. Have you heard of talking therapy before?
Explain concept of treatment-resistant depression	If, after adjusting the dose of your second antidepressant to an appropriate dose, you still have not shown any response, it could indicate that you have treatment-resistant depression. Have you heard of treatment-resistant depression before?	Treatment-resistant depression usually occurs when an individual has not shown an adequate response to an adequate dose of two different antidepressants that have been tried for an adequate duration of time (usually about 6 weeks).	There are still many other alternatives if your depression is indeed treatment resistant. We could consider enhancing the effects of your existing antidepressant using either another antidepressant or other medications.
Clarify use of ECT	ECT might be one of the other alternatives if you do not show much response to antidepressants.		I understand that I have shared quite a lot of information with you today. Do you have any questions for me?

Common pitfalls

a. Failure to identify reasons leading to poor response (poor medication compliance, existing stressors, high expressed emotions in family, etc.).
b. Failure to discuss alternatives before recommending ECT. (In this case, the existing antidepressant medication dose could be adjusted first and augmentation strategies could be tried first prior to ECT.)

You will need to know the various augmentation techniques in management of treatment-resistant disorders.

Quick recall*

Pharmacological treatment for depressive disorder

Clinical response	If improvement is not occurring on the first antidepressant after 2–4 weeks, check that the drug has been taken as prescribed. If antidepressant has been taken as prescribed, increase the dose based on the summary of the product recommendation. If there is improvement after 4 weeks, continue treatment for another 2–4 weeks. Consider switching antidepressants if the response is considered inadequate, there is the presence of side effects or the patient requests to change drug.
Switching antidepressant	Consider a different SSRI or better tolerated new-generation antidepressant. Normally switch within 1 week for drugs with short half-life. Consider a 2-week washing period when switching from fluoxetine to other antidepressants, from paroxetine to TCA (because of anticholingeric side effects), from other antidepressants to new serotonergic antidepressant or monoamine oxidase inhibitor (MAOI) and from a nonreversible MAOI to other antidepressants.

For possible treatment-resistant depression, options include the following:

- Offer other treatments such as ECT or psychotherapy such as CBT or interpersonal therapy (IPT) with medication.
- Discuss augmentation with another antidepressant. Alternatives include SSRI + bupropion, SSRI + venlafaxine or SSRI + mirtazapine.
- Discuss augmentation with other agents:
  a. Add lithium (effective in 50% of cases).
  b. Add T3.
  c. Consider second-line agents:
     1. Add lamotrigine.
     2. Combine olanzapine and fluoxetine.
     3. Combine MAOI and TCA.
     4. Add tryptophan.

STATION 27: OCD (HISTORY TAKING)

Information to candidates

Name of patient: Stephen

Stephen has been referred by his GP to the mental health service for excessive handwashing.

Task

Please speak to Stephen and obtain a detailed history to arrive at a diagnosis. Please also rule out other comorbidity.

---

* Adapted from B.K. Puri, A. Hall and R. Ho (2014). *Revision Notes in Psychiatry*. London, UK: CRC Press, p. 391.

Outline of station

You are Stephen, and you have been having increased fears of contamination ever since a laboratory accident that happened 6 months ago, where there was a chemical leakage. Ever since then, you realized that due to your constant fears, you always needed to wash your hands multiple times to reduce the fears. You do not have other comorbid anxiety or depressive symptoms. This has affected your life significantly, as you are always late for appointments and are contemplating quitting your job at the lab.

CASC construct table

The CASC construct table is formatted such that candidates will be able to cover adequately both the range and the depth of the assessment required in this station.

Starting off: 'Hello, I am Dr Melvyn, one of the psychiatrists from the mental health unit. I have received some information from your GP regarding the difficulties that you have been having. Would you mind telling me more?'			
Core OCD symptoms	**Origin of thoughts** Can you tell me more about those worries that you have been having? How long have you been having them? Do those thoughts come from within your mind or are they imposed by outside persons or influences? **Nature of thoughts** Are those thoughts that you have repetitive in nature? Are they bothering you consistently even though you do not wish to have them?	**Exploration of other obsessional thoughts** Are you also concerned about needing to arrange things in a special way? Do you also have thoughts, images or doubts that keep coming to your mind? **Exploration of compulsions** Tell me more about how you have been dealing with those obsessional thoughts. How do you feel after performing the rituals?	**Exploration of other compulsions** Do you find yourself needing to check very frequently? Do you find yourself needing to perform other rituals to prevent something bad from happening? When did your symptoms start? *Assess circumstances of onset of symptoms and progression (any worsening?).*
Current functioning	**Impact of illness** Can you tell me how these rituals have impacted your life?	Have they affected other areas of your life, such as your relationships, etc.? Water bills?	Any medical complications from your symptoms? For example, dermatological problems from excessive handwashing? *(Offer to check the skin if the patient has this problem.)*

(Continued)

Other symptoms	Assessment for depressive symptoms How has your mood been? Are you still interested in things you used to enjoy?	How have you been sleeping? How has your appetite been? Have these mood symptoms come on before your OCD symptoms?	Are there other worries that you have been having?
Coping mechanisms	It has been a difficult time for you. Have you used alcohol to help you get through these difficult times?	Have you used any other drugs to help you cope with this difficult time?	

Common pitfalls

a. Failure to cover the range and depth of the OCD symptoms
b. Failure to assess the impact of the symptoms

Assess for characteristics of 'obsession' and 'compulsion' in the interview, and explore other themes and types of obsession and compulsions, respectively.

Quick recall: OCD*

Epidemiology: Lifetime prevalence of around 1.9%–3.0%
Affects males and females equally
Usual onset either between the age of 12 and 14 years or between the age of 20 and 22 years

Diagnostic criteria adapted from *ICD-10*:

a. Has to be present for at least 2 weeks.
b. Obsessional symptoms are recognized as one's own.
c. There must be at least one act or thought that cannot be resisted.
d. The thoughts of carrying out the compulsion are not pleasurable.
e. Thoughts, images and impulses are experienced as being unpleasant in nature.
f. There must be interference in existing functioning.

Most common obsessions (in descending order)

a. Fear of contamination
b. Doubting
c. Fear of illness, germs or bodily symptoms
d. Symmetry
e. Sexual or aggressive thoughts

* Adapted from B.K. Puri, A. Hall and R. Ho (2014). *Revision Notes in Psychiatry*. London, UK: CRC Press, pp. 418–420.

Most common compulsions (in descending order):

a. Checking
b. Washing
c. Counting

Suggested References: NICE guidelines for OCD and BDD. http://guidance.nice.org .uk/CG26; J.L. Kolada, R.C. Bland and S.C. Newman (1994). Obsessive-compulsive disorder. *Acta Psychiatr. Scand.* (Suppl. 376): 24–35.

STATION 28: OCD (EXPLAIN MEDICATIONS)

Information to candidates

Name of patient: Stephen

Stephen has been previously referred by his GP to the local mental health service to seek treatment for his OCD. He has been previously referred to the psychologist to receive psychological treatment. After his undergoing several sessions of psychological treatment, his symptoms have not improved. He has been recommended to try fluoxetine, an antidepressant to help him with his symptoms. You are the core trainee in charge of the anxiety disorder clinic in your service, and you have been asked by your consultant to speak to him.

Task

Please speak to Stephen and explain to him more about the recommended medications. Please also address all his concerns and expectations.

Outline of station

You are Stephen, and you have been having increased fears of contamination ever since a laboratory accident happened 6 months ago, when there was a chemical leakage. Ever since then, you realized that due to your constant fears, you always needed to wash your hands multiple times to reduce the fears. You do not have other comorbid anxiety or depressive symptoms. This has affected your life significantly as you are always late for appointments and are contemplating quitting your job at the lab. You have seen the psychiatrist previously, and he recommended that you see a psychologist to receive what is commonly known as CBT. You have been consistent with the sessions arranged, but you have not had much improvement. During the last outpatient review you had with the consultant, he recommended that you try an antidepressant known as fluoxetine. You are having doubts about being on medication. You have searched online and are concerned about the antidepressant being addictive. You are glad to be able to speak to someone who can address all your concerns and expectations.

CASC construct table

The CASC construct table is formatted such that candidates will be able to cover adequately both the range and the depth of the assessment required in this station.

Starting off: 'Hello, I am Dr Melvyn, one of the psychiatrists from the mental health unit. I have received some information from the consultant you have been seeing. I understand you have some concerns. Can we have a chat about this?'			
Explain and clarify indications for SSRIs	I understand from the consultant that he previously recommended you for psychological treatment. How have the sessions been for you? I'm sorry to hear that the sessions have not helped you with your symptoms.	OCD is a very common mental health disorder that could be treated using psychological treatment, medications or both. Have you heard about the medications that might be helpful for OCD?	The medication that we feel will help you with your condition belongs to the group of antidepressants called SSRIs. It helps in the regulation of the chemical known as serotonin, which has been implicated for both OCD and depression. The dosage of the medications used for OCD is usually higher for OCD compared with the dosage used for depression. SSRIs such as fluvoxamine, fluoxetine, paroxetine and sertraline are commonly used.
Explain effectiveness and side effects of SSRIs	The success rates for patients with OCD who are on medications is around 50% to 80%.	Like all medications, SSRIs do have some side effects. The common side effects include nausea, gastric discomfort, headaches and dizziness. These side effects are usually related to the dosages of the medications that are prescribed. We will monitor you closely with regard to the side effects and adjust the dosages accordingly.	We usually need you to continue on the medications for some time, until your symptoms are in control.

(Continued)

Address concerns	I need to clarify that antidepressants are not addictive in nature. Sometimes, we do prescribe sleeping pills or anxiolytics to help you when you first start on the antidepressant. Only those anxiolytics are addictive.	The chance of having a relapse is high if you were to discontinue the medications abruptly. We recommend that you discuss with us if you have any concerns pertaining to the medications, and we will advise you accordingly.	In the event that SSRIs still do not help you with your symptoms, we could try switching you over to another medication called clomipramine or, for treatment-resistant cases, adding an antipsychotic to enhance the efficacy of the antidepressant.
Address need for inpatient treatment	I am hopeful that with the commencement of an antidepressant, it will greatly help you with your symptoms.	An inpatient stay might not be necessary at this stage, as your symptoms are not so severe and life-threatening.	In addition, we have also not tried all the recognized forms of therapy.

Common pitfalls

a. Over-emphasizing on the side effects of the medications and forgetting to tell the patient more about the clinical efficacy of the medication

Quick recall: OCD*

Pharmacotherapy:

- Antidepressants are effective in the short-term treatment of OCD.
- SSRIs such as fluvoxamine, fluoxetine, paroxetine, and sertraline are commonly used.
- Clomipramine and SSRIs have greater efficacy than antidepressants with no selective serotonergic properties.
- Concomitant depression is not necessary for serotonergic antidepressants to improve symptoms.
- The success rates are around 50%–79%.
- Relapse often follows the discontinuation of treatment.
- For treatment-resistant OCD, there is some evidence that adding quetiapine or risperidone to antidepressant would increase efficacy.

---

* Adapted from B.K. Puri, A. Hall and R. Ho (2014). *Revision Notes in Psychiatry.* London, UK: CRC Press, pp. 418–420.

Psychological treatment:

- The NICE guidelines recommend either evoked response prevention (ERP) or CBT for OCD and body dysmorphic disorder.
- For the initial treatment of OCD, ERP (up to 10 therapist hours per client), brief individual CBT using self-help materials and by telephone, and group CBT should be offered.
- For adults with OCD with mild-to-moderate functional impairment, more intensive CBT (including ERP) (more than 10 therapist hours per client) is recommended.
- For children and young people with OCD with moderate-to-severe functional impairment, CBT (including ERP) is the first-line treatment.

Physical treatment:

- Psychosurgery may be indicated for chronic unremitting OCD of at least 2 forms of therapy.
- Open, uncontrolled studies show that 65% of patients with OCD are improved or greatly improved with cingulotomy plus bifrontal operations.
- Deep brain stimulation at the anterior limb of the internal capsule may be an option for treatment-resistant OCD.

If the patient asks about the prognostic factors for OCD, the following should help to determine the prognosis:

Favourable prognostic factors	Poor prognostic factors
• Mild symptoms	• Males with early onset
• Predominance of phobic ruminative ideas, absence of compulsions	• Symptoms involving the need for symmetry and exactness
• Short duration of symptoms	• Presence of hopelessness, hallucinations or delusions
• No childhood symptoms or abnormal personality traits	• Family history of OCD
	• Continuous, episodic or deteriorating course

STATION 29: POST TRAMATIC STRESS DISORDER (PTSD) STATION

Information to candidates

Name of patient: Mr Jones

Mr Jones has been referred by his local GP to the mental health service. He was deployed for his military service in Iraq and was sent back prematurely, as his commanders noted that he was not able to keep up with his work demands. The referral letter from the GP stated that Mr Jones currently has no intentions to go back to Iraq to continue his job. The letter also states that there was an occasion in which Mr Jones needed to seek medical help in Iraq, after being involved in an intense crossfire with the enemy forces.

Task

Please speak to Mr Jones with the aim of clarifying the history that the GP has provided. Please also perform an MSE with the aim to come to a diagnosis. It is also pertinent during the clinical interview to rule out other psychiatric disorders.

Outline of station

You are Mr Jones, and you have been previously deployed for military duties in Iraq. You have served and functioned in your duties without any issues since deployment 6 months ago. Unfortunately, you and your colleagues were involved in an intense crossfire with the enemy forces just 1 month ago. You witnessed how your best friend succumbed in that intense crossfire. This has affected you much, and you broke down that very night. You found yourself crying continuously and the commanders asked the local medical doctor to see you. He gave you some pills to calm you down. However, since then, you have been having a lot of difficulties. You find yourself not being able to perform in your job and tend to avoid the place in which the crossfire took place. Your colleagues have commented that your mood seems more irritable lately. Your concentration has been poor, and you have been bothered by flashbacks and nightmares of the incident and have been finding yourself getting startled very easily. It has been a tough time for you, but you have not resorted to coping by using any alcohol or street drugs. You are desperate for help.

CASC construct table

The CASC construct table is formatted such that candidates will be able to cover adequately both the range and the depth of the assessment required in this station.

Starting off: 'Hello, I am Dr Melvyn. I have received some information from your GP. I understand that you have been undergoing a very difficult time. Can we have a chat about this?'			
Clarification of the incident/event	Would you mind sharing with me more about what has happened? Can you tell me when did this incident take place? At that time, did you really think that you could have died? Any physical injuries sustained? Head injury?	I'm sorry to hear of the incident. Can you tell me who was involved? Do you know what happened to your colleague? Any survivor guilt?	It has indeed been a difficult time for you. How did you feel immediately after the incident?
Elicit core symptoms of PTSD – intrusions	How have things been since you have returned?	Are there times when you get flashbacks of the incident? Or times when you feel that you are reliving the incident again? Can you tell me more?	How has your sleep been? Have there been any nightmares that have been bothering you?

(Continued)

Elicit core symptoms of PTSD – hyper-arousal	How has your mood been? Do you find yourself more irritable than usual?	Have there been times in which you feel easily startled or edgy? Can you tell me more?	How has your concentration been? What about your memory?
Elicit core symptoms of PTSD – avoidance	I understand that you have since been back to the United Kingdom. Do you have thoughts of returning back to Iraq?	After the incident, have you been back to the place where it has occurred? Any avoidance?	
Elicit core symptoms of PTSD – emotional numbing	How do you feel if you come across news or events similar to what you have experienced?	Do you find it tough to experience normal experiences? Or to talk about how you feel?	Have you ever felt like the people around you (derealization) or yourself (depersonalization) is not real?
Assess for compensation/legal involvement and rule out other comorbidities	Are you currently involved in any legal suits or compensation claims in view of the incident? Any history of experiencing traumatic events? Any history of mental illness?	Do you find yourself having interest in things you previously liked to do? How has your appetite been? Sometimes when people undergo stressful experiences, they do have unusual experiences. Does that sound like you?	Are there times in which you feel very anxious or have worries about everyday events? I'm sorry to hear that this has been such a distressing experience for you. Have you used any alcohol or any other substances to help you cope?

Common pitfalls

a. Failure to empathize with the patient adequately, and hence failure to elicit the necessary information pertaining to the incident
b. Failure to cover the range and the depth of the symptoms of PTSD
c. Failure to ask and assess for compensation and other legal issues

Quick recall: OCD*

Diagnostic criteria adapted from *ICD-10*:

- PTSD arises within 6 months as a delayed and or protracted response to a stressful event of an exceptionally threatening nature. The symptoms include repeated reliving of the trauma. Repetitive, intrusive memories (flashbacks), daytime imagery or dreams of the event must be present.

---

* Adapted from B.K. Puri, A. Hall and R. Ho (2014). *Revision Notes in Psychiatry*. London, UK: CRC Press, pp. 427–429.

- Emotional detachment, persisting background numbness and avoidance of stimuli reminiscent of original events are often present but not essential.
- Autonomic disturbances (hyper-arousal) with hyper-vigilance, enhanced startle response, and insomnia and mood disorder contribute to the diagnosis but are not essential.

Overview of the management of PTSD:

Psychological therapy	Cognitive techniques would include challenging underlying automatic thoughts that accidents or disasters will occur again and the associated cognitive distortions.
	Cognitive restructuring, distraction thought replacement and thought stopping have been shown to be useful.
	Psycho-education should offer an explanation of the PTSD symptoms.
	Behaviour techniques include relaxation training, in vivo and in vitro scenes, rehearsal, as well as assertiveness or social skill training.
	The NICE guidelines recommend the following:
	a. Trauma-focused CBT should be offered to people with severe PTSD within 3 months of the trauma with fewer sessions in the initial first month after the trauma.
	b. The duration of trauma focused CBT is 8–12 sessions with one session per week.
	Eye movement desensitization reprocessing:
	• Involuntary multi-saccadic eye movements occur during disturbing thoughts. It has been believed that inducing these eye movements whilst experiencing the intrusive thoughts stops the symptoms of PTSD.
Pharmacotherapy	Fluoxetine, sertraline, paroxetine, venlafaxine and escitalopram are beneficial in PTSD. These drugs tend to need up to 8 weeks' duration before the effects are evident.
	To reduce the hyper-arousal and the intrusive symptoms, carbamazepine, propranolol and clonidine could be used.
	Fluoxetine and lithium are effective towards improving mood and reducing the explosiveness. Buspirone may lessen fear-induced startle; it may play an adjunctive role.

STATION 30: MINI-MENTAL STATE EXAMINATION (MMSE)

Information to candidates

Name of patient: Mr Joel

Mr Joel has been missing from home for the past 2 days. He was found wandering in a shopping centre by the police and has been brought into the emergency services by them. The medical team has done the necessary lab work and everything thus far has been normal. You are the core trainee on call and have been asked to assess Mr Joel.

Task

Please speak to Mr Joel and perform a detailed cognitive assessment. Please do not take any history or perform an MSE.

Outline of station

You are Mr Joel, and you wandered out of your house 2 days ago. You then could not remember the way back home. Your memory has been failing you for the past year, and you have been having a lot of difficulties lately due to your poor memory. You do not have hearing or visual impairment and are willing to cooperate and perform the tasks that the core trainee asks you to perform.

CASC construct table

The CASC construct table is formatted such that candidates will be able to cover adequately both the range and the depth of the assessment required in this station.

Starting off: 'Hello, I am Dr Melvyn. I understand that the police have brought you in to the emergency services. I need to ask your some questions to test your memory. Is that alright?'			
Assess for orientation	Before we begin, can I check whether you have any visual or hearing impairment? Can you see and hear me clearly? What is your highest education level?	Do you know where we are at the moment? What level are we on? Which part of the county is this? What is the greater country that we are in?	Do you know what time it is at the moment? Do you know what year this is? Can you tell me what season, month and the day and date today?
Assess for registration	I will like you to remember three objects, which I will ask you to repeat immediately and 5 minutes later.	The three objects I would like you to remember are 'apple, table and penny'.	Can you repeat the three objects that I have told you?
Assess for attention and calculation	Can I trouble you to spell the word 'world' for me?	Can you please spell the word 'world' backwards for me?	(If the patient is unable to spell, assessment could be done using calculation/numbers instead)
Assess for recall, naming, repetition, comprehension	Can you tell me the three objects that I asked you to remember earlier?	Can you name these objects for me? (Show the patient a pen and a watch.)	Can you please repeat this phrase: 'No, ifs, ands or buts'. Please listen to my instructions and follow my instructions. I would like you to take this piece of paper with your right hand, fold it in half and place it on the floor.

(Continued)

Assess for reading, writing and copying	(Write 'close your eyes' on a piece of paper) Can you please read this sentence and do what it says?	Can you help me to write a complete sentence that has a subject and a verb?	(Draw two intersecting pentagons) Can you please help me to copy this figure?

Common pitfalls

a. Failure to ask the patient whether he has visual or hearing impairment prior to the start of the assessment
b. Failure to remember all the steps in the MMSE and perform a complete MMSE

Quick recall: MMSE*

The core components and domains being tested using the MMSE include the following:

- Orientation
- Registration and recall
- Attention and calculation
- Language
- Visuospatial ability
- Praxis

The MMSE does not assess for frontal lobe symptoms.

The normal score should be more than 24. The score is determined by education. For patients with only primary school education, the following cut-offs are used:

Age 18–69 years: Median MMSE score: 22–25
Age 70–79 years: Median MMSE score: 21–22
Age over 79 years: Median MMSE score: 19–20
To make the diagnosis for mild cognitive impairment, the normal score is over that of 24.

STATION 31: FRONTAL LOBE ASSESSMENT

Information to candidates

Name of patient: Mr Green

Mr Green has been having personality changes after a head injury, which he suffered 2 years ago. His wife has accompanied him today, and they want some help from your specialized mental health service.

---

* Adapted from B.K. Puri, A. Hall and R. Ho (2014). *Revision Notes in Psychiatry*. London, UK: CRC Press, p. 689.

Task

Please speak to Mr Green and perform a detailed cognitive assessment looking for features suggestive of frontal lobe dysfunction. Please do not take a history and do not perform an MSE.

Outline of station

You are Mr Green, and you suffered a head injury following a fight at the local pub around 2 years ago. Since then, your wife has been complaining that you are no longer the same person she once knew. She claims that you have been more irritable than usual. She also claims that your memory is not as good as it was before. This you allude to, as you realize you can no longer function in your finance job and have since left the company for which you have been working for the past 20 years. You finally agree for an assessment by a psychiatrist today after much persuasion by your wife. You agree to cooperate with whatever tests that the psychiatrists want you to answer.

CASC construct table

The CASC construct table is formatted such that candidates will be able to cover adequately both the range and the depth of the assessment required in this station.

Starting off: 'Hello, I am Dr Melvyn, one of the psychiatrists from the mental health service. Thanks for coming to see us today. Would it be alright for me to ask you to do some memory tests?'			
Verbal fluency assessment	Before we start, can I ask whether you have any visual or hearing impairment? Please do feel free to stop me at any time if you do not understand me.	I would like you to say as many words as possible starting with the letter F in 1 minute, without naming any names of people. Can we begin?	Alternatively, I would like you to say as many animals as you can within 1 minute. Can we begin?
Abstract thinking assessment	Can you tell me your understanding of this proverb: 'A stitch in time saves nine'?	Can you tell me the similarities between an apple and an orange? (Alternatively, use a table and chair as example.)	Can you tell me what is the average height of an Englishman? Can you tell me the approximate distance (in miles) between London and Manchester?
Assessment of coordinated movements	Please have a look at this diagram (alternate sequence of squares and triangles). Can you copy this diagram for me?	I would like you to place your index finger on the table. Please raise your index finger once when you feel a single tap, and do not raise it when you feel two taps. Can we try this?	Now, I am going to reverse the rule. Please do not raise your index finger when you feel a single tap, and raise it when you feel two taps. Can we try this?

(Continued)

Assessment for response inhibition	I am going to show you a sequence of hand movements. (To demonstrate to the patient: specific sequence of a fist, then placing the edge of the palm and then a flat palm on the table)	I would like you to follow my sequence of hand actions.	Do you think you could show me the sequence?
Primitive reflexes	Now, I am going to test some of your reflexes.	I would need to place my hands and gently tap between your eyebrows. Are you fine with this?	Next, I will need to gently stroke your palm. Are you fine with this? I need to use the spatula to gently tap on your lips. Are you fine with this? Thanks for your cooperation.

Common pitfalls

a. Failure to ask the patient whether he has visual or hearing impairment prior to the start of the assessment
b. Failure to remember all the steps in the frontal lobe assessment battery
c. Failure to ask the patient for permission before testing for the primitive reflexes

Quick recall: Frontal lobe lesions and assessment*

A frontal lobe lesion might cause any one of the following:

a. Personality changes: dis-inhibition, reduced social and ethical control, sexual indiscretions, poor judgement, elevated mood, lack of concern for the feelings of other people and irritability
b. Perseveration
c. Utilization behaviour
d. Impairment of attention, concentration and initiative
e. Slowed psychomotor activity
f. Motor fits
g. Urinary incontinence
h. Contralateral spastic paresis
i. Aphasia
j. Primary motor aphasia
k. Motor agraphia
l. Anosmia
m. Ipsilateral optic atrophy

* Adapted from B.K. Puri, A. Hall and R. Ho (2014). *Revision Notes in Psychiatry*. London, UK: CRC Press, p. 110.

Assessments done in frontal lobe assessment	Impairments detected in patients with frontal lobe impairment
Word fluency	The patient can only mention a few words. Very often, they tend to repeat those words that they have already mentioned. Finally, the person stops and cannot provide more words or items.
Abstract thinking	The patient would not be able to appreciate the deeper meaning and just focus on the words superficially. It is also not uncommon to find that a patient might be talking about the differences between two objects as it seemed to be easier compared with the similarities.
Cognitive estimates	The answer given by the patient is obviously beyond the normal estimates.
Luria's hand test	Patients with frontal lobe impairment may not be able to appreciate that there are three different hand positions and cannot alternate from one to another as a result of motor perseveration.
Alternative sequence test	Patients with frontal lobe impairment will continue with the last shape. The failure to appreciate the alternative pattern is a result of perseveration.
Primitive reflexes	Patients with frontal lobe impairment show emergence of primitive reflexes.

STATION 32: SUICIDE RISK ASSESSMENT (PAIRED STATION A: HISTORY TAKING)

Information to candidates

Name of patient: Ms Valarie

Ms Valarie is a 25-year-old university student who has been admitted to the accident and emergency department following an overdose of 20 tablets of medication. The medical doctors have done the necessary tests, and currently she is considered to be medically stable. The medical consultant has requested for her to be seen by a psychiatrist in view of the recent overdose.

Task

Please speak to Ms Valarie and obtain a further history pertaining to the recent overdose. Please also perform a relevant suicide risk assessment. Please take note that in the next station, you are due to discuss the case with your consultant, so please note down pertinent points to facilitate the discussion.

Outline of station

You are Ms Valarie, a 25-year-old university student. You were found unconscious in your hostel room by your hostel-mate and brought into the hospital. You had just overdosed on 20 tablets of a combination of medications. Your recent stressor was that you had failed a major university examination. This was your first failure in life.

You felt disappointed and felt that there was no longer a reason to live on, as your opportunities to find your dream job had been compromised. You made a deliberate plan and attempt to end your life, and you are now upset that you were found.

CASC construct table

The CASC construct table is formatted such that candidates will be able to cover adequately both the range and the depth of the assessment required in this station.

Starting off: 'Hello, I am Dr Melvyn, one of the psychiatrists from the mental health unit. I have some information regarding what happened this morning. Can we have a chat?'			
Assess suicide plan and intent	I have some limited information about what happened this morning. It must have been a very difficult time for you. Can you tell me more about why you took the 20 tablets of medication? Were you troubled by any significant life events recently?	Was the overdose planned? Have you considered or contemplated it for long? How did you manage to have access to those medications? What did you think would happen if you took all of the medications?	Have you thought and hoped that you would take your own life by taking the overdose?
Assess circumstances of the suicide attempt	Where did you take the medications? Was anyone else there, or were you likely to have been found? Did you lock the door or take any precautions to avoid discovery?	Did you take other medications beside these tablets? Did you mix the medications with alcohol? Did you harm yourself by other means?	Did you leave a suicidal note? Did you send an SMS or email to say good-bye to your partner or family members?
Assess events after suicide attempt	How did you manage to come to the accident and emergency department? Did someone else discover you?	Can I understand whether the overdose led to any physical discomfort? Did you have a period of blackout?	How do you feel about it now? Do you regret your suicide attempt? Would you do it again?
Assess for the presence of risk factors or protective factors	Have you attempted suicide previously? If yes, when was it? How many times have you done so? Did you try other methods like hanging, stabbing yourself, jumping from heights or drowning?	Do you have any history of any mental health disorder, such as depression? Are you suffering from any other illnesses? Any family history of mental illness/suicide?	We have spoken quite a lot about the overdose and some of your stressors. I understand that it has been a difficult time for you. Are there things in life you are looking forward to?

(Continued)

Common pitfalls

a. Failure to cover the range and depth of the information required for this station

Quick recall*

- Suicide is not only more common in men than women but also more common for those who are over 45 years.
- The highest rates are those who are divorced, single or widows and in social classes I and V.
- Suicide is associated with unemployment and retirement.
- There seems to be a seasonable variation in the rates of suicide.
- There is evidence that the availability of method affects the gross suicide rates as well as the choice of the methods.

Positive association with suicide in the general population include the following:

a. Being male in gender
b. Being elderly
c. Having suffered loss or bereavement
d. Being unemployed
e. Being retired
f. Childlessness
g. Living alone in a big, densely populated town
h. Having a broken home in childhood
i. Mental or physical illness
j. Loss of role
k. Social disorganization: overcrowding, criminal history in the family, drug and alcohol misuse

- Effects of psychiatric disorders and suicide:
  a. Schizophrenia: Approximately 10% mortality from suicide. Those who commit suicide tend to be young, male, unemployed and often with chronic relapsing illness. The suicide rates are higher immediately postdischarge, with good insight.
  b. Affective psychosis: Approximately 15% mortality from suicide. Those who are at increased risk include older men, separated, widowed or divorced, living alone and not working. For women, they tend to be middle-aged, middle class with a history of para-suicide and having made threats in the last month.
  c. Neurotic disorders: Approximately 90% have a history of para-suicide, and a high proportion have threatened suicide in the preceding month.
  d. Alcoholism: 15% mortality from suicide. Usually tends to occur later in the course of the illness and those affected also tend to be depressed.
  e. Personality disorder: High-risk factors are labile mood, aggressiveness, impulsivity and associated alcohol and substance misuse.

---

* Adapted from B.K. Puri, A. Hall and R. Ho (2014). *Revision Notes in Psychiatry*. London, UK: CRC Press, pp. 398–400.

- Life events and suicide: Compared with psychiatric controls, patients who commit suicide tend to have experienced interpersonal loss more frequently. The risk of suicide does increase, more amongst males than females, usually in the first 5 years following the passage of a parent or spouse.

Assessment of the individual for suicide:

- It is pertinent to ask for suicidal ideations as part of routine MSE. The majority of people who have committed suicide have told somebody beforehand of their thoughts. Two-thirds have seen their GP in the previous month. One-fourth have been psychiatric outpatients at the time of death, and half of them have seen a psychiatrist in the preceding week.
- A high degree of suicidal intent is indicated by the following:
  a. The act being planned and prepared for
  b. Precautions have been taken to avoid discovery
  c. The person did not make any effort to seek help immediately after the act
  d. The act involved a dangerous method
  e. There were final acts such as making a will or leaving a suicide note.
- In the assessment, the presence of psychiatric disorders should be looked for, and any previous history of suicide attempts should be asked about. Social and financial support should be detailed. It is important to ask about suicidal ideations and intent.

STATION 33: SUICIDE RISK ASSESSMENT (PAIRED STATION B: MANAGEMENT)

Information to candidates

Name of patient: Ms. Valarie

Ms Valarie is a 25-year-old university student who has been admitted to the accident and emergency department following an overdose of 20 tablets of medication. The medical doctors have done the necessary tests, and currently she is considered to be medically stable. The medical consultant has requested for her to be seen by a psychiatrist in view of the recent overdose. You have been tasked to speak to Ms Valarie to get a history about the suicide attempt in the previous station, as well as to perform a current suicide risk assessment. In this station, the on-call consultant has heard about this case and is awaiting your call to discuss with him more details about the case.

Task

Please speak to Dr Thomson, the on-call consultant, to discuss more about the circumstances surrounding the overdose and to discuss the management of the case, given the risks involved.

Outline of station

You are Dr Thomson, the on-call consultant. You have learnt about this case and understand that your core trainee has been tasked to assess the patient. You are expecting a consultation by your core trainee. You wish to know more about the circumstances surrounding the overdose. You expect that the core trainee has performed a comprehensive suicidal risk assessment and wish to know the current risk. You will then proceed to discuss with the core trainee more about the specific management plans.

CASC construct table

The CASC construct table is formatted such that candidates will be able to cover adequately both the range and the depth of the assessment required in this station.

Starting off: 'Hello, I am Melvyn, one of the core trainees. Can I discuss a case with you?'			
Brief formulation of the case	Dr Thomson, I have been asked to see a 25-year-old university student in the Emergency Department. She was found and taken to the hospital by her friends following an overdose on a variety of 20 medications in total.	I have spoken to her and the current stressor contributing to the overdose seemed to be that of a recent failure in her academics. There are no other stressors that I could identify.	The medical team doctors have treated her for the overdose and have asked us for an evaluation.
Evaluation of the suicidal intent and the seriousness of the attempt	I understand from her that she had made plans for the overdose and had accumulated the medications over a total duration of 3 days. She left a suicide note for her parents and made an attempt to conceal the attempt by locking the doors and making sure her friends were not at home.	She was fully aware of the seriousness of the attempt and wanted to end it all entirely by taking the pills. She is currently expressing regrets with regard to her being rescued by her friends.	She has not taken other adjunctive medications and has not consumed alcohol together with the medications.
Current risk assessment	When I spoke to her, she was still vocalizing that she has thoughts of suicide. She claimed that there was nothing to stop her from attempting something more lethal and was determined to make it a success.	She does not have any past psychiatric disorders, and she does not have a family history of any psychiatric conditions. This is the first time she has overdosed on medications.	My current suicide risk assessment would place her at high risk given the circumstances of the recent overdose, as well as her current suicide ideations.

(Continued)

Management plans	Given the current risk, I would like to suggest that she should be admitted to the inpatient unit for further observation and stabilization. In the short term, we need to observe her closely and place her on the necessary suicide caution.	We might consider starting an antidepressant if her mood is clinically low, only when she is medically stable and her labs are normal.	I feel that she would benefit from further engagement with a psychologist, who could teach her some coping strategies as well as engage her in some form of therapy. We might need to consider other supports that she could be engaged in whilst at school. Do you have any questions for me?

Common pitfalls

a. Failure to cover the range and depth of the information required for this station

Quick recall*

Management of suicidal ideation:

- If there is a serious risk of suicide, the patient should be admitted to the hospital.
- Any psychiatric disorder from which the patient suffers from should be treated adequately.
- If the person is suffering from severe depression, ECT may be required.
- Patient with manic depression have a mortality of up to three times that of the general population.
- For patients with manic depression and treated with lithium prophylaxis, cumulative mortality does not differ from that of the general population. A minimum of 2 years of lithium treatment is needed to reduce the high mortality resulting from manic depression. It is proposed that lithium does have anti-suicide effects.

Management of para-suicide:

- The individual should be treated medically as appropriate.
- Assess fully the individual.
- It is important to reduce the immediate risk and treat the underlying causes.
- If the patient suffers from a psychiatric disorder, this should also be treated appropriately.

---

* Adapted from B.K. Puri, A. Hall and R. Ho (2014). *Revision Notes in Psychiatry*. London, UK: CRC Press, pp. 398–400.

- It is important to allow the individual to ventilate. Talking out avoids acting out. It is important to strike a bargain on medication. Ask whether the person can cope with the responsibility of a bottle of tablets. If no, then admit to hospital.
- It is important to assess a list of problems areas and establish possible practical help. Allow for an underestimate of the true risk.

Prevention includes the following:

- Recognizing high-risk cases and taking them seriously
- Asking patient about their suicidal ideas
- Not removing hope
- Prescribing the safest drugs
- Treating underlying illness well

STATION 34: GRIEF REACTION

Information to candidates

Name of patient: Ms Davis

Ms Davis, a 60-year-old female, has been referred by her GP, as her GP has noted that her mood has been low for the past couple of months since the passage of her husband. The GP is concerned that she might be depressed and hopes that she could benefit from being seen and being managed by a mental health specialist.

Task

Please speak to Ms Davis to take a history of her presenting symptoms with the aim of establishing a diagnosis.

Outline of station

You are Ms Davis, a 60-year-old female who has been referred by your GP for your mood symptoms. Your mood has been low since the sudden passage of your husband 6 months ago. He died from a heart attack, which was totally unexpected. You do not have any dependants and hence are currently staying alone in your home. You did manage to attend your late husband's funeral. Previously, you were feeling emotions of denial, anger and had bargained why God had been so unfair towards you. Recently, in the past month or so, you have noticed that your mood has been low and have been more emotional. You do not have any interest and have been confining yourself at home and have been having poor appetite and sleep. You do not have any perceptual disturbances and do not have any suicidal ideations.

CASC construct table

The CASC construct table is formatted such that candidates will be able to cover adequately both the range and the depth of the assessment required in this station.

Starting off: 'Hello, I am Dr Melvyn, one of the psychiatrists from the mental health unit. I understand that your GP has referred you to see us. Can we have a chat today?'			
History of presenting complaint/nature of husband's death	I received some information from your GP. I'm sorry to hear of all that has happened recently. I understand that it must have been a very difficult time for you. It would be helpful if I could understand a bit more about your husband's recent passage. Would you mind sharing with me more about what happened?	I'm sorry to hear that. You mentioned that it was unexpected and sudden. Were you with him when it happened? What happened thereafter? Can you tell me how long ago was this?	Was there any form of closure for you? Did you manage to attend the wake? How were you coping then? Have you been to his burial place since? How was your relationship with your husband?
Exploration of her current stage of grief/ assessment for comorbid depressive symptoms	Sometimes, when people experience the loss of their loved ones, they do experience a whole range of emotions. It is clear that you have lost someone significant and recently you have been feeling quite emotional about it.	Have you ever felt angry? Do you blame anyone for causing the death? Were there times in life in which you started to bargain, wishing that it were you instead of your husband?	How have you been feeling in your mood recently? Do you feel that your mood is low, and you have been very emotional? Are you able to enjoy and partake in activities which you used to enjoy previously? How are your energy levels? How is your sleep? What about your appetite? Are you able to concentrate and focus on things you wish to do? Do you think you have come to terms with your recent loss?
Exploration for symptoms suggestive of atypical grief	For some individuals who have lost their loved ones, they tend to leave their loved ones' belongings as if they were still around. Does that sound like you?	Are there times in which you felt as if you could hear your husband still?	Do you feel responsible for his death? Are you feeling guilty about anything? Have you felt that life has lost its meaning? Do you feel that life is not worth living anymore? Have you ever have plans to take your own life?

Common pitfalls

a. Failure to cover the range and depth of the information required for this station

It is important to ascertain the circumstances of the loss and relationship between the deceased and the patient. For younger patients, you will also need to check for any dependants, which may potentially be a risk factor for abnormal grief, as one may not be able to fully express the grief.

Quick recall*

- Grief usually has three phases.
- The stunned phase lasts from a few hours to a few weeks. This gives way to the mourning phase, with intense yearning and autonomic symptoms.
- After several weeks, the phase of acceptance and adjustment takes over.
- Grief reaction typically lasts about 6 months.
- Atypical grief is divided into the following:
  a. Inhibited grief: absence of expected grief symptoms at any stage
  b. Delayed grief: avoidance of painful symptoms within 2 weeks of loss
  c. Chronic grief: continued significant grief-related symptoms for 6 months
- It is important to understand the differences between depression and bereavement. The following features are more common in depression but not in bereavement:
  a. Active suicidal ideations
  b. Depressive symptoms which are out of proportion with loss
  c. Feelings of guilt not related to the deceased
  d. Marked functional impairment for longer than 2 months
  e. Preoccupation with worthlessness
- Management:
  a. Grief is usually managed in the outpatient setting but inpatient setting is indicated for patients who are at high suicidal risk.
  b. Psychiatrist needs to assess and distinguish normal grief from that of abnormal grief.
  c. Grief work is supportive psychotherapy which allows expression of the loss and its meaning and working through the issues. It also provides a secure base, identifies factors that block natural grief and addresses social isolation and spiritual issues.
  d. Family involvement and psycho-education.
  e. If psychotropic drug is indicated, careful dosing is required to avoid side effects. Maintenance treatment is required for severe prolonged grief.
  f. Rehabilitative efforts emphasize on stage-appropriate tasks such as developing vocational and social skills.

---

* Adapted from B.K. Puri, A. Hall and R. Ho (2014). *Revision Notes in Psychiatry.* London, UK: CRC Press, p. 381.

STATION 35: BODY DYSMORPHIC DISORDER

Information to candidates

Name of patient: Mr Thomas Smith

You have been tasked to speak to Mr Thomas Smith, a 30-year-old man. He is a taxi driver and has been referred by his GP to see you in the mental health service. From the referral memo, you gathered that he has visited his GP recently, requesting for a specialist referral to a plastic surgeon. The GP has stated that Mr Thomas Smith has been insistent on a referral to a plastic surgeon for correction of a deformity of his nose. The GP has not identified anything abnormal, and hence he is hoping that you could evaluate him prior to him being referred and possibly undergoing any corrective surgery.

Task

Please speak to Mr Smith to get a better understanding of his current problems. Please take sufficient history to formulate a clinical diagnosis.

Outline of station

You are Mr Thomas Smith and are a taxi driver. You have been troubled by your nose problem since you were a teenager. You always remember how your peers used to tease you and bully you in school previously. You firmly believe that there is something abnormal about your nose, in terms of the way it is shaped. Because of this deformity, even though you have managed to graduate from university with a business degree, you are not able to work in an office job. You have resorted to working as a taxi driver, as you do not need to face people that much. As a result of your nose problem, you do not have many friends and have yet to be in a relationship. You cannot help checking in the rear-view mirror at times due to your concerns about your nose deformity. You avoid going out for events, and there have been times in which you needed to resort to some special way of grooming to hide the deformity. You are keen for immediate help. You do not understand why you have to see the psychiatrist, when all you want is for the GP to refer you to the plastic surgeon for a definitive surgery to correct the defect. You have watched some videos online and feel that if the doctors are not going to help you, there might be a chance you might take things in your own hands and correct it yourself. You do not have other psychiatric history of note.

CASC construct table

The CASC construct table is formatted such that candidates will be able to cover adequately both the range and the depth of the assessment required in this station.

Starting off: 'Hello, I am Dr Melvyn, one of the psychiatrists from the mental health unit. I understand that you have been referred by your GP. Can we have a chat?'			
History of presenting complaint	I understand that you have been to your GP recently to request for a referral to a plastic surgeon. Can I understand more about that? I'm sorry to hear the distress that you have had. It is not uncommon for us to speak to patients prior to them undergoing a procedure.	You mentioned that you have been troubled by your nose deformity. Can I understand from you when did this all first start? Was it just recently? When did you first notice that you had such a problem? Apart from you noticing it, what have others said?	It seems like this has been a chronic problem that has troubled you for many years. Do you feel increasingly more concerned about it recently? Was that any trigger that caused you to feel this way recently? It seems to me that you are very concerned about the shape of your nose. Do you have any other concerns about any other bodily parts?
Assessment of strength of beliefs and challenging beliefs	You mentioned that you feel that there is something wrong with your nose. However, it seems to me that other people have not commented so.	Can it be that there is really nothing wrong with your nose? How convinced are you that there is something wrong with your nose?	If the plastic surgeon tells you that there is really nothing wrong with your nose, and that no surgery is required, would you be amenable to his suggestion?
Impact of illness	I'm sorry to hear that this has been a problem that has been bothering you for many years. I understand that you are really keen to have a quick fix of your problem. Before we discuss more about how best we could help you with your problem, can I understand how this problem has affected you over the years?	Has it affected your work? Has it affected your relationships with your family members? Has it affected your relationships with your peers? Do you tend to avoid certain situations due to the defect of your nose?	Are you very concerned about the deformity of your nose that you would spend a lot of time looking at it, say in a mirror? How much time do you spend daily? How frequently do you check? Have you resorted to camouflaging your deformity in the event you have a social gathering to attend to?
Risk assessment	Are you so distressed by your nose issue that you have ever felt that life has no meaning for you? Have you contemplated or entertained thoughts of suicide before?	Have you done anything to your nose before? What are your plans if the surgeon is not willing to do the surgery for you?	Do you have any plans to correct the deformity yourself? Can you tell me more about what you have in mind with regard to what you might do to yourself?

(Continued)

| Ruling out other comorbid psychiatric disorders | How has your mood been recently? Do you still have interest in things you used to enjoy doing? | How has your sleep been? What about your appetite? Can you still function at work? Sometimes, when people are undergoing stressful experiences, they do report having unusual experiences. Do you have similar experiences? | Have you seen a psychiatrist before? Is there anyone in the family who has a mental health history? |

Common pitfalls

a. Failure to cover the range and depth of the information required for this station

It is important to ascertain whether the patient is dissatisfied with more than one body part.

Quick recall*

- The prevalence of this disorder amongst the general population ranges from 1% to 2%.
- In dermatological and cosmetic surgery patients, the prevalence is from 2.9% to 16%.
- Aetiology: In terms of genetics, there might be a family history of BDD, OCD and mood disorder. In terms of neurochemistry, there are reduced serotonin levels. In terms of the psychodynamic theory, there is displacement of the conflict onto body component. In terms of development, there might be rejection previously in childhood as a result of body image problem and possibly disharmony in the family. Cultural influence might play a part as well, as in some culture, beauty means a perfect body.
- The *DSM-5* criteria state the following:
  a. Preoccupation with perceived defects or flaws in physical appearance that is not observable to others.
  b. The person performs repetitive behaviours or mental acts (such as comparing their appearance with others) in response to the appearance concerns.
  c. Specifiers include muscle dysmorphia, good or fair insight and absent insight.
- The common behavioural problems include self-harm in 70%–80%, social avoidance in 30% and suicide in 20%.
- The common rituals include camouflage, mirror check and compulsion in 90% and skin pick in 30%.

---

* Adapted from B.K. Puri, A. Hall and R. Ho (2014). *Revision Notes in Psychiatry.* London, UK: CRC Press, pp. 422–423.

- Most common body sites concerned include hair (63%), nose (50%), skin (50%), eye (30%), face (20%), breast (less than 10%) and neck, forehead and facial muscle (less than 5%).
- The differences compared with patients with OCD are that patients with OCD are less likely to suffer from social phobia, less likely to attempt suicide, less likely to be involved in substance abuse, have better insight and have better relationships.
- The common associated psychiatric conditions include social phobia, substance abuse, suicide, OCD and depression.
- With regard to management options, the following could be tried:
    a. Antidepressants: SSRIs – 50% of patients respond to SSRIs.
    b. Antipsychotics: If patient does not respond to SSRIs, the psychiatrist could augment with second-generation antipsychotics.
    c. Other pharmacological agents such as clomipramine and lithium.
    d. For patients with BDD with moderate functional impairment, more intensive CBT (including ERP) is recommended based on the NICE guidance.

STATION 36: SLEEP DISORDERS – INSOMNIA

Information to candidates

Name of patient: Mr Tom Foster

You have been asked to see Mr Tom Foster. He has been referred by his GP for sleeping difficulties. He does not have any other chronic medical conditions, aside from hypertension.

Task

Please speak to Mr Foster and elicit a history to come to a potential diagnosis.

Outline of station

You are Mr Tom Foster and have visited your GP a couple of days ago, as you have been having difficulties falling asleep. You do not have any other medical conditions, apart from hypertension. You do not have a family history of any mental health condition and have not seen a psychiatrist before. You are married, but recently, there has been increasing stress due to relationship issues. You are employed at the moment and are just coping with the job that you have been assigned. You have done routine blood investigations, and they are all normal. You will provide the psychiatrist with a copy of the results. Your GP has not prescribed you any medications but has advised you on sleep hygiene methods. You have tried them, but you are still having much difficulty with initiation of sleep. You hope the psychiatrist can explain to you what is wrong with you and suggest a treatment for your condition.

CASC construct table

The CASC construct table is formatted such that candidates will be able to cover adequately both the range and the depth of the assessment required in this station.

Starting off: 'Hello, I am Dr Melvyn. I received some information from your GP. Can we have a chat about it?'			
Explore sleep issue and rule out medical causes	I understand from the memo from your GP that you have been having some difficulties with your sleep. I'm sorry to hear that, and I know that it must be difficult for you. Can you please tell me more about your problem? When did this first start? Is it a problem with falling asleep or staying asleep?	Can you take me through a typical day of yours? Can you tell me more about your routine before bedtime? How has this problem affected you? Has this been a problem for you previously?	Can you tell me if you have any physical or medical conditions that I need to know of? Any obstructive sleep apnoea (snoring)? Are you on any medications for your hypertension? What sort of work do you do? Any shift work? Assess *patient's current sleep hygiene.*
Explore current mental state	How has your mood been recently? Do you find yourself feeling low? How would you rate your mood currently? Is there variation in your mood in a day? Do you find yourself being able to enjoy things that you used to enjoy?	Apart from your sleep difficulties, have you been experiencing issues with your appetite as well? How do you find your energy levels to be? Are you able to concentrate on doing things that you used to enjoy?	Can you tell me if there is anything that is particularly stressful for you at the moment? Can you tell me more? Have you ever felt that life is meaningless? Have you ever entertained thoughts of ending your life? Have you ever had any strange experiences, such as hearing voices when no one is there?
Explore personal history	Have you seen a psychiatrist before? Can I ask if there is anyone in the family who has a mental health condition?	Do you use any substances such as alcohol? What about drugs?	How would you describe yourself in terms of your personality?

(Continued)

Explain management plans	I understand that your GP has given you some sleep hygiene advice previously. I'm sorry to learn that it did not seem to have helped you with your condition. Based on my assessment, your mood is not clinically depressed.	I would recommend that we try the sleep hygiene tips that were shared previously. Would you want me to go over them again?	If these techniques still do not work, we could consider starting you on a low dose of some sleeping medications. We will aim to use these for a short duration of time as I am concerned about their inherent addictive potential.
Address concerns and expectations	Do you have any questions for me?		

Common pitfalls

a. Failure to cover the range and depth of the information required for this station

Quick recall*

- Insomnia is the disturbance of normal sleep pattern and characterized by an insufficient quantity or quality of sleep.
- The prevalence of insomnia is between 1% and 10% in the general population.
- The estimated 1-year prevalence in adults ranges between 15% and over 40%.
- Prevalence is particularly high in the elderly.
- Females tend to have this disorder more often than males.
- The clinical features include the following:
  a. The patient has a history of being a light sleeper with easily disturbed sleep.
  b. The patient usually is concerned about sleep duration and quality. This often leads to increased cognitive, physiological and emotional arousal prior to sleep. Their overconcerns and poor sleep often form a viscous cycle.
  c. The main result of insomnia is daytime tiredness or napping, low mood, decreased attention and concentration, low energy level and fatigue.
- In terms of the diagnostic criteria, the *ICD-10* states the following:
  a. The sleep disturbance occurs nearly every day for at least 1 month and causes marked distress or interference with personal functioning in daily living.
  b. A complaint of excessive daytime sleepiness or prolonged transition to fully aroused state upon awakening.

---

* Adapted from B.K. Puri, A. Hall and R. Ho (2014). *Revision Notes in Psychiatry*. London, UK: CRC Press, pp. 609–612.

c. Absence of narcolepsy or sleep apnoea (nocturnal breath cessation).

d. Absence of any organic factor, psychoactive substance–use disorder or effect of medication.

- Differential diagnosis for the condition includes depressive disorders, mania, anxiety disorders, substance misuse and dependence and organic disorders.
- Management (non-pharmacological):

  a. Sleep hygiene education: a moderate intake of easily digested warm food; a comfortable bed; avoid caffeine, nicotine, alcohol and excessive fluid intake in the evening; keep a regular sleep schedule and regular daytime exercise; limit time in bed and remove clock from bedroom to avoid excessive monitoring.

  b. Sleep restriction therapy: The patient should keep a sleep log that records the total sleep duration, bedtime and wake-up time. The time allowed in bed is reduced to the total sleep duration, and the patient is advised to increase the time in bed by 15 minutes on a weekly basis by adjusting the bedtime.

  c. Stimulus control therapy: Arise at the same time every morning, avoid daytime napping, go to bed only when sleepy, use the bed only for sleep, leave the bed when unable to sleep, reduce the lighting and level of noise in the bedroom.

  d. Cognitive therapy aims at correcting cognitive distortions and unrealistic expectations.

  e. Behaviour therapy would include progressive muscle relaxation techniques for any associated anxiety.

- Management (pharmacological)

  a. The NICE guidelines recommend that doctors should consider offering non-pharmacological treatments first. If they think that pharmacological treatment is the appropriate way to treat severe insomnia that is interfering with normal functioning, they should prescribe one hypnotic agent for only short periods and strictly according to the license for the drug.

  b. Doctors are advised to consider non-benzodiazepine hypnotic agents.

  c. Benzodiazepines are only indicated for short-term usage (less than 4 weeks).

  d. Treatment should be changed from one of these hypnotics to another if side effects occur that are directly related to the medicine. If treatment with one of the benzodiazepines or benzodiazepines receptor agonist does not work, the doctor should not prescribe one of the others.

- Course and prognosis:

  a. Insomnia typically occurs in young or middle adulthood. Chronic insomnia may last through to old age.

  b. Previous insomnia is the most significant predictor for future insomnia.

  c. Fifty to seventy-five per cent of patients have insomnia that lasts for more than 1 year.

  d. Insomnia caused by life event or stressor usually has a limited course to a period of less than 1 year.

STATION 37: CAPACITY ASSESSMENT (INFORMED CONSENT FOR PROCEDURE)

Information to candidates

Name of patient: Mr Charlie Brown

You have been tasked to assess Mr Charlie Brown. He has been admitted to the medical ward, as he has had two prior episodes of vomiting out blood. The medical consultant wishes to schedule him for an urgent endoscopy to find out the cause of the bleed. The team has noted that he has had a history of schizophrenia. They are concerned whether he is fit to sign on the pre-operation consent forms. They have thus called in the psychiatrists to assess his capacity to provide consent.

Task

Please speak to Mr Brown and determine whether he has capacity to provide consent for the endoscopy that the medical team has scheduled him for.

Outline of station

You are Mr Charlie Brown and have been admitted to the medial ward. You have had two episodes in which you vomited out fresh blood. The medical team has seen you and advised that you should undergo further evaluation, which includes that of an endoscopy evaluation. You have a rough idea of the procedure that is involved. The team has informed you of the potential complications as well. You have decided not to go ahead, as you feel strongly that the surgeons might attempt to implant another chip in you.

CASC construct table

The CASC construct table is formatted such that candidates will be able to cover adequately both the range and the depth of the assessment required in this station.

Starting off: 'Hello, I am Dr Melvyn. I received some information from the medical doctors who have seen you. They have requested that I come to do a quick evaluation of your condition. Can we have a chat about your condition?'			
History of current issues	I understand that you have been recently admitted to the hospital. Can you tell me more about what has been happening? How long have you had this problem for?	Is the problem getting worse? Can you tell me more?	What do you think is wrong with you?

(Continued)

Mental state evaluation	I understand that you have a pre-existing mental health disorder. Can you tell me more about what condition you have had? How long have you had this condition for? In the past, did you require any inpatient hospitalizations for your mental health condition? Are you currently on any medications for this condition? Have you been compliant with the dose of mediations prescribed?	Over the past month, how has your mood been for you? Do you find yourself losing interest in things that you previously used to enjoy? Are there any difficulties with your sleep or appetite? Have you had any unusual experiences? By that I mean, do you hear voices or see anything unusual when you are alone?	Do you feel that there are others out there who are trying to harm you? Do you feel in control of your thought processes? Do you feel in control of your emotions and actions?
Assessment of mental capacity – ability to understand information	Can you share with me your understanding of what is wrong with you? What has the medical team told you with regard to your current condition?	Did they tell you what they think might be the cause of the problem? Have they suggested that you need to be further evaluated?	Can you tell me more about your understanding of what they have told you with regard to the further evaluation?
Assessment of mental capacity – ability to retain information	Did the medical doctors tell you what the advantages of doing the endoscopy would be?	Did the medical doctors inform you about the risks associated with the procedure? Are there other life-threatening complications that they have informed you about?	Please allow me to explain why the medical doctors have recommended this procedure for you. Please also allow me to explain the potential complications that might arise from the procedure.
Assessment of mental capacity – ability to weigh information and come to a decision	Can you tell me once again why the doctors have made such a recommendation?	Can you tell me once again what complications the procedure is associated with?	Can you tell me your decision with regard to the procedure? Can you tell me the reasons why you are refusing the treatment? Is this your final decision?
Summarize and communicate that the best decision is not made	It seems to me that you are worried about the procedure as you feel that the surgeons might implant a device within you. This is despite the fact that the team has clearly told you the rationale for the procedure.	Unfortunately, this does not seem to be the best possible decision in the current situation. Please give me some time to discuss with the rest of your medical team.	Would it be alright for me to return to speak to you about it again?

Common pitfalls

a. Failure to cover the range and depth of the information required for this station

Quick recall*

- Capacity is a clinical concept and refers to the mental ability to make a rational decision based on understanding and appreciating all relevant information.
- A valid consent has the following properties:
  a. A consent is classified as an implicit consent (verbal consent for blood-taking) or an explicit consent (written consent to participate in a clinical trial).
  b. The presence of capacity in a person so that he or she must be able to understand the information and appreciate the foreseeable consequences of a decision and be able to communicate such decision.
  c. Informed with clear information (diagnosis, purpose of proposed treatment, risks and benefits, alternatives and associated prognosis).
  d. Voluntary and without coercion or persuasion.
  e. Specific to the issue involved.
- It is the responsibility of the doctor to judge whether the patient has the capacity to give a valid consent. The doctor has a duty to provide information in a language understandable by a layperson about a condition, the benefits and the risks of a proposed treatment and alternatives to a treatment. The high court has held that an adult has capacity to consent to a medical or surgical treatment if he or she can do the following:
  a. Understand and retain the information relevant to the decision in question.
  b. Believe in the information.
  c. Weigh the information in balance to arrive at a choice. The person has the right to refuse treatment even though the refusal is contrary to the views of most other people. The decision should be consistent with the individual value system.

STATION 38: CAPACITY ASSESSMENT FOR SOCIAL CARE NEEDS (PAIRED STATION A)

Information to candidates

Name of patient: Stephen

You have been tasked to speak to Stephen. He has a history of vascular dementia and has been recently admitted to the hospital following a recurrent vascular infarct. The medical team has optimized his medications and arranged for him to undergo rehabilitation whilst he is in hospital. The physiotherapist and

---

* Adapted from B.K. Puri, A. Hall and R. Ho (2014). *Revision Notes in Psychiatry*. London, UK: CRC Press, pp. 609–612.

occupational therapist have provided their inputs about his social functioning, regarding which they have both recommended that he would need more social care support at home. The team has since recommended this option to Stephen, but he has rejected the need for increased support. Given his history of dementia, the team has decided to call you, the psychiatry trainee on call, hoping that you could help in the evaluation of his decision- and capacity-making ability.

Task

Please speak to Stephen and determine whether he has the capacity to make care arrangements, given that he has a background history of vascular dementia.

Outline of station

You are the patient, Stephen. You are 68 years old, and you were diagnosed with vascular dementia 5 years ago. You needed inpatient hospitalization recently, as you woke up one day to find that there was weakness on your left side. The medical doctors have diagnosed you with a recurrence of stroke. You have been asked to participate in rehabilitation programs organized during the inpatient stay, which you have duly participated in. You were surprised when the team informed you that you would need further social care support when you're back home. You are not receptive towards having more people in your home.

CASC construct table

The CASC construct table is formatted such that candidates will be able to cover adequately both the range and the depth of the assessment required in this station.

Starting off: 'Hello, I am Dr Melvyn. I received some information from the medical doctors who have seen you. They have requested that I come to do a quick evaluation of your condition. Can we have a chat about your condition?'			
MSE	I understand that you have a pre-existing mental health disorder. Can you tell me more about what condition you have had? How long have you had this condition for? In the past, did you require any inpatient hospitalizations for your mental health condition? Are you currently on any medications for this condition? Have you been compliant with the dose of mediations prescribed?	Over the past month, how has your mood been for you? Do you find yourself losing interest in things that you previously used to enjoy? Are there any difficulties with your sleep or appetite? Have you had have any unusual experiences? By that I mean, do you hear voices or see anything unusual when you are alone?	Do you feel that there are others out there who are trying to harm you? Do you feel in control of your thought processes? Do you feel in control of your emotions and actions?

(Continued)

Assessment of ability to understand	I understand that you have been through the rehabilitation program recommended by your doctors.	Have they told you their assessment of your condition? What do you know about your current condition?	
Assessment of ability to appreciate risks and benefits and retaining information	Have the doctors told you their rationale for recommending social care support for you? Can you tell me more about what they have explained to you?	Have the doctors told you the dangers and risks involved if you do not have enhanced social care support?	I'd like to re-explain to you the advantages and the disadvantages of having increased social support.
Assessment of mental capacity – ability to weigh information and come to a decision	Can you tell me once again why the doctors have made such a recommendation?	Can you tell me once again what risks that might be if you do not have enhanced social care support?	Can you tell me your decision with regard to this? Can you tell me the reasons why you are refusing the recommendations of your doctor? Is this your final decision?
Summarize and communicate that the best decision is not made	Thanks for speaking to me. Let me reassure you that the team is very concerned about your condition and hence after careful evaluation, they have decided to make such a decision and recommendation.	The team is trying their best to help you with your condition whilst you are at home. I would like to re-discuss your case with the team of doctors who are caring for you once again.	Would it be ok for me to return to speak to you about this again?

Common pitfalls

a. Failure to cover the range and depth of the information required for this station

Do not appear to be paternalistic and force the patient into accepting social service support. Ascertain reasons why he refuses the recommendation.

It may be worthwhile to ask some quick screening questions about his memory in the middle of the interview, e.g., three-item registration and recall orientation. This will come in helpful to explain to the family about his cognitive ability in the next station (especially if they ask you about it).

The patient in this station may either have no capacity to make a decision or have the capacity but is not making the best-informed decision.

Quick recall*

Management of financial affairs:

- Mental disorder from whatever cause can restrict person's ability to handle financial affairs and is more common in the elderly, particularly amongst those who are suffering from dementing conditions.
- Various options exist to help deal with the financial affairs of people who are unable to do so themselves because of mental disorder.

Further information about the court of protection:

- This is an office of the Supreme Court. It exists to protect the property and affairs of persons who, through mental disorder, are incapable of managing personal financial affairs. The court's power is limited to dealing with the financial and legal affairs of the person concerned. Only on medical certificate is required, from a registered medical practitioner who has examined the patient. Guidance to medical practitioners accompanies the certificate of incapacity.
- The court appoints somebody to manage the patient's affairs on his or her behalf. This person is called the receiver. It may be a relative, friend, solicitor or other persons. The receiver must keep accounts and spend the patient's money on things that will benefit the patient. The court must give permission before the disposal of capital assets such as property.

STATION 39: CAPACITY ASSESSMENT FOR SOCIAL CARE NEEDS (PAIRED STATION B)

Information to candidates

Name of patient: Stephen

You have been tasked to speak to the son of Stephen. You have previously done an assessment of Stephen in the previous station and have assessed his capacity for social care services. His son is keen to find out more about the assessment. He has some questions for you as well.

Task

Please speak to Mr Jonathan Smith, Stephen's son, and explain the outcomes of your assessment. Please address all his concerns and expectations.

Outline of station

You are Mr Jonathan Smith, the son of Stephen, and have heard from the medical team that your father needs to have enhanced social care in place if he were

---

* Adapted from B.K. Puri, A. Hall and R. Ho (2014). *Revision Notes in Psychiatry*. London, UK: CRC Press, p. 718.

to return home after his recent recurrent stroke. You are keen for your father to receive more social support when he returns home as you have just been promoted to a new position and hence will have less time to take care of his needs. You understand that the medical team has referred your father to the psychiatry team for an assessment. You are keen to find out more about the assessment made by the psychiatrist. You also wish to understand whether it would be legal for you to go against his wishes in the event that he is not making the best possible decision.

CASC construct table

The CASC construct table is formatted such that candidates will be able to cover adequately both the range and the depth of the assessment required in this station.

Starting off: 'Hello, I am Dr Melvyn. I understand that you have some concerns about your father. I have just seen him and done an assessment of his condition. Can we have a chat?'			
Explanation of assessment	I hear that you have some concerns about your father's condition. I'd like to take this opportunity to tell you more about my assessment. I'd have just seen him, as the team wanted my inputs about his condition. They wanted to know whether he has capacity to make decisions with regard to his social care.	In assessing whether he has capacity, I evaluated whether he understood what the team had told him. In addition, he was asked to recall the indications for the enhanced social care as well as the disadvantages associated with it, if he does not have access to the enhanced care. He demonstrated to me that he has the full understanding of the information. In addition, he demonstrated the ability to recall not only the indications but also the disadvantages of having the enhanced care.	When asked what his decision was in consideration of the risks against the benefits, he told me that he would still prefer not to have the enhanced social care. I have told him that it seemed that he has not made the wisest decision in consideration of the risks against the benefits. Nevertheless, he was adamant that he did not want the enhanced care. There seemed to be no other obvious mental state abnormalities that might have caused him to make such a decision.
Address concerns and expectations	I understand that it would be very difficult for you to manage him, given that you now have a new position.	I could try to re-explain the indications and the risks associated with his decision again and do a re-evaluation in due course. Some modifications that can be done at home: Involve the occupational therapist to do home assessment, include anti-slip mat, grip bars etc., to improve his functional capability at home.	Are there other concerns that you have currently?

(Continued)

Clarification about legal issue	I understand that you would want him to receive social support. I also understand that you are worried about the legal issues involved in this process. If I did not misunderstand you, you are concerned whether it would be legal for us to provide care against his wishes?	At times, there are exceptions in which we need to do so in consideration of the best interest of the patient.	
Address any other concerns	Do you have any other questions for me?		

Common pitfalls

a. Failure to cover the range and depth of the information required for this station

Quick recall*

Management of financial affairs

- Mental disorder from whatever cause can restrict a person's ability to handle financial affairs and is more common in the elderly, particularly amongst those who are suffering from dementing conditions.
- Various options exist to help deal with the financial affairs of people who are unable to do so themselves because of mental disorder.
- Further information about the court of protection:
- This is an office of the Supreme Court. It exists to protect the property and affairs of persons who, through mental disorder, are incapable of managing personal financial affairs. The court's power is limited to dealing with the financial and legal affairs of the person concerned. Only one medical certificate is required, from a registered medical practitioner who has examined the patient. Guidance to medical practitioners accompanies the certificate of incapacity.
- The court appoints somebody to manage the patient's affairs on his or her behalf. This person is called the receiver. It may be a relative, friend, solicitor or other persons. The receiver must keep accounts and spend the patient's money on things that will benefit the patient. The court must give permission before the disposal of capital assets such as property.

---

* Adapted from B.K. Puri, A. Hall and R. Ho (2014). *Revision Notes in Psychiatry*. London, UK: CRC Press, p. 718.

STATION 40: BREAKING BAD NEWS

Information to candidates

Name of patient: Mr Lionel

Mr Lionel is an 80-year-old male who has been admitted to the psychiatric ward for an acute change in his mental state. Prior to this, he has been well and does not have any chronic medical conditions. He does not have any underlying pre-existing psychiatric disorders. The team has evaluated his condition and has done some baseline blood investigations and brain scan. All the blood investigations were within normal limits. The radiological investigations (a computed tomography scan of his brain) did reveal a suspicious lesion. The neurologist has been called in for a further evaluation, and they feel that the lesion is most likely that of a meningioma. His daughter, who is his main caregiver, is currently here and hopes to find out more about his condition.

Task

Please speak to his daughter and explain more about his current condition. Please address all her concerns and her expectations.

Outline of station

You are the daughter of Mr Lionel. You are his main caregiver and have been increasingly stressed about his condition. Your father has been healthy up until 4 months ago. You noticed that he has been having personality changes. You are very concerned that last night, he appeared to very confused and hence you decided to send him in for an extensive evaluation. You understand from the nursing staff that some baseline investigations have been done for your father. You hope to be able to speak to the team to understand more about his condition. You are devastated to learn of the fact that he has a brain lesion. You wish to know more about the prognosis of his condition. In addition, you hope to be able to obtain from the team their inputs with regard to the possible treatment options. You hope to be able to bring him back home as soon as possible and would highlight this request to the team of doctors. You hope that the team doctor can provide you with further information with regard to the treatment plans and options.

CASC construct table

The CASC construct table is formatted such that candidates will be able to cover adequately both the range and the depth of the assessment required in this station.

Starting off: 'Hello, I am Dr Melvyn. I understand that you wish to get some updates about your father's current condition. Can we have a chat about this?'			
Introduction and establishing what carer has known	I understand that it has been a very difficult time for you. I hear that you wish to have an update about his current condition. Before that, can you please share with me more about what happened prior to the current admission?	Have you managed to visit your father before speaking to me? What do you understand about his current condition?	I wonder whether anyone has updated you with regard to his current condition.
Gradually break the bad news	In view of the acute changes in his mental state, upon his admission, the team decided to perform a variety of tests, which included baseline blood tests and radiological scans. Thus far, the blood work that we have done seems to be fine.	I would like to share with you more about the results of the brain scan that we have done. Would it be alright for me to go on? Unfortunately, we noticed that there is a lesion in his brain when we did the scan. Are you alright with me going on?	*(Allow carer to have some time to accept the bad news)* The brain lesions might have accounted for the acute changes in his current mental state. I'm sorry that I need to be informing you of this news. Do you have any questions for me at the moment?
Discuss expectations and concerns	I understand that you are concerned with regard to the further treatment options. We have actually referred your father to the neurologist, who has since taken a look at the radiological scan.	Based on my understanding, there are several treatment options, which usually include surgery, radiotherapy or even chemotherapy. However, I would not be in the best position to comment which of these modalities of treatment is the best indicated currently, as I am not the specialist in this area. I'm hoping my neurology colleague will get back to us as soon as possible, and we will arrange a joint session to discuss treatment options.	I hear your request that you wish to take him home. However, it might not be the best decision currently. We might need to run further investigations and tests to help in our diagnosis, and hence it would be better for him to stay in the hospital. Also, I understand that you have had a difficult time managing him at home. We hope that we could help you in this aspect as well. We hear your concerns with regard to whether your father will be in pain. Please be assured that we will get our multidisciplinary team on board. We might give him some medications to help him with the pain that he is experiencing.
Summarize discussion	I know that we have given you a lot of information. Do you have any questions for me?	Do you need me to speak to anyone in the family?	

Common pitfalls

a. Failure to cover the range and depth of the information required for this station
b. Use of jargon and giving too much information without checking understanding of the family member

STATION 41: EXPLAIN NEUROLEPTIC MALIGNANT SYNDROME

Information to candidates

Name of patient: Joel

Joel, a 22-year-old university student, was admitted to the inpatient unit 2 days ago. He was admitted after his roommate found him behaving abnormally. Since admission, the team has managed to acquire further history and has diagnosed him with first-onset psychosis. Joel has a positive family history of mental health disorders. In addition, he has been using cannabis since the age of 15 years old, on a regular basis. The team has decided to start him on a course on antipsychotics, as he was experiencing significant positive symptoms. However, he was noted to be spiking a high temperature this morning. The on-call core trainee who examined him found him to be rigid as well. The attending consultant suspects that he might have developed neuroleptic malignant syndrome and has since transferred him to the intensive care unit. Joel's father is here now and is demanding to find out more about the condition of his son.

Task

Please speak to Joel's father and address all his concerns and expectations. Please also provide him with an explanation of what has happened to his son.

Outline of station

You are the father of Joel. You are very concerned to know that Joel needed admission to the psychiatry unit and are devastated to know that your son is suffering from first-episode psychosis. You hoped for the inpatient stay to be as short as possible and were initially hoping that your son could get back to his baseline functioning as soon as possible. You are shocked to learn of the fact that your son is now being transferred over to the intensive care unit. You demand an explanation from the doctor in charge of him. You also wish to know the further prognosis of his condition. You also want to know what the plans are with regard to the further management of his condition.

CASC construct table

The CASC construct table is formatted such that candidates will be able to cover adequately both the range and the depth of the assessment required in this station.

Starting off: 'Hello, I am Dr Melvyn. I understand that you wish to get some updates about your son's condition. Can we have a chat?'			
Explain rationale for medications	I'm sorry to inform you that your son has been transferred to the medical intensive care unit. I understand that you're very concerned about his current condition. The team is also very concerned about his current condition.	As your son was experiencing florid symptoms of his psychosis, we needed to start him on a course of antipsychotics to help him with his symptoms. The team has commenced him on a low dose of antipsychotic (olanzapine).	This antipsychotic is commonly used for most patients, and most patients do not experience acute side effects after commencement.
Explain likely diagnosis – neuroleptic malignant syndrome and clinical features of the condition	It is very likely that your son has developed a condition known as neuroleptic malignant syndrome (NMS). Have you heard about this condition before?	Would it be alright for me to explain more about this condition? This is a rare condition that occurs in approximately every 1 in 100 individuals.	In this condition, it is not uncommon for individuals to have unstable vitals (heart rate and blood pressure). They might also spike a temperature. Clinically, on examination, these individuals are usually relatively rigid in their extremities. It is a medical emergency, and hence we have transferred your son to the medical intensive care unit for more intensive monitoring.
Explain likely causes for NMS	The most likely cause for this condition is the antipsychotic medication that we have just commenced.	As said, this is an unpredictable and rare side effect of an antipsychotic medication.	Of course, there are other medical conditions that might present in the same way. We have done some basic laboratory investigations, and the findings are suggestive of NMS. It is usually more common if patients are prescribed with the older generation of antipsychotics.

(Continued)

Explain further management	Given that neuroleptic malignant syndrome is considered to be a medical emergency, we have immediately arranged for a transfer to the medical intensive care unit. The medical team is also currently on board to help us with the acute management of your son's condition.	We have since stopped the antipsychotics that we had recently introduced. We are monitoring his vitals very clearly and making sure that we are providing him with adequate hydration. The medical team might consider the usage of other agents to help him with his condition.	We will routinely do blood tests, and in particular, we will trend a blood test result known as creatinine phosphokinase. We will continue to monitor his condition, and we will provide you with regular updates.
Address concerns	Currently, the medical stability of your son's condition is of utmost importance.	We have since stopped the likely offending agent and have also reported that your son has an adverse reaction to that particular medication.	Once he is clinically more stable, we will try to re-challenge him with another antipsychotic medication, as it would be helpful for his symptoms.
Address complaints procedure	I would like to apologize for this. As said, NMS is a very rare condition, and it's difficult for us to know who would and would not acquire it.	I understand that you have some concerns which you would like to bring up to the hospital. Would you like me to guide you on the procedure?	I know that I have provided you with quite a lot of information today. Do you have any other questions for me?

Common pitfalls

a. Failure to cover the range and depth of the information required for this station
b. Use of jargons and giving too much information without checking understanding of the family member

It is important to address the anger and frustration raised by the family member. Apologize for what the family has gone through, but remember not to apologize for causing this to happen (there is a huge difference in this!).

It may be helpful to use reflective statements especially at the start of the interview. For example, 'I can see that you are very angry at this point . . . It is very understandable for you to experience this . . .'

Remember to address family member's complaint and guide him to the appropriate channel. Do not push blame on anyone – it is important to maintain collegiality towards colleagues.

Quick recall*

- Neuroleptic malignant syndrome is characterized by the following features:
  a. Hyperthermia
  b. Changing levels of consciousness
  c. Muscular rigidity
  d. Autonomic dysfunction
  e. Tachycardia
  f. Labile blood pressure
  g. Pallor
  h. Sweating
  i. Urinary incontinence

Laboratory investigations commonly, but not invariably, demonstrate the following:

- Increased creatinine phosphokinase
- Increased white blood count
- Abnormal LFTs

Neuroleptic malignant syndrome requires urgent medical treatment.

STATION 42: URINE DRUG TEST

Information to candidates

Name of patient: Mr Charlie Brown

You have been tasked to speak to Mr Charlie Brown. He is a 30-year-old male with a history of paranoid schizophrenia and has just been admitted to the inpatient unit following a relapse of his condition. As he has been more settled in terms of his mental state, he was allowed on home leave. He has since returned from his home leave and the nursing staff has contacted you. You are the on-call core trainee. During the interview, you noticed that Mr Brown appeared to be very distractible, and at times, he was observed to be mumbling to himself. You have discussed the case with your attending consultant, who recommended that you acquire a sample of the patient's urine, as he has been known to have abused cannabis previously as well.

Task

Please speak to Mr Brown and persuade him to provide you with a sample of his urine for testing. Please do not perform an MSE.

Outline of station

You are the patient, Mr Charlie Brown. You have a history of paranoid schizophrenia and have been admitted to the inpatient unit on several occasions. You recently got admitted again as you have not been concordant with the medications that you were prescribed in the outpatient setting. Before admission, you harboured

---

* Adapted from B.K. Puri, A. Hall and R. Ho (2014). *Revision Notes in Psychiatry*. London, UK: CRC Press, p. 253.

paranoid ideations, which led you to be cooped up at home, as you were afraid that others out there might harm you. With the current inpatient treatment, you have gradually recovered and are currently better. You have been granted Section 17 home leave over the weekend. You are worried about returning home, and hence you spend your time at the nearby park instead. You did meet up with your friends, and they did offer you some weed to try. You are reluctant to share this history, as you know that it would lead to a longer stay in the hospital. Also, those paranoid ideations and auditory hallucinations have since returned as well.

CASC construct table

The CASC construct table is formatted such that candidates will be able to cover adequately both the range and the depth of the assessment required in this station.

Starting off: 'Hello, I am Dr Melvyn. I understand that you have just been back from your home leave. Can we have a chat?'			
Explain indications for assessment	I understand that you have just been back from your home leave. The nurses are quite concerned about how you have been since you returned back and hence requested for me to see you. Would it be alright for me to have a chat with you?	I would like to understand from you how your home leave was. Would you be able to tell me more about it?	
Explain rules and regulations of Section 17 home leave	Is this the first time you are allowed on home leave? Are you able to tell me what your previous home leaves were like? What happened after you returned from your previous home leave?	One of the rules when our patients are under Section 17 home leave is that they might be asked to provide a sample of their urine after they return back to the ward. Had the team told you about this before you went on home leave?	We hope you could cooperate with us and provide the necessary sample. It would help us in the further management of your condition. We hope that you could get well and be discharged sooner.
Explore concerns about provision of urine sample	It seems to me that you are quite reluctant to provide us with your urine sample. Is there any reason why?	Did you spend your home leave at home? If not, where were you?	Can you tell me more about what happened? Was there a chance you were offered or used any drugs or alcohol during your scheduled home leave? We do need to know this, as this will affect the medications we have prescribed and it will also affect how we help you with regard to your current condition.

(Continued)

Exploration of possible psychotic symptoms	It seems to me that you have appeared to be very distracted throughout the interview. Is there anything bothering you?	Do you feel that there might be others out there who are plotting against you, or who might harm you?	Do you have any strange experiences, such as hearing voices or seeing things that are not there? Do you feel in control of your thought processes? Do you feel in control of your emotions and actions?

Common pitfalls

a. Failure to cover the range and the depth of the information required for this station

For the patient in this station, it may helpful to ask in an indirect and non-threatening manner circumstances of the home leave and his reasons for refusing a urine drug screen. Do not be overly fixated on insisting he go for the screening. It is important to address his concerns and alleviate his anxiety about the fear of being convicted if the drug screen comes back positive.

Quick recall*

In this station, it is important to not only know the common drugs of abuse but also the local colloquial names. It is important and essential to have an appreciation of the length of time the drugs could be detected in the urine sample as well.

Drug	Colloquial name	Length of time detected in the urine
Amphetamines	Speed, Whizz	48 hours
Barbiturates	Downers	24 hours for short-acting and as long as 3 weeks for long-acting
Cannabinoids	Grass, hash, ganja, pot	3 days to 4 weeks
Cocaine	Snow, coke, girl, lady	6–8 hours (metabolites 2–4 days)
Heroin	Smack	36–72 hours
LSD	Acid	12–24 hours
MDMA	Ecstasy, XTC, Adam, E	48 hours
PCP	Angel dust, peace pill	8 days
Temazepam	Jellies	6–48 hours

---

* Adapted from B.K. Puri, A. Hall and R. Ho (2014). *Revision Notes in Psychiatry*. London, UK: CRC Press, p. 529.

STATION 43: DEALING WITH ANGRY RELATIVES – CLOZAPINE CASE

Information to candidates

Name of patient: Mr Charlie Brown

You have been tasked to speak to the mother of Mr Charlie Brown. Charlie was diagnosed with schizophrenia at the age of 20 years, with the aetiology most likely due to chronic usage of cannabis since the age of 15 years. He has had multiple relapses that previously required inpatient admission and treatment under Section 2. Recently, he relapsed again due to him being nonconcordant with medications, and he has since been in the ward for the past 2 months.

The team has tried him on at least three typical and atypical antipsychotics and have commenced him on clozapine, as he fulfils Kane's criteria for treatment-resistant schizophrenia. His mother is here today and is demanding to see a member of the team. She is particularly upset that her son would still require prolonged hospitalization and is also worried about the clozapine that he has been started on. She has read up more about the medication (clozapine) on the Internet and has learnt of significant adverse effects.

She wishes to bring him home today.

Task

Please speak to the mother of Mr Charlie Brown and attempt to de-escalate the situation and explain the rationale for her son being started on clozapine. Please address all her concerns and expectations.

Outline of station

You are the mother of Charlie and are very upset with the management of the team. Charlie has had multiple admissions to the hospital within this year. You understand that the team has since started him on clozapine. You are upset that no one from the team has sought your perspectives about it. You have done some research about it and know that it is associated with dangerous side effects. You do not want Charlie to have more medical problems in addition to to his pre-existing psychiatric disorder and are upset with the rate of the progression of his condition. You do not find that it is helpful for him to remain in the hospital and wish to bring him home today. If the core trainee does not allow you or recommend you to do so, you will ask for a discharge against medical advice.

CASC construct table

The CASC construct table is formatted such that candidates will be able to cover adequately both the range and the depth of the assessment required in this station.

Starting off: 'Hello, I am Dr Melvyn. I understand that you have some concerns about your son. Can we have a chat?'			
Introduction, using empathetic statements to calm relative down	Thanks for coming today. I hope we can make use of this opportunity to clarify any concerns that you might have about your son's condition.	I'm sorry and I do apologize for the fact that the doctors in the team did not inform you that your son has been commenced on clozapine.	Please let me speak to them to find out what has actually happened. However, I hope that I can try my best to address all your concerns. I understand that it has been a difficult time for you, given your son's multiple readmission and prolonged admission. I hope you understand that we are both trying our best to help your son with his psychiatric issues.
Explanation of rationale for clozapine	I hear your concerns about clozapine. Your son has had a trial of multiple antipsychotics, including the newer generation as well as the older generation of antipsychotics.	During this admission, we have adjusted the dosing of the medications accordingly, and we have tried administrating the maximum possible doses to your son. Unfortunately, it did not seem to help your son with his condition.	Given that, the team's opinion during our multidisciplinary meeting is that your son most likely has a condition known as treatment-resistant schizophrenia. Have you heard of this before? Can I take some time to explain to you what we mean and refer to as treatment-resistant schizophrenia? Treatment-resistant schizophrenia is diagnosed when a patient fails to respond to a trial of three antipsychotics of different classes, using an adequate dose of antipsychotic for an adequate duration.
Discuss side effects and monitoring procedures	I hear your concerns about the side effects of clozapine. Prior research has indeed shown that clozapine could cause agranulocytosis, so regular blood counts are necessary.	Hence, when your son was started on clozapine, we also organized regular blood tests for him. In the first 18 weeks, we are required to determine his full blood count on a weekly basis. In addition, we also monitor closely the other side effects associated with the medication, such as hyper-salivation.	We have started your son on the lowest dose of clozapine and have gradually increased the dose accordingly. We have done so to make sure that his body is able to gradually adapt to the effects of the medications.

(Continued)

Discuss management options	Despite the fact that we have already initiated your son on a course of clozapine, I'm sorry to inform you his progress of recovery on the medication has been relatively slow.	Hence, we have kept him in the hospital, so that we can adjust the dosing accordingly and monitor his condition more closely. I hear that you are concerned about him being admitted for so long, but our team is trying our best to help him using the new medication (clozapine).	In addition, one of the other concerns we have had was that upon admission, we noticed that your son's LFTs were abnormal. Is there a possibility that he has been drinking prior to admission? Can you tell me more?
Advice against discharging against medical advice	I understand your concerns about the prolonged hospitalization. I hope we are better able to help your son during this admission, so that his rates of relapse would be reduced. I hear that you wish to consider a discharge against medical advice. However, I hope that you can reconsider that.	One of our concerns about your son's condition lies with the fact that he might potentially be using alcohol. It is not recommended for him to be using alcohol when he is also using clozapine. We might need to refer him to the dual diagnosis unit to help him should your son have an alcohol problem as well.	I hear that you might want to raise a complaint against the team and the hospital. If I could help, I could direct you to the appropriate procedure. Do you have any other concerns that you would like to discuss today?

Common pitfalls

a. Failure to cover the range and the depth of the information required for this station

Quick recall*

- Clozapine should be introduced if schizophrenia is inadequately controlled despite the sequential use of two or more antipsychotics (one of which should be a typical antipsychotic) each for at least 6–8 weeks.
- Treatment-resistant schizophrenia could be diagnosed based on Kane's criteria.

---

* Adapted from B.K. Puri, A. Hall and R. Ho (2014). *Revision Notes in Psychiatry*. London, UK: CRC Press, pp. 366–367.

- If a patient failed to respond to a trial of three antipsychotics of different classes, using an adequate dose for an adequate duration, an atypical agent such as clozapine can be tried. Clozapine can cause agranulocytosis, so regular blood counts are necessary. The incidence is 0.8% at 12 months and 0.9% at 18 months, with a peak risk in the third month. It is higher in women and older patients.
- Prior research has shown that clozapine was significantly better than chlorpromazine in the treatment of schizophrenia previously resistant to haloperidol. Improvement was observed in both positive and negative symptoms.
- In the United Kingdom, patients receiving clozapine are required to have their full blood counts monitored at regular intervals.

At baseline, the following actions are required:

1. Perform assessment and discuss with patients and carers.
2. Information and advice regarding swapping to clozapine from another antipsychotic should be sought from the pharmacy.
3. Decide whether it is an inpatient or outpatient initiation. Inpatient initiation is indicated for elderly and adolescents, and those with concurrent medical problems.
4. Register the patient with the CPMS and obtain an initial FBC.
5. Start clozapine at 12.5 mg once a green blood result is issued by the CPMS.
6. For inpatient treatment, physical monitoring is required every hour for 6 hours, and the patient needs to be accompanied by a carer.
7. For outpatient treatment, patient and carer must be provided with emergency contact details for the first 24 hours.
8. Inform his or her GP on the start date.
9. Baseline physical examination: weight, temperature, pulse and BP (both lying and standing).
10. For patients with diabetes, HBA1c at baseline; for patients without diabetes, fasting blood glucose.

Physical Examination Stations
- Candidates should take note that in the CASC examination, physical examination stations do appear.
- The common physical examination stations include the following:
  a. Examination for extra-pyramidal side effects
  b. Examination of thyroid gland following chronic and long-term lithium usage
  c. Neurological examination of upper extremities or lower extremities
  d. Examination of cerebellar system
  e. Cardiovascular system examination
  f. Ability to read and interpret ECG
  g. Examination of cranial nerves
- Candidates are recommended to refer to other basic medical books for physical examination techniques. A brief overview of the techniques will be covered in this book.
- In our book, we will focus on a variety of clinical psychiatric case scenarios with detailed explanation and step-by-step approach with tips and common pitfall analysis. This is the aim of our book.

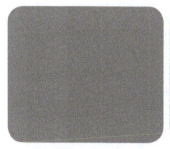

TOPIC 2
PHYSICAL
EXAMINATIONS

STATION 44: EXAMINATION FOR EXTRA-PYRAMIDAL SIDE EFFECTS

In this station, candidates are typically asked to assess for a variety of extra-pyramidal side effects. The common side effects include the following:

Pseudo-parkinsonism (lesions in nigrostriatal pathway)	**Epidemiology:** Incidence (20%). **Risk factors**: More common in older women, particularly those with neurological damage, and may persist for many months. **Onset:** After a few weeks of usage and develop gradually. **Symptoms**: Mimicking Parkinson's disease, with akinesia (generalized slowing and loss of movements, particularly the involuntary movements of expression), rigidity and tremor. Rigidity and akinesia develop more frequently than tremor. **Management:** Gradually reducing the dose can reduce the symptoms. Otherwise change to second-generation antipsychotic. Anticholinergic agents (e.g., benzhexol or artane 2 mg BD) have been shown to be effective in reducing the severity of EPSEs and may be prescribed to patients experiencing these side effects.
Acute dystonia (lesions in nigrostriatal pathway)	**Epidemiology:** Incidence (10%). **Risk factors**: Young men are at highest risk. High-potency antipsychotic in schizophrenia patients who are antipsychotic naïve is also a risk factor. **Onset:** Occur within a few hours of antipsychotic administration. **Symptoms:** The classic example includes oculogyric crisis (fixed upward or lateral gaze), but torsion dystonia and torticollis occur, as well as spasms of the muscles of the lips, tongue, face and throat. Acute dyskinesia (involuntary movements), with grimacing and exaggerated posturing and twisting of the head, neck or jaw, can also occur. Trismus refers to the dystonic reaction to antipsychotic medication affecting the jaw muscles. **Management:** Intramuscular anticholinergics (e.g. IM congentin 2 mg stat) in oculogyric crisis and torsion dystonia.

(Continued)

Akathisia (lesions in nigrostriatal pathway)	**Epidemiology:** Incidence (25%–50%). **Risk factors:** Acute forms are related to rapid increases in antipsychotic dose. **Onset:** Most commonly after the fifth day of initiation of dopamine receptor antagonists. **Symptoms:** The patient may become irritable or unsettled, complains of needing to go out or may try to leave for no clear reason. **Management:** Acute akathisia may respond to anticholinergics. Chronic akathisia responds poorly to anticholinergics but may respond to benzodiazepines. The best-established treatment for either form of akathisia is propranolol.

Tardive dyskinesia (lesions in nigrostriatal pathway)	**Epidemiology:** 5% after 1 year of treatment; 20% after chronic treatment.
	Risk factors:
	
	  1. Elderly women, those with affective disorder, organic brain disorder and history of EPSE
	  2. Long exposure to antipsychotics
	  3. Precipitated by anticholinergic
	
	Pathology: Tardive dyskinesia (TD) is caused by supersensitivity of D_2 receptors.
	Symptoms: Typical TD includes lip smacking, chewing, 'fly catching' tongue protrusion, choreiform hand pill rolling movements and pelvic thrusting
	Management:
	Change to second-generation antipsychotics.
	Vitamin E.

Please seek consent from the patient before you start off with the examination. Please ask the patient whether he has pain in any particular region of his body. Make sure you make use of the alcohol rub before starting off with the examination. The patient could be seated down for the examination. Please inform the patient that the examination will involve looking at his mouth, moving his upper and lower limbs and getting him to walk.

Candidates are encouraged to start off the examination by observing the patient at rest. Observe and look for any movement abnormalities in his limbs and trunk. Please ask the patient whether he has anything in his mouth before asking him to open his mouth. In the event that the patient is wearing dentures, please get the patient to remove them. You will have to ask the patient to open his mouth twice. You need to observe whether there are any abnormal movements of his mouth at rest. Subsequently, you need to ask the patient to repeat the above again, but this time with him sticking out his tongue. Please observe for any movement abnormalities of his tongue. Thereafter, you can examine the patient's upper extremities for Parkinsonism-like features. Please observe whether the patient has any baseline tremors by getting him to hold both his arms in front of him. Next, proceed to manipulate his arms and check for both lead-pipe rigidity as well as cog-wheeling. Please ask the patient to gently tap his thumb with each of his fingers and observe whether he appears to have any difficulties with these movements.

Subsequently, get the patient to sit at rest and observe whether there are any abnormal bodily movements. Get the patient to place both his arms in-between his legs and observe once again for any abnormal movements. You could then get the patient to stand up and get him to walk. Whilst you are with the patient and he is walking, please observe his gait. Also take note of whether there is a reduction in his arm swing.

STATION 45: EXAMINATION OF THE THYROID GLAND

Suggested Reference: G. Douglas, F. Nicol, C. Robertson (2013). *Macleod's Clinical Examination* (13th edition). Edinburgh, UK: Churchill Livingstone.

STATION 46: NEUROLOGICAL EXAMINATION

Suggested Reference: A. Barnett and T. Bannister (2014). *Pocket Clinical Examiner* (1st Edition). Boca Raton, FL: CRC Press, pp. 37–58.

STATION 47: EXAMINATION OF THE CEREBELLAR SYSTEM

Suggested Reference: A. Barnett and T. Bannister (2014). *Pocket Clinical Examiner* (1st Edition). Boca Raton, FL: CRC Press, pp. 37–58.

STATION 48: CARDIOVASCULAR SYSTEM EXAMINATION

Suggested Reference: A. Barnett and T. Bannister (2014). *Pocket Clinical Examiner* (1st Edition). Boca Raton, FL: CRC Press, pp. 9–17.

STATION 49: READING ECG

Suggested Reference: A. Barnett and T. Bannister (2014). *Pocket Clinical Examiner* (1st Edition). Boca Raton, FL: CRC Press.

STATION 50: FUNDOSCOPY

Suggested Reference: G. Douglas, F. Nicol, C. Robertson (2013). *Macleod's Clinical Examination* (13th edition). Edinburgh, UK: Churchill Livingstone.

STATION 51: EXAMINATION OF CRANIAL NERVES

Suggested Reference: A. Barnett and T. Bannister (2014). *Pocket Clinical Examiner* (1st Edition). Boca Raton, FL: CRC Press, pp. 37–58.

STATION 52: OLD AGE PSYCHOSIS (LINKED STATION A)

Information to candidates

Name of patient: Mrs Thomas

Mrs Thomas has been arrested by police officers following a confrontation with her neighbours, and is sent to the emergency department for further medical and psychiatric assessment. You are the core trainee 3 on call and are tasked to speak to her to determine whether she has any psychiatric condition which might necessitate invoking the appropriate sections to keep her in the hospital.

Task

Please speak to Mrs Thomas and perform a mental state examination.

Outline of station

The purpose of providing an outline of the station is to allow candidates to be familiar with the structure of the station. This outline could also be helpful when candidates practice for the MRCPsych, joining with their colleagues to act out the station.

Please note that the outlines provided are based on the experiences of the authors. There may be variations in the actual examination.

You are Mrs Thomas and are frustrated as to why you're the one in the hospital and not your neighbours. Your neighbours have been troubling you for the past year or so, ever since they moved into a nearby apartment. You frequently hear them speaking about you, and they often make demeaning remarks about you. You know that they are doing so, as they want to get rid of you, so they can occupy your apartment. You hear them most clearly at the wall separating your apartment from theirs. You believe that the food you cook in the house tastes strange, and you believe that your neighbours have poisoned it. You have to go out and buy your packaged food as you do not feel safe cooking at home. You have previously complained to the police but they took no action. You have approached your local district council, but the officer did not believe you. You have been feeling increasingly troubled and have decided that you need to do something about this issue. You have decided to confront your neighbours today. You have used your

walking stick to threaten them and have told them not to bother you further.
At the start of the interview, you are frustrated that you have been arrested and not your neighbours. You do not wish to speak to a psychiatrist, as you believe you do not have any mental health condition.

CASC construct table

The CASC construct table is formatted such that candidates will be able to cover adequately both the range and the depth of the assessment required in this station.

Approach: Be prepared for a patient who might be frustrated and not willing to share more information. Demonstration of empathy is crucial towards eliciting the symptomatology.			
Starting off: 'Hello, I am Dr Melvyn, one of the psychiatrists from the mental health unit. I understand that the police have brought you in today. Can we have a chat about this?'			
Clarification of history of presenting complaint	It does sound like you have been having a very difficult time. Can you tell me more so that I can better understand your situation?	I'm sorry to learn about the difficult circumstances that you have been through.	Can you tell me for how long you feel your neighbours have been troubling you? Have you sought any form of help?
Exploring auditory hallucinations/ exploring delusional beliefs	Can you tell me more about the voices that you have been hearing? Are they as clear as our current conversation? What do they say?	Do they speak directly to you? Can you give me examples of what they have been saying to you?	Do they refer to you as he or she or do they call you by your name? Do they comment on what you are doing? Do they give you commands as to what to do? Could there be any alternative explanations that could help account for these experiences that you have been having?
Eliciting hallucinations in all other modalities	Have you noticed that your food or drink seems to have a different taste recently? Has there been anything wrong with your sense of smell?	Have you had any strange experiences or feelings in your body recently?	Have you been able to see things that other people cannot see? What kind of things can you see? Can you give me an example?
Elicit thought disorders	Do you feel that your thoughts are being interfered with? Who do you think is doing all this?	Do you have thoughts in your head that you feel are not your own thoughts? Where do you think these thoughts come from?	Do you feel that your thoughts are being broadcasted, such that others would know what you are thinking? Do you feel that your thoughts are being taken away from your head by some external forces?

(Continued)

Elicit passivity experiences	Do you feel in control of your own actions and emotions?	Do you feel that someone or something is trying to control you?	Who do you think this would be?
Impact of symptoms on mood and coping mechanisms	It has been a difficult time for you. How have you been coping? How has your memory been? Any visual or auditory impairment?	How has this affected your mood? Are you still interested in things that you used to enjoy? Are there any difficulties with your sleep or appetite?	Have you made use of any substance, such as alcohol, to help you to cope? What about street drugs?
Risk assessment	Can you tell me more as to why the police have been involved today?	Do you currently still have any plans or thoughts to confront your neighbours?	Are you so stressed by all these experiences that you might have thoughts of ending it all?

Common pitfalls

a. Failure to be empathetic enough to engage the frustrated patient
b. Failure to cover the range and depth of the task – need to demonstrate to the college examiner that you have explored all the other modalities of hallucinations and also make an attempt to elicit the rest of the first-rank symptoms

Quick recall: Geriatric psychosis/paraphrenia*

Paraphrenia is a terminology used to describe a psychiatric condition that is characterized by relatively late age of onset, chronic delusions and hallucinations and the preservation of volition and a lack of personality deterioration. Studies have shown that there is an annual incidence of late paraphrenia of 17–26 per 100,000 individuals. The condition is more common in females than males. Those with late-onset psychosis tend to be unmarried and have a lower reproductive rate compared with controls.

Aetiology

a. There is an increased risk of schizophrenia in the first-degree relatives of paraphrenics, but it is less than the risk to the relatives of younger-onset schizophrenics.
b. Long-standing paranoid personalities tend to predispose to the development of paraphrenia in the elderly.
c. Hearing impairment is associated with the development of paranoid symptoms. The characteristics most strongly associated include early age of

---

* Adapted from B.K. Puri, A. Hall and R. Ho (2014). *Revision Notes in Psychiatry*. London, UK: CRC Press, p. 712.

onset of hearing impairment and long duration and profound hearing loss. Auditory hallucinations are more consistently associated with hearing loss.

d. Those with late-onset psychosis also tend to have significantly larger cerebral ventricles compared with controls.

Clinical features

a. Most individuals have at least one type of delusion. The most common delusion includes that of persecution, self-reference, thought broadcast, sin, guilt and grandiosity.

b. Forty-six per cent of individuals have at least one first-rank symptom.

c. Eighty-three per cent of individuals had some hallucinatory experience, most commonly auditory, but some also visual, somatic and olfactory.

d. Thought disorder and catatonic symptoms are almost never seen.

e. Inappropriate affect was not seen.

f. Negative symptoms are seen frequently, but mostly mild.

g. Other common symptoms include worry, irritability, poor concentration, self-neglect and obsessive features.

STATION 53: OLD AGE PSYCHOSIS (LINKED STATION B)

Information to candidates

Name of patient: Mrs Thomas

Mrs Thomas has been assessed by the medical team and deemed to be medically well. She has been seen by the consultant psychiatrist and deemed to have late-onset psychosis. She has been commenced on an antipsychotic called olanzapine at a dosage of 5 mg at night. Her brother, Mr Smith, has called in requesting to speak to the team as he has some concerns about his sister's condition.

Task

Please speak to Mr Smith and address all his concerns and expectations.

Outline of station

You are Mr Smith, the brother of Mrs Thomas. Your sister was widowed 2 years ago, and you are her only relative. You have previously learned about the police arresting her and have learned that following the arrest, she was transferred to a hospital and is currently being sectioned for treatment. You are keen to know more about her diagnosis and the potential causes for her current condition. You understand that your sister has been commenced on a medication, but you are also wondering whether there are other alternatives apart from medications. You want to know more about the medication (olanzapine) and also wish to know more about the longer-term treatment. You wish to know if she needs an alternative housing or placement.

CASC construct table

The CASC construct table is formatted such that candidates will be able to cover adequately both the range and the depth of the assessment required in this station.

Starting off: 'Hello, I am Dr Melvyn, one of the psychiatrists from the mental health unit. I understand that you have some concerns about your sister's condition? Can we have a chat?'			
Clarification about diagnosis	I understand that it must be a difficult time for you. I'm here to explain and to clarify any doubts that you have.	With the symptoms that your sister has shared with us, it seemed like what she has is late-onset psychosis. Have you heard about it before?	Late-onset psychosis is actually the same as schizophrenia. Schizophrenia is a common mental health disorder that affects the way one thinks, feels and behaves.
Explain aetiological causes	There are many causes for this condition. It is tough to identify the exact cause in your sister's condition.	If there is a known family history of schizophrenia, your sister might be predisposed to it.	Often, those with paranoid personality disorders as well as hearing impairments might be predisposed as well.
Explain treatment options	You're right to mention that there are both inpatient and outpatient treatment options.	To determine which is more suitable, we need to perform an assessment of risks. In your sister's case, there is an element of risk as she has confronted her neighbours.	As your sister did not have much insight into her condition, there is thus a need for the team to detain her under the Mental Health Act.
Explain pharmacological treatment	I'm sure you're aware that your sister has been started on a medication known as olanzapine. Have you heard about it before?	Olanzapine is one of the commonly used anti-psychotic medications. It works for patients with late-onset psychosis by regulating the amount of chemicals such as dopamine in the brain.	Like all medications, antipsychotics do have their own side effects. The common side effects include sedation and weight gain. We usually would recommend a continuation of the medications for at least 6 months.
Explain alternative treatments	Apart from medication, the other alternative form of treatment would be that of psychological or talking therapies. Have you heard of that before?	Cognitive behavioural therapy could be helpful for your sister when she is more settled, as she would be able to learn techniques to cope with her symptoms.	If sensory impairments are a concern, we could refer your sister to our specialist colleagues to help her with impairments.

(Continued)

Explain long-term management	In the long term, we hope that we could get your sister our multidisciplinary team involvement.	We hope that our community psychiatric nurse could help support her and watch her medication adherence in the community.	If you do have concerns about her current accommodation, we could also consider alternatives, such as shelter housing. Alternatively, we may recommend that your sister attend day centres to keep her engaged.

Common pitfalls

a. Failure to explain the rationale as to why the patient needs sectioned treatment
b. Failure to explain other non-pharmacological management, such as looking into and helping the patient with her sensory impairments
c. Failure to cover and explain the long-term management of the patient

One helpful method in psychoeducation of illness is to link the patient's experiences with the characteristics of the disorder. This will make the discussion more relevant to the patient/family member.

Quick recall: Geriatric psychosis linked station – Discussion*

- The treatment of metabolic disorders or other physical conditions may bring about an improvement in the mental state.
- The treatment of hypertension may prevent deterioration if the change in mental state is caused by a silent cardiovascular disease.
- Antipsychotic medication may bring about an improvement. Antipsychotics with low anti-cholinergic, low-hypotensive potential are recommended for the elderly.
- The first-line treatment includes risperidone (1–3 mg/day).
- The second-line treatment includes olanzapine (2.5–7.5 mg/day) and quetiapine (50–300 mg/day).
- A significant proportion shows no significant response, and about one-quarter shows a full response to treatment.
- Treatment response is associated with improved compliance, the use of depot medication, an involvement of a community practice nurse (CPN) and lower medication doses.
- With regard to non-pharmacological treatment, day-care centre attendance may be helpful in increasing socialization.
- If sensory impairment is present, there is evidence that the condition can improve upon treatment of the underlying deficit (for example, providing a hearing aid for a deaf person).

* Adapted from B.K. Puri, A. Hall and R. Ho (2014). *Revision Notes in Psychiatry*. London, UK: CRC Press, pp. 712–713.

- With regard to prognosis, some patients have little or no response to treatment.
- Others do have a full response.
- Long-term contact with psychiatric services is required.

STATION 54: BEHAVIOURAL AND PSYCHOLOGICAL SYMPTOMS IN DEMENTIA (LINKED STATION A)

Information to candidates

Name of patient: Mr Johnson

Mr Johnson has been a resident in the nursing home for the previous 6 months. Recently, over the past week or so, the nursing staff noted that Mr Johnson had been increasingly agitated during the day. There was an episode in which Mr Johnson attempted to hit one of the staff as well as another resident in the nursing home. The support worker has been informed about his changes in behaviour.

Task

Please speak to Mr Johnson's support worker to obtain more collateral information to arrive at a possible diagnosis.

Outline of station

You are Sarah, the support worker of Mr Johnson. You have known him since the day he was transferred to your nursing home. Over the past week or so, you have heard from the staff that he has increasingly difficult behaviours. You have not identified any specific triggers prior to the episodes of aggression. You know that Mr Johnson has a history of Alzheimer's dementia, and he was last seen by the geriatric psychiatrist around 3 months ago. Per the memo from the specialist, there is no worsening of his symptoms, and the specialist also does not feel that there are any associated comorbid psychiatric disorders. You know that Mr Johnson has not been sick recently. You understand from the staff that there have been two new residents in the nursing home over the past week. In addition, due to Mr Johnson's wife being sick, she has not visited him for the past 2 weeks. You are keen to share as much information as possible with the doctor, as you hope that Mr Johnson's condition can improve, or else it will be tough for the nursing home to continue having him.

CASC construct table

The CASC construct table is formatted such that candidates will be able to cover adequately both the range and the depth of the assessment required in this station.

Starting off: 'Hello, I am Dr Melvyn, one of the psychiatrists from the mental health unit. I understand that you have some concerns about Mr Johnson, one of your residents in your home, due to changes in his behaviours. Can we have a chat about this?'			
Clarification of behavioural changes	I understand that it has been a difficult time for you and your nursing staff. Can you please tell me more about the difficulties? How long have you noticed these changes?	Have you noticed any changes in his mood? You mentioned that there are times in which he seems more irritable. Are there specific triggers?	Has he been verbally or physically violent towards your staff or any of the other residents? Can you tell me more? Are his behaviours progressively getting worse?
Exploration of psychiatric symptoms	Can you share with me the reasons as to why he needed a placement in your nursing home? What was the diagnosis that was given to Mr Johnson previously?	Has he been regular with his follow-up appointments with the psychiatrist? Has the psychiatrist started him on or changed any of his medications? What did the psychiatrist say about his condition during the latest follow-up appointment?	Does he appear to be more emotional than usual? Is he still able to enjoy things that he used to enjoy? Are there times in which your staff have noticed him to be responding to things or talking to himself?
Exploration of physical symptoms	Has he been unwell recently? Any medical conditions?	Did he spike a temperature in the past week or so? Did he have any recent falls?	Is he in any form of pain? Is he able to clear his bowels and pass urine without any issue?
Exploration of environmental changes	Have there been any changes in your nursing home?	Are there new staffs in your nursing home? (Or) Are there new staffs attending to his needs?	Have there been any changes to the regular routine in the nursing home? Have there been any changes in the structured activities usually conducted in the home?
Exploration of social changes/lack of visitors	How does he usually spend his time in the nursing home?	Has his family visited him recently?	

Common pitfalls

a. This might seem to be an easy station as basically candidates only need to elicit information from the support worker. However, candidates need to have a structure as to what information they need to gather from the support worker.

b. Candidates need to adequately cover the range and the depth of the task – they need to explore the psychiatric symptoms, rule out physical problems and assess environmental changes as well as changes in the social environment. They also need to check whether there have been changes in the structured activities in the home.

STATION 55: BEHAVIOURAL AND PSYCHOLOGICAL SYMPTOMS IN DEMENTIA (LINKED STATION B)

Information to candidates

Name of patient: Mr Johnson

Mr Johnson has been a resident in the nursing home for the previous 6 months. Recently, over the past week or so, the nursing staff noted that Mr Johnson had been increasingly agitated during the day. There was an episode in which Mr Johnson attempted to hit both one of the staff and another resident in the nursing home. The support worker has been informed about his changes in behaviour. You have obtained further information from the support worker in the previous station. Mr Johnson's son now demands to speak to you. He is very upset that the team has started his father on an antipsychotic medication called olanzapine.

Task

Please speak to Mr Johnson's son and address all his concerns and expectations.

Outline of station

You are Tom, Mr Johnson's son. You have heard about the issues in the nursing home. You understand that the team has decided to start your father on a medication known as olanzapine. You have read up on the medication on the Internet, and it seemed to be a very dangerous medication for use in the elderly. You are frustrated that the team went ahead and started the medication without informing you. You are very concerned about the increased risk of stroke from the medication. You wonder how long the team will be continuing the medications. You are not very keen for your father to be on medications. You expect the core trainee to talk with you about other options, apart from medications.

CASC construct table

The CASC construct table is formatted such that candidates will be able to cover adequately both the range and the depth of the assessment required in this station.

Starting off: 'Hello, I am Dr Melvyn, one of the psychiatrists from the mental health unit. I understand that you have some concerns about your father, Mr Johnson. I am hoping we can have a chat about this'.

Clarification of chief concerns	I apologize that the team should have kept you informed that your father has been commenced on an antipsychotic medication.	I hear that you have some concerns about the medication olanzapine. Can you tell me more?	(Or) Can you share with me your understanding about olanzapine?
Explain rationale for commencement of antipsychotics	I understand that you're deeply concerned about your father's condition. Can I tell you more as to why the team has come to such a decision?	As you know, your dad has Alzheimer's dementia, and this is a condition that affects his cognitive functioning as well as his behaviours. In Alzheimer's dementia, there is deterioration in one's cognition and daily functioning gradually. This is at times accompanied by behavioural changes, such as aggression and agitation.	I hope you understand that there was a situation last week in which the safety of your father and others was compromised. Despite the staff's efforts to calm him down, he was still quite agitated and aggressive and hence the team needed to start him on olanzapine, to calm him down.
Clarification of side effects of antipsychotics and duration of use	I understand that you have much concern about the side effects of the medications. Like all medications, olanzapine also has its side effects.	It is true that the medication does predispose your father to an increased chance of strokes. In addition, the other common side effects of the medications include sedation and weight gain.	Prior to the commencement of any medication, the team usually weighs the risk/benefit ratio before starting. In your father's case, the benefits clearly outweigh the risks of him injuring himself. We have started him on the lowest possible dose of medication and will monitor him closely for side effects. The team is not planning to continue the medication on a long-term basis. Once your father has calmed down and has shown response to other interventions, the team will consider discontinuation of the treatment.

(Continued)

| Explain non-pharmacological options | Apart from the usage of medications, the team is hoping that other forms of treatments may be useful for your father. This includes reality orientation – which involves the consistent usage of orientation devices to remind patients of their environment. | Reminiscent therapy – this involves reliving the past experiences using old television sets and radios. Art therapy, aromatherapy, pet therapy and music therapy might be helpful as well. | We will speak to our multidisciplinary team and try to organize a schedule of activities for your father to keep him consistently engaged. We would recommend that your mother visits him regularly as it would be helpful for him as well. In the meantime, we will make sure that we have more staff, as well as ensure he has more supervision from the staff. Do you have any questions for me? |

Common pitfalls

a. Failure to engage with an angry relative by demonstrating adequate empathy and understanding of his concerns
b. Failure to explain clearly why the team has decided for commencement of antipsychotic medications (need to mention the specific risks and that the team has considered the risk/benefit ratio)
c. Failure to explain alternatives to pharmacological treatment

Quick recall: Behavioural and psychological symptoms in dementia (Linked station B)*

Management of behavioural and psychological symptoms of dementia

- A small amount of antipsychotic medication may be needed in those patients who are agitated, distressed and aggressive or who have sleep wake reversal.
- If antipsychotic medication is ineffective, cognitive enhancers could be considered.
- According to the National Institute for Health and Care Excellence (NICE) guidelines, intramuscular lorazepam could be used as a single agent (but not diazepam or chlorpromazine).
- It is of importance to note that those with Alzheimer's dementia are predisposed to developing depression, which may require treatment with antidepressant medication, preferably using preparations with few antiadrenergic and anti-cholinergic side effects.

---

* Adapted from B.K. Puri, A. Hall and R. Ho (2014). *Revision Notes in Psychiatry*. London, UK: CRC Press, p. 698.

Non-pharmacological interventions that may be useful include the following:

- Reality orientation involves the consistent use of orientation devices to remind patients of their environment.
- Reminiscent therapy involves reliving the past experiences using old TV sets, radios and home environment.
- Validation therapy empathizes with the feelings and meanings hidden behind their confused speech and environment.
- Art therapy (painting and drawing), aromatherapy (lavender), pet therapy and music therapy may be useful.

STATION 56: GENETICS IN ALZHEIMER'S DEMENTIA: COUNSELLING

Information to candidates

Name of patient: Mr Mitchell

Mr Mitchell is a 75-year-old gentleman who has been recently diagnosed with Alzheimer's dementia. He has been started on anti-dementia medications to help slow down the progression of his symptoms. Brian, his son, has accompanied him today for his routine follow-up. Brian is turning 50 years old this year, and he is very concerned after learning that his father has been diagnosed with Alzheimer's dementia. He is worried about acquiring the illness himself. He would like to clarify his concerns with a doctor.

Task

Please speak to Mr Mitchell's son and address all his concerns and expectations.

Outline of station

You are Brian, the son of Mr Mitchell. You understand from the doctor that recently your father has been diagnosed with Alzheimer's dementia. You are very concerned about him being given this diagnosis. You wonder what the difference is between Alzheimer's dementia and dementia. You would like to know more about how your father will progress as the condition worsens. In addition, you are very worried about your acquiring the same disorder. You want to hear the doctor more clearly explain more about the genetic risk of acquiring the disorder. In addition, you want to know all the causes of the disorder. If there is an underlying genetic linkage, you wish to ask if blood and genetic testing would help. You want to check with the doctor whether other specific lifestyle changes, such as eating a special diet, would reduce your risks.

CASC construct table

The CASC construct table is formatted such that candidates will be able to cover adequately both the range and the depth of the assessment required in this station.

Starting off: 'Hello, I am Dr Melvyn, one of the psychiatrists from the mental health unit. I understand that you have some concerns about your father, Mr Mitchell. I am hoping we can have a chat about this'.

Clarifications about the diagnosis for the patient	I'm sorry to be informing you that your father has been diagnosed with Alzheimer's dementia. We have since started him on some medications to help with slowing down of the progression of memory loss.	Have you heard about Alzheimer's dementia before? Alzheimer's dementia is the commonest type of dementia. The terminology 'dementia' is a general term, and there are various types of dementia.	In essence, dementia refers to a condition that usually starts off with memory difficulties. In time to come, it might get worse as other areas of the brain are involved. There might be impairments and difficulties with coping with daily tasks.
Address main concern about risk	I understand that you are concerned about your chances of acquiring the same disorder.	Generally speaking, the risk would be approximately three to four times higher for children whose parents have dementia.	It's hard to predict whether you will acquire dementia. In a small minority of individuals, dementia appears to be transmitted from generation to generation. However, this is rare and accounts for 1% of all cases of Alzheimer's dementia.
Address concerns about blood and genetic testing	Apo-lipoprotein E has been discovered to be responsible for one's susceptibility towards getting the disorder.	I understand that you are concerned whether there are blood tests or genetic tests that could tell whether there's a chance you would get the disorder.	Unfortunately, the current blood test and genetic testing are not diagnostic and have a limited role in predicting whether you would acquire the same disorder.
Clarifications about other factors that would predispose to Alzheimer's dementia	The chances of one having Alzheimer's dementia increase as one gets older.	Individuals with a previous history of head injury, previous episode of depression and lower education are more susceptible towards acquiring dementia.	In addition, individuals with Down's syndrome are more susceptible towards acquiring Alzheimer's dementia.
Address any other concerns	There has not been much evidence regarding smoking and how it might protect against Alzheimer's dementia.	Also, there is no concrete evidence about special diets and their protective effect against dementia.	

Common pitfalls

a. Failure to explain Alzheimer's dementia in a non-technical way
b. Failure to explore all the concerns of the relative
c. Failure to state specifically the exact increment in risk of acquiring dementia

Quick recall: Genetics in Alzheimer's dementia: Counselling*

Explanation of the concept of dementia

- Dementia is defined as a global deterioration or worsening in brain function, in clear consciousness, that is usually progressive and irreversible.
- It results in the deterioration of all higher brain functions including memory, thinking, orientation, comprehension, calculation, the capacity to learn, language and judgement.
- At times, this is also associated with deterioration in emotional control, behaviour and motivation.
- Dementia usually becomes more prevalent with increasing age.
- The most common dementia is Alzheimer's dementia.

Alzheimer's dementia: Genetic factors

- Genetic factors might account for the disease in some patients.
- It tends to be familial in some families, especially for those whose age of onset is early (under 65, with pre-senile dementia).
- The following genes are involved:
  a. Apo-lipoprotein (APP) gene on chromosome 21 (which accounts for 20% of early-onset Alzheimer's disease [AD]).
  b. Presenilin 1 (PS1) gene on chromosome 14.
  c. PS2 gene on chromosome 1.

Risk factors predisposing to dementia:

Modifiable risk factors	Non-modifiable risk factors
Endocrine: history of diabetes	Advanced age and female gender
Lifestyle: exposure to pesticides, lack of physical activity, repetitive head injury and smoking	Genetics: apo-lipoprotein E4 on chromosome 19, abnormalities in chromosomes 1, 14 and 21 and family history of dementia
Psychiatry history of depressive disorder	Low intelligence and limited education
Vascular: hypertension, hyperlipidaemia, stroke	History of mild cognitive impairment

---

* Adapted from B.K. Puri, A. Hall and R. Ho (2014). *Revision Notes in Psychiatry*. London, UK: CRC Press, pp. 693–694.

STATION 57: HISTORY TAKING – DEMENTIA

Information to candidates

Name of patient: Mr Casey

Mr Casey has been referred to your service by his local general practitioner (GP) as he has been having problems with his memory over the past year or so. He is here today with his wife, Sandra.

Task

Please speak to his wife, Sandra, and obtain a history to arrive at a possible diagnosis.

Outline of station

You are Sandra, the wife of Mr Casey. You have noticed that over the past year, your husband has been having increasing memory difficulties. It has been progressively worsening over the past 2 months, and you are increasingly concerned as you are the only caregiver staying with him. He seems to have a lot of trouble with his short-term memory. He muddles up dates and times. He has difficulties at times recognizing your grandchildren as well. In addition, you have noticed that over the past 2 months, he has been having difficulties with finding the right words during conversation. He is still able to dress and groom himself. You are concerned that over the past 2 months, he is increasingly forgetful, and that has led to some issues. He once forgot his way back home after his early morning walk. In addition, there was an occasion when he forgot to turn off the kettle, as he could not remember that he had boiled some water. Thus far, there have not been other behavioural issues such as any aggression or self-harm episodes.

CASC construct table

The CASC construct table is formatted such that candidates will be able to cover adequately both the range and the depth of the assessment required in this station.

Starting off: 'Hello, I am Dr Melvyn, one of the psychiatrists from the mental health unit. I understand that you have some concerns about your husband. I am hoping we can have a chat about this'.			
Clarification about presenting complaint	I understand that the GP has referred your husband to us, as there have been some concerns about his memory difficulties. Can you please tell me more?	Can you tell me when these memory difficulties first started? (Or) How long have there been difficulties with his memory?	How have things been recently? I'm sorry to hear that it has been getting worse. It must be a very difficult time for you.

(Continued)

Exploration of memory difficulties	Have there been any problems with his short-term memory? By that I mean are there times in which he misplaces things? Have there been times he forgets his meals?	What about his memories for things in the past? Can he still remember things that happened years ago?	Onset and progression of symptoms – gradual or sudden? Any previous head injury? Any medical problems (e.g., high blood pressure, high cholesterol, stroke/transient ischaemic attacks)? Any low mood prior to memory problems (pseudodementia)?
Exploration of orientation and visuo-spatial dysfunction	Does he seem to get muddled up with the day and dates?	Have there been times in which you noticed that he seemed very confused?	Is he able to recognize his loved ones? What about distant relatives that he hardly meets?
Exploration of language, communication and recognition difficulties	Have there been times in which he has difficulties finding the right words in a conversation?	Are there times in which he seems to have great difficulties with understanding a normal conversation?	Is he able to recognize and identify everyday objects? Can he find the right words to name those objects?
Exploration of functioning	Is he still able to manage himself? Can you tell me more about the difficulties that he has been having?	Does he need additional help with any of the following? • Dressing • Washing • Toileting • Ambulation	Does he need additional help with any of the following? • Finances • Shopping • Food preparation • Transportation
Risk assessment	Have there been any other concerns with regard to his behaviour of late?	Has he wandered out of the house previously? Has he ever gotten lost when he was out of the house? Any fire/flooding accidents (from failing to turn off stoves/taps)? Any financial exploitation by others? Any abuse from caregivers?	Has he been aggressive verbally or physically at home? Has he accidentally hurt himself recently?

Common pitfalls

   a. Failure to demonstrate empathy when the caregiver shares the history and the account of the difficulties she has been experiencing
   b. Failure to cover the range and the depth of the task

It would be worthwhile to try to distinguish whether the symptoms are due to AD or of a vascular nature.

Quick recall: History taking – Dementia*

Diagnostic criteria for Alzheimer's dementia:

International Statistical Classification of Diseases and Related Health Problems, 10th revision (ICD-10) criteria for dementia
• A decline in memory that is most evident of learning new information: Recall of learnt information is affected in severe cases. This impairment applies to both verbal and non-verbal materials.   • A decline in judgement, thinking, planning and organizing.   • Awareness of the environment and consciousness are preserved.   • Decline in emotional control and motivation (emotional lability, irritability, apathy and coarsening of social behaviour).   • Dementia is classified as mild (able to live independently), moderate (dependent on others in activities of daily living [ADL]) and severe (unable to retain information and absence of intelligence).   • Other causes of dementia should be excluded.   • ICD-10 classifies dementia of Alzheimer's type to be early onset (less than 65 years old) and late onset (more than 65 years old).

STATION 58: ANTI-DEMENTIA DRUGS

Information to candidates

Name of patient: Mr Brown

Mr Brown has been recently referred by his GP to the geriatric psychiatry service as he has been having increasing difficulties with his memory over the past year. The geriatric consultant has decided to start Mr Brown on one of the anti-dementia drugs known as donepezil. His son Jonathan is here today and wants to discuss more about the medication that Mr Brown has started taking. Jonathan has read about the medication on the Internet and is concerned about the side effects of the medication.

Task

Please speak to his son, Jonathan, and address all his concerns and expectations.

Outline of station

You are Jonathan, the son of Mr Brown. Your father has been diagnosed with Alzheimer's dementia recently, and he has since been started on an anti-dementia medication known as donepezil. You have read about the medication on the Internet, and you are concerned about the side effects associated with the medication. You wish to know the duration of treatment and the effectiveness of this medication for patients. You wish to know more about the outpatient follow-up as well as investigations that are required during each visit. You are concerned about the effects the medication might have on the liver, and you are also concerned about the cost of the medication. You have read on the Internet that

---

* Adapted from B.K. Puri, A. Hall and R. Ho (2014). *Revision Notes in Psychiatry*. London, UK: CRC Press, pp. 693–694.

psychiatric medications are addictive, and you do not want your father to be on any addictive medication.

CASC construct table

The CASC construct table is formatted such that candidates will be able to cover adequately both the range and the depth of the assessment required in this station.

Starting off: 'Hello, I am Dr Melvyn, one of the psychiatrists from the mental health unit. I understand that you have some concerns about your father. I am hoping we can have a chat about this'.			
Clarification about anti-dementia drugs	I understand that you have some concerns about the medication that we have started your father on. The medication we have started is called donepezil. It is one of the anti-dementia drugs. Have you heard about it before?	Thanks for sharing with me your understanding and your concerns about the medications. Unfortunately, the anti-dementia drug will not cure your father of his dementia.	However, it could help to slow down the progression of his current condition. It could help him with his mood, motivation and alertness.
Explain duration of treatment and efficacy	Anti-dementia drugs work on chemicals in the brain. When an individual has dementia, there is a reduction in the amount of a particular brain chemical known as acetylcholine.	Anti-dementia drugs help to increase the levels of this chemical. It is thus hoped that increasing the levels of this chemical would help to stabilize the memory and the functioning of your father.	Previous research has shown that approximately 40%–50% of individuals do respond to the medication. We will monitor your father's cognition and memory regularly using memory tests and decide whether he would benefit from the drug.
Explain side effects of donepezil	Like any other medication, anti-dementia drugs do have their side effects as well. Before starting the medication, we need to consider the medical history of the patient. Donepezil is contraindicated for patients with asthma.	The most common side effects include feeling of nausea, diarrhoea and urinary incontinence. Some patients might complain of insomnia. Other side effects might include the risk of slowing down the heart rate.	

(Continued)

Clarify follow-up required and investigations needed	We usually start patients on the lowest dose of the medications and aim to get them early in our outpatient clinic to see whether they can tolerate the medication.	If they are tolerating well, we might gradually increase the dosage. We would aim to see your father every 6 months.	During the subsequent visitations, we will perform a memory test known as the mini–mental state examination (MMSE). This test helps us understand the extent of cognitive deficits. We will continue the medications if the test scores are more than 10/30.
Address concerns	Do you have any other concerns regarding the medications or donepezil in particular? I do wish to inform you that the costs of the medications are covered by the National Health Service (NHS).	Thanks for highlighting your concerns. Anti-dementia medications are not addictive. They usually do not affect the liver functioning.	The advantage of donepezil is that the frequency of administration is once per day. In the event that your father does not wish to take the tablets, we might need to consider alternative medications that are available in the form of patches. I know that we have discussed quite a lot today. I would like to offer you some leaflets.

Common pitfalls

a. Failure to determine and establish the baseline understanding that the caregiver might have
b. Failure to cover the range and the depth of the task

Quick recall: Anti-dementia drugs*

Recommendations:

- For patients suffering from moderate Alzheimer's dementia (MMSE score of 10–20 points or score >20 but with significant impairments in functions or learning disability), the NICE guidelines recommend that the specialist prescribe acetyl-cholinesterase inhibitors.
- The three major benefits of using these medications are that it could help to stabilize the cognitive decline, improve the ADL and reduce the behavioural problems.
- Treatment needs to be commenced in a specialist clinic.

---

* Adapted from B.K. Puri, A. Hall and R. Ho (2014). *Revision Notes in Psychiatry*. London, UK: CRC Press, pp. 693–694.

- The NICE guidelines recommend patient-centred care, and the specialist has to consider issues relating to informed consent to pharmacological treatment.
- The specialist should also seek the carer's view on the patient's functions at baseline. Medications are broadly similar in efficacy, and they are chosen largely based on their costs, side effect profiles and patient's preferences.
- The specialist should consider an alternative medication if adverse events or drug interactions occur.
- MMSE, global, functional and behavioural assessment should be performed every 6 months.
- Treatment will be continued if either the MMSE score remains at or above 10 points or global, functional and behavioural conditions indicate worthwhile effects.
- The common side effects include excessive cholinergic effects such as nausea, diarrhoea, dizziness, urinary incontinence and insomnia. Other side effects include headache, parasympathetic stimulation and bradycardia.
- Donepezil is contraindicated for individuals with asthma.
- Rivastigmine is safe for individuals with asthma and chronic obstructive pulmonary disease.

STATION 59: VASCULAR DEMENTIA: HISTORY TAKING

Information to candidates

Name of patient: Mr Steven

Mr Steven has been referred by his GP to the specialist memory clinic. His son, Joseph, reports that his father has been having difficulties with his memory for the past year.

Task

Please speak to his son, Joseph, and obtain as much history as possible to arrive at a diagnosis.

Outline of station

You are Joseph, the son of Mr Steven. You have noticed that over the past year, your father's memory has been declining. He has been having problems with immediate recall of information and especially with his short-term memory. He cannot recognize your distant relatives at times. Otherwise, he is still able to care for himself, but perhaps not as well as before, as it seems that he needs more assistance from your mother. You know that he has a long-standing history of poorly controlled blood pressure and diabetes mellitus. He had a minor cerebrovascular event around 2 years ago, in response to which his neurologist recommended that Mr Steven be maintained on lifelong warfarin treatment.

CASC construct table

The CASC construct table is formatted such that candidates will be able to cover adequately both the range and the depth of the assessment required in this station.

Starting off: 'Hello, I am Dr Melvyn, one of the psychiatrists from the mental health unit. I understand that you have some concerns about your father. I am hoping we can have a chat about this'.			
Clarification about presenting complaint	I understand that the GP has referred your father as there have been some concerns about his memory difficulties. Can you please tell me more?	Can you tell me when these memory difficulties first started? (Or) How long has there been difficulties with his memory?	How have things been recently? I'm sorry to hear that it has been getting worse. It must be a very difficult time for you.
Exploration of memory difficulties	Have there been any problems with his short-term memory? By that I mean are there times when he misplaces things? Are there times when he forgets his meals?	What about his memories for things in the past? Can he still remember things that happened years ago?	
Exploration of orientation and visuo-spatial dysfunction	Does he seem to get muddled up with the day and dates?	Have there been times when you noticed that he seemed very confused?	Is he able to recognize his loved ones? What about distant relatives that he hardly meets?
Exploration of language, communication and recognition difficulties	Have there been times when he has difficulty finding the right words in a conversation?	Are there times when he seems to have great difficulties with understanding a normal conversation?	Is he able to recognize and identify everyday objects? Can he find the right words to name those objects?
Exploration of functioning	Is he still able to manage himself? Can you tell me more about the difficulties that he has been having?	Does he need additional help with any of the following? - Dressing - Washing - Toileting - Ambulation	Does he need additional help with any of the following? - Finances - Shopping - Food preparation - Transportation
Clarify medical history	Does your father have any chronic medical conditions that I need to know of?	Thanks for sharing with me. Can I know more about his control of his medical conditions? Did his doctor tell you how his medical conditions were?	Has he had a stroke before? Have there been scans done previously? How has he been since the onset of his stroke? Has his stroke led to any functional impairment?

(Continued)

Risk assessment	Have there been any other concerns with regard to his behaviour of late?	Has he wandered out of the house previously? Has he ever gotten lost when he is out of the house?	Has he been aggressive verbally or physically at home? Has he accidentally hurt himself recently?

Common pitfalls

a. Failure to ask for adequate information to cover the range and the depth of the station.
b. Failure to ask for previous history of medical conditions.
c. Failure to ask for residual impairments after the onset of his previous cerebrovascular accident.

Quick recall: Vascular dementia*

- Vascular dementia is characterized by a stepwise deteriorating course with a patchy distribution of neurological and neuropsychological deficits. There is evidence of vascular disease on physical examination (hypertension, hypertensive changes on fundoscopy, carotid bruits, enlarged heart and focal neurological signs suggestive of cerebro-vascular accident [CVA]).
- Three presentations typically occur: (1) dementia following a stroke, (2) dementia gradually following multiple asymptomatic cerebral infarcts and (3) neuropsychiatric symptoms gradually becoming evident.
- It is important to distinguish between vascular dementia and Alzheimer's dementia, which could be difficult. A more insidious onset with a continuous rather than a stepwise course, less insight, fewer affective symptoms and lack of hypertension or neurological signs is more suggestive of the latter.
- Vascular dementia is more likely than Alzheimer's dementia to produce co-existent depression, delusion, anxiety and emotional disturbances.
- The *ICD-10* criteria (WHO, 1992) emphasize the unevenly distributed cognitive impairment and signs of focal brain damage (unilateral spastic weakness, unilateral increased tendon reflexes, an extended plantar response and pseudobulbar palsy). In multi-infarct dementia, the onset is gradual with minor ischaemic episode.
- In acute-onset vascular dementia, the onset of dementia is within 1 month of the cerebrovascular dementia.
- In subcortical vascular dementia, there is evidence of deep white-matter lesions.
- National Institute of Neurological Disorders and Stroke and Association Internationale pour la Recherché et l'Enseignement en Neurosciences (NINDS-ARIEN) criteria (Roman et al., 1993): A relationship between the

---

* Adapted from B.K. Puri, A. Hall and R. Ho (2014). *Revision Notes in Psychiatry*. London, UK: CRC Press, p. 699.

aforementioned dementia and CVAs manifested or inferred by the presence of one or more of the following: amnesia and cognitive impairment in at least one domain with resultant disability; focal sign and image findings; onset of dementia within 3 months following a recognized stroke and abrupt deterioration in cognitive functioning. Clinical features that are consistent with the diagnosis include early presence of a gait disturbance, history of unsteadiness and frequent unprovoked falls, early urinary symptoms not explained by neurological disease, pseudobulbar palsy, mood changes or abulia.

STATION 60: VASCULAR DEMENTIA: EXPLANATION

Information to candidates

Name of patient: Mr Steven

Mr Steven has been referred by his GP to the specialist memory clinic. His son, Joseph, reports that his father has been having difficulties with his memory for the past year. He has had been assessed by the psychiatrist, and the necessary blood work as well as radiological imaging has been done. The blood results are normal. However, the radiological imaging (computed tomography [CT] scan) showed progressive subcortical vascular encephalopathy and enlarged ventricles, likely secondary to infarction in the hemispheric white matter.

Task

Please speak to Mr Steven's son, Joseph, to explain the diagnosis and clarify your management plans. Please address any concerns and expectations that his son might have.

Outline of station

You are Joseph, the son of Mr Steven. You have noticed that over the past year, your father's memory has been declining. He has been having problems with immediate recall of information and especially with his short-term memory. He cannot recognize your distant relatives at times. Otherwise, he is still able to care for himself, but perhaps not as well as before, as it seems that he needs more assistance from your mother. You know that he has a long-standing history of poorly controlled blood pressure and diabetes mellitus. He had a minor cerebrovascular event around 2 years ago, in response to which his neurologist has recommended that he be maintained on life-long warfarin treatment. In this station, the candidate will inform you about the blood test results as well as the results of the brain imaging. You need the candidate to explain the results to you without using medical jargon. You want to know about the medications that might help and how else you can help your father. In addition, you wish to know the prognosis of the condition. You do have concerns about your father's safety and his potential to be agitated if his demands are not met at home, and you hope the candidate will address these concerns.

CASC construct table

The CASC construct table is formatted such that candidates will be able to cover adequately both the range and the depth of the assessment required in this station.

Starting off: 'Hello, I am Dr Melvyn, one of the psychiatrists from the mental health unit. I understand that you have some concerns about your father. I hope that I could take some of your time to explain what we think your father has and answer any questions that you might have'.			
Clarification of diagnosis and possible aetiological causes	I'm sorry to hear that it must be a very difficult time for you. Can I share the results of your father's blood test with you? Is it okay if I go on to explain his brain scan results?	I'm sorry to inform you that the brain scan shows that your father is likely to have had multiple blocked vessels that might have affected the blood supply to his brain. This might account for his memory difficulties.	From our opinion, he is likely to have a form of dementia known as vascular dementia. Have you heard of vascular dementia before? Vascular dementia is actually a relatively common dementia and is the second most common dementia worldwide, aside from Alzheimer's dementia. There are multiple factors that might results in the development of vascular dementia. The most common risk factors are having medical problems such as hypertension, diabetes and high cholesterol.
Explain likely progression and prognosis	I'm sorry to inform you that vascular dementia is a progressive disorder.	This means that over time, it is likely that your father's memory difficulties might worsen.	In addition, some individuals who have vascular dementia are more predisposed towards developing other psychiatric conditions such as depression, delusions, anxiety and emotional disturbances.

(Continued)

Explain management plans (pharmacological)	Thanks for sharing your understanding about anti-dementia medications. The local NICE guidelines do not recommend the usage of these medications for vascular dementia.	Despite the fact that we cannot start anti-dementia medications to slow down the progression of the memory difficulties, we would like to help your father gain better control of his underlying medical conditions (for example, better control of his blood pressure, cholesterol problems and diabetes). The local GP who is following up on your father's condition could help by prescribing appropriate medications to help better optimize his medical conditions.	In the event that your father develops other psychiatric disorders, such as depression, usage of other medications, such as antidepressants, might be helpful.
Explain management plans (non-pharmacological)	Apart from medications, we hope we can slow down the progression by encouraging your father to modify his lifestyle.	We like to recommend that he participate in regular exercises, as well as cut down on smoking or drinking (if he is doing so).	In addition, it will be helpful if he could eat more healthy food.
Address concerns	Thanks for allowing me to share more about your father's condition. Do you have any other questions for me?	I hear your concern about the possibility of your father forgetting to take his medications. We recommend the usage of a pill box to help him remember.	

Common pitfalls

a. Failure to discuss non-pharmacological options to help with the management of the condition
b. Failure to address all other concerns and expectations

Quick recall: Vascular dementia: Explanation*

- Aetiology: There is an excess of vascular dementia in males, which is probably caused by an increased prevalence of cardiovascular disease in men. Hypertension is the most frequent risk factor amongst those with vascular dementia (contributing to 50% of vascular dementia cases). Risk factors known to increase the risk of stroke also increase the risk of vascular dementia: for example, smoking, heart disease, homocystinuria, hyperlipidaemia, metabolic syndrome, low levels of high-density lipoprotein, moderate alcohol consumption and sickle-cell anaemia.
- Investigation: CT and magnetic resonance imaging (MRI) may show infarcts, lacunes and leukoaraiosis. Single-photon emission computed tomography (SPECT) and positron emission tomography (PET) scans may show patchy hypoperfusion.
- Management: The NICE guidelines do not recommend the use of anti-dementia medications for cognitive decline. Donepezil may be beneficial, but it is not licensed for usage. It is worth attempting to treat the underlying cardiovascular condition to slow or halt the progression of vascular dementia. The treatment of hypertension is especially helpful. In the event that the individual has depression, it might be beneficial to start an antidepressant.
- Prognosis: The prognosis of vascular dementia is worse than that of Alzheimer's dementia. The mean survival of Alzheimer's dementia is 6 years, whilst the mean survival of vascular dementia is only 3 years. Poor prognostic factors include severity of dementia, being bedridden and the presence of urinary incontinence.

STATION 61: LEWY BODY DEMENTIA (LBD) (PAIRED STATION A)

Information to candidates

Name of patient: Mr Thompson

Mr Thompson is a 75-year-old retired teacher who was diagnosed with Parkinson's disease 6 months ago. His family members have noted that, in addition to the symptoms of Parkinson's disease that he is suffering from, his memory has declined over the past few months. A recent DaTscan was done, which showed features consistent with that of Lewy body dementia.

Task

Please speak to his daughter, Sally, to clarify the diagnosis and to explain the treatment options for this condition.

---

* Adapted from B.K. Puri, A. Hall and R. Ho (2014). *Revision Notes in Psychiatry*. London, UK: CRC Press, pp. 699–700.

Outline of station

You are Sally, the daughter of Mr Thompson. You do not live with your father, but you are aware that he was diagnosed with Parkinson's disease 6 months ago, following a fall at home. He has multiple features of Parkinson's disease. However, you have noticed that his memory has not been as good as previously. He is not able to remember the name of your daughter, despite her visiting him frequently. Your mother has mentioned that he is especially bad with recall of immediate events and things discussed. At times, your mother has noticed that he responds to hallucinations. This has been a cause of concern for all. You want to know the exact diagnosis that your father has. You have queries as to whether the doctors might have misdiagnosed, and this might just be Parkinson's disease–related dementia (based on your own research, you have found out that individuals with Parkinson's disease do have dementia as well). You are curious as to what will be the best choice in terms of medications for your father. You are especially concerned about falls, and you will share this only if the candidate remembers to ask for your other concerns and expectations.

CASC construct table

The CASC construct table is formatted such that candidates will be able to cover adequately both the range and the depth of the assessment required in this station.

Starting off: 'Hello, I am Dr Melvyn, one of the psychiatrists from the mental health unit. I understand that you have some concerns about your father. I am hoping we can have a chat about this'.			
Clarification of diagnosis	I understand that it must be a very difficult time for you and your family.	Based on the specialized scan results, your father has a form of dementia known as Lewy body dementia.	Have you heard about this particular form of dementia before? It is actually the third most common cause of late-onset dementia and commonly affects more men than women.
Explain common clinical manifestations	This form of dementia has three classical symptoms, which include falls, fluctuating cognition and visual hallucinations.	With regard to cognition, individuals with the disorder tend to have fluctuating cognition, and short-term memory is less affected in the early stages. The common non-cognitive features include depression, hallucinations (usually complex visual hallucinations) and delusions.	There might be other associated changes such as progressive loss of facial expression, changes in strength and tone of the voice, slowness, muscle stiffness, trembling of the limbs, a tendency to shuffle when walking.

(Continued)

Explain possible aetiological causes	The exact cause is still uncertain.	The memory impairments and the changes are likely to be due to the presence of Lewy bodies in the brain.	It is believed that the presence of these deposits influences the action of some of the important chemicals in the brain.
Clarification of the differences with Parkinson's disease dementia	Thanks for sharing with me your understanding about Parkinson's disease and its associated memory problems.	Based on the clinical history and the results of the brain scan, our team is not inclined to think that this is Parkinson's disease dementia.	For Parkinson's disease–related dementia, the cognitive symptoms tend to occur at least 1 year after the development of extra-pyramidal signs.
Explain management options	Antipsychotics are usually not used due to the risk of severe adverse reactions.	Anti-dementia medications are usually considered for patients with significant non-cognitive symptoms that have led to significant distress or challenging behaviours. Rivastigmine has the best-researched evidence to date and could help with the cognitive symptoms, the delusions and the hallucinations.	Antiparkinsonian medications could be used to help with the motor symptoms. We would like to work closely with the neurologist to adjust the doses of the medications accordingly.
Address concerns	I know that I have shared a lot today. Do you have any questions for me?	I hear your concerns about the risk of falls for your father.	I would like to recommend that he be referred to our multidisciplinary team. The occupational therapist could help to look into environmental modifications to reduce the risk associated with falls.

Common pitfalls

a. Failure to explain in depth with regard to the clinical manifestation of LBD
b. Failure to clearly clarify the differences between Parkinson's disease–related dementia and that of LBD
c. Failure to elicit other concerns and address them accordingly

Quick recall: LBD*

- This particular form of dementia is the third most common cause of late-onset dementia and a less common cause of early-onset dementia. It frequently occurs in combination with Alzheimer's dementia. It most commonly affects men more than women.
- There is little atrophy in the early stages of this form of dementia. Lewy bodies are located in the cingulate gyrus and the cortex as well as the substantia nigra.
- In terms of the differences between dementia of Lewy bodies and that of Parkinson's disease, the cognitive and extrapyramidal signs develop concurrently in Lewy body dementia (LBD). However, for Parkinson's disease–related dementia, the cognitive symptoms occur at least 1 year after the development and onset of extrapyramidal signs in Parkinson's disease dementia.
- The common clinical features include (a) cognitive symptoms, (b) non-cognitive symptoms and (c) extrapyramidal signs and parkinsonism.
- The cognitive symptoms include enduring and progressive cognitive impairment with impairments in consciousness, alertness and attention. Cognition is noted to be fluctuating, and short-term memory is not affected in the early stage. Patients suffering from LBD tend to have less episodic amnesia and more executive dysfunction.
- The common non-cognitive features include apathy, depression, hallucinations (complex visual hallucinations occur 80% of the time, with auditory hallucinations 20% of the time) and delusions (paranoid ideations 65% of the time).
- Extrapyramidal signs and parkinsonism include loss of facial expression, changes in strength and tone of the voice, slowness, muscle stiffness, trembling of the limbs and a tendency to shuffle when walking.
- It is important to note serious clinical events, which include neuroleptic sensitivity (in approximately 60% of the patients), falls, syncope and spontaneous loss of consciousness.
- With regard to radiological investigations, DaTscan is able to differentiate LBD from AD; 90% of patients with LBD also tend to have electroencephalographic (EEG) abnormalities.
- For management: Antipsychotics are not indicated in mild-to-moderate non-cognitive symptoms, due to the enhanced risk of adverse reactions. If an antipsychotic needs to be used, quetiapine could be considered, but it is also essential to monitor for its associated side effects.
- Anti-dementia medications could be considered for patients with LBD who have non-cognitive symptoms causing significant distress or leading to behaviour that challenges. Rivastigmine currently has the best research evidence for improvement of cognitive functions in LBD. It could also help to improve cognitive symptoms, delusions and hallucinations.

---

* Adapted from B.K. Puri, A. Hall and R. Ho (2014). *Revision Notes in Psychiatry*. London, UK: CRC Press, pp. 702–703.

- For patients with difficulties with sleep, chlormethiazole is usually used for night sedation.
- Additional notes about Parkinson's disease dementia: It is actually very difficult to distinguish dementia specifically associated with Parkinson's disease from other causes of dementia, which are likely to occur coincidentally in elderly people suffering from Parkinson's dementia.

STATION 62: LBD (PAIRED STATION B)

Information to candidates

Name of patient: Mr Thompson

Mr Thompson is a 75-year-old retired teacher who was diagnosed with Parkinson's disease 6 months ago. His family members have noted that, in addition to the symptoms of Parkinson's disease he is suffering from, his memory has declined over the past few months. A recent DaTscan was done which showed features consistent with that of Lewy body dementia. His daughter, Sally, has been told of his diagnosis. Her husband, Bobby, is here today and hopes to see the doctor as soon as possible, as he needs help with managing his father-in-law. Mr Thompson was started on rivastigmine (3 mg daily) previously and became better. However, in the past couple of weeks, his condition has deteriorated. He is noted to be increasingly confused and responding to visual hallucinations.

Task

Please speak to his son-in-law, Bobby, and address all his concerns and expectations.

Outline of station

You are Bobby, the son-in-law of Mr Thompson. You have learnt more about his diagnosis from your wife around 1 year ago. You know that your father-in-law was started on medications, and the medications were helpful for his symptoms previously. However, in the past few weeks or so, you have noticed that his condition has taken a drastic turn for the worse. He is increasingly confused and has sleep–wake reversal. At times, in the middle of the night, he becomes very agitated whilst responding to visual hallucinations. Sally, your wife is out of town and you are the only caregiver for the next couple of weeks. You want to know what you could do to help your father-in-law with his condition. You wish to know the possible reasons for his current condition. In addition, you are hoping that the doctor could adjust or start him on new medications, such as antipsychotics, to help him with his condition. You also wish to know what else could be beneficial for him. You desperately need answers and hope that the candidate can understand the difficulties you are facing.

CASC construct table

The CASC construct table is formatted such that candidates will be able to cover adequately both the range and the depth of the assessment required in this station.

Starting off: 'Hello, I am Dr Melvyn, one of the psychiatrists from the mental health unit. I understand that you have some concerns about your father-in-law. I am hoping we can have a chat about this'.			
Establishing rapport	I'm sorry to learn about what has been happening. It must be a very difficult time for you.	I'm hoping that we can do our best to help you with the care needs of your father-in-law.	Do you think you will be willing to undergo a carer assessment? (Or) We would like to discuss your father-in-law's case with the rest of the members of our multidisciplinary team. Our community psychiatric nurse could help by visiting your home and offering some interventions. How does that sound for you?
Establish likely causes for changes in behaviour	Can you tell me more about how he has been? How long have you noticed these changes? Are these behaviours new in nature, or have you noticed them before? Sometimes when there is a progression of the underlying dementia, there might be worsening of these symptoms.	Has the neurologist seen him recently? Have there been any recent adjustments in his Parkinson's medications?	Has he been taken ill recently? Has there been any change or decline in his physical functioning and physical health recently?
Discuss pharmacological treatment options	At times adjustment of medications might help with his behavioural difficulties. Did he previously respond well to the anti-dementia medication? We could consider increasing the dose of the anti-dementia medication to help him with his current condition.	If his neurologist has recently changed his antiparkinsonian medication, it might be worthwhile for him or her to do an early review. Sometimes adjustment of the medication could result in behavioural changes as well.	I understand that you feel a sleeping medication might help him with his behaviour. However, we would not recommend it, given that there is a high risk of falls associated with the usage of these medications. In addition, chronic usage might lead to dependency.
Discuss non-pharmacological treatment options	Apart from medications, there are other techniques that might be beneficial and helpful to deal with the current behavioural difficulties that you are facing.	Such techniques might include the usage of aromatherapy as well as regular re-orientation.	

(Continued)

Address all other concerns	We have spoken a lot today. Do you have any questions for me?	I think your concern about the usage of an antipsychotic is valid. Usually we would not consider using an antipsychotic in view of the adverse effects associated with its use.	If the behaviours are indeed severe and distressing and all other measures have failed, we might consider a very low dose of quetiapine. However, we need to watch carefully for side effects as patients with LBD are prone to side effects as they are more sensitive to these neuroleptics.

Common pitfalls

a. Failure to empathize and discuss with the relative alternatives management plans to help him with the care arrangement of his father-in-law
b. Failure to consider other causes for the acute changes in behaviour (hence failing to cover the range and the depth needed for the station adequately)
c. Failure to consider titration of the dose of the antiparkinsonian medications (as changes in the dose of the medications might cause behavioural changes)
d. Failure to consider and explain non-pharmacological alternatives

Quick recall: Lewy body dementia: Management*

- For management: Antipsychotics are not indicated in mild-to-moderate non-cognitive symptoms due to the enhanced risk of adverse reactions. If an antipsychotic needs to be used, quetiapine could be considered for usage, but it is also essential to monitor for its associated side effects.
- Anti-dementia medications could be considered for patients with LBD who have non-cognitive symptoms causing significant distress or leading to behaviour that challenges. Rivastigmine currently has the best research evidence for improvement of cognitive functions in LBD. It could also help to improve cognitive symptoms, delusions and hallucinations.
- For patients with difficulties with sleep, chlormethiazole is usually used for night sedation.

---

* Adapted from B.K. Puri, A. Hall and R. Ho (2014). *Revision Notes in Psychiatry*. London, UK: CRC Press, pp. 702–703.

STATION 63: FRONTO-TEMPORAL DEMENTIA

Information to candidates

Name of patient: Mr Johnson

Mr Johnson, a 60-year-old man, has been referred by his GP to the geriatric psychiatry service. His family shared that there has been progressive worsening of his memory over the past year. In addition, there are times in which they noted that he has sexually inappropriate behaviours. His wife, the main caregiver, is extremely distressed by his condition and wants some help from your service.

Task

Please speak to his wife, Sally, and take a history to come to an eventual diagnosis.

Outline of station

You are Sally, the wife of Mr Johnson. Over the past year, you have noticed that your husband's memory has been failing. On several occasions, he seemed unable to recall conversations that you just had had with him. In addition, there have been occasions in which he has exhibited sexually inappropriate behaviours. On one occasion, you were attending a church service with him, and he openly made inappropriate sexual remarks to another female there. In addition, you have noticed that he has difficulties recognizing your distant relatives. He also has difficulties finding the right words in his conversations. He does seem to need more help with regard to his daily activities. There was an occasion in which he wandered out of the house and could not find his way back. You are very worried about his condition and wonder how best you can help him. You are very distressed and will share more only if the candidate is empathetic towards you.

CASC construct table

The CASC construct table is formatted such that candidates will be able to cover adequately both the range and the depth of the assessment required in this station.

Starting off: 'Hello, I am Dr Melvyn, one of the psychiatrists from the mental health unit. I understand that you have some concerns about your husband. I am hoping we can have a chat about this'.			
Clarification about presenting complaint	I understand that the GP has referred your husband as there have been some concerns about his memory difficulties and the changes in his behaviours. Can you please tell me more?	Can you tell me when these memory difficulties and behavioural difficulties first started? (Or) How long has there been difficulties with his memory?	How have things been recently? I'm sorry to hear that it has been getting worse. It must be a very difficult time for you.

(Continued)

Exploration of memory difficulties	Have there been any problems with his short-term memory? By that I mean are there times when he misplaces things? Have there been times when he forgets his meals?	What about his memories for things in the past? Can he still remember things that happened years ago?	
Exploration of orientation and visuo-spatial dysfunction	Does he seem to muddle up the day and dates?	Have there been times in which you noticed that he seemed very confused?	Is he able to recognize his loved ones? What about distant relatives that he hardly meets?
Exploration of language, communication and recognition difficulties	Have there been times in which he has difficulties finding the right words in a conversation?	Are there times in which he seems to have great difficulties with understanding a normal conversation?	Is he able to recognize and identify everyday objects? Can he find the right words to name those objects?
Exploration of functioning	Is he still able to manage himself? Can you tell me more about the difficulties that he has been having?	Does he need additional help with any of the following? • Dressing • Washing • Toileting • Ambulation	Does he need additional help with any of the following? • Finances • Shopping • Food preparation • Transportation
Clarification of frontal lobe symptoms	I'm sorry to hear how distressing it has been for you. Can you describe to me how your husband has been in terms of his personality previously?	Has he done anything embarrassing recently or anything that is sexually inappropriate? Can you tell me more?	Is he able to plan what he wants to do for the day? How has his mood been? Have you noticed that he has been more irritable and annoyed recently? Has he been more impulsive recently? Does he seem to keep repeating particular words or actions? Is he able to shift from task to task easily?
Risk assessment	Have there been any other concerns with regard to his behaviour of late?	Has he wandered out of the house previously? Has he ever gotten lost when he was out of the house? Does he still drive a vehicle now?	Has he been aggressive verbally or physically at home? Has he accidentally hurt himself recently?

Common pitfalls

a. Failure to empathize with the caregiver at the start of the interview. Rapport building is essential in this station.
b. Failure to ask about frontal lobe symptoms such as disinhibited behaviours, executive planning and organization and mood changes.
c. Failure to ask about risky behaviours.

Quick recall: Fronto-temporal lobe dementia information*

- Dementia of the frontal lobe type and Pick's disease both mainly affect the frontal and anterior temporal areas of the brain.
- Fronto-temporal lobe dementia (FTD) is associated with cortical and striatal serotoninergic deficits but not cholinergic deficit.
- Patients with FTD have younger age of onset, more severe apathy, disinhibition, reduction in speech output, loss of insight and coarsening of social behaviour but less spatial disorientation compared with patients with AD. Primitive reflexes such as grasp, pour and palm mental reflexes often appear in FTD.
- Patients who suffer from AD have more impairment in calculation and constructions, lower MMSE scores and higher prevalence of depression (20%), compared with patients with FTD.
- Both AD and FTD have an insidious onset.
- It is important to note the following syndrome: Kluver–Bucy syndrome, which consists of emotional placidity, hyperorality, hypersexuality and tendency to place things in the mouth, which may occur concurrently with AD or FTD.
- In terms of investigations, psychometry will show characteristic impairments in higher executive function, verbal fluency and agnosia. Structural imaging may show characteristic lesion in the early stage, and functional imaging shows anterior hypo-perfusion. EEG is usually normal in FTD.
- With regard to management, there is no specific pharmacological intervention for cognitive impairments in FTD. Selective serotonin reuptake inhibitors (SSRIs) or other antidepressants are indicated for non-cognitive features. Psychosocial interventions are often useful.
- With regard to prognosis, the mean duration of dementia of the frontal lobe type is 8 years, and that of Pick's disease is around 11 years.
- Diogenes syndrome is associated with frontal lobe dysfunction and compulsive collecting.

---

* Adapted from B.K. Puri, A. Hall and R. Ho (2014). *Revision Notes in Psychiatry.* London, UK: CRC Press, pp. 700–702.

STATION 64: MILD COGNITIVE IMPAIRMENT (PAIRED STATION A)

Information to candidates

Name of patient: Norman

Norman is a 75-year-old male who has been having increasing difficulties with his memory over the past 6 months. He has been misplacing things, and at times he gets confused and lost in a conversation. He decided to check in with his GP last week, who referred him over to your specialized service for further assessment and management.

Task

Please speak to him to elicit more history about his memory difficulties and also perform a relevant cognitive examination.

Outline of station

You are Norman, a 75-year-old male who has been having increasing difficulties with your memory over the past 6 months. You have been misplacing things, as well as getting confused and lost in a conversation. You have no difficulties with your long-term memory and you are able to recall memories in the past. You have no difficulties with finding the right words in conversation and no difficulties with recognition of distant relatives. You do not muddle up the days of the week. You are still able to handle your daily activities independently. You have not been involved in any risky behaviour. You do not have any visual and hearing impairment and agree to the cognitive examination that the candidate wants you to do. You have difficulties only with delayed recall.

CASC construct table

The CASC construct table is formatted such that candidates will be able to cover adequately both the range and the depth of the assessment required in this station.

Starting off: 'Hello, I am Dr Melvyn, one of the psychiatrists from the mental health unit. I understand that you have been referred by your GP as you have some concerns about your memory. Can we talk about this today?'			
Clarification about presenting complaint	Can you please tell me more about your memory difficulties?	Can you tell me when these memory difficulties first started?	How have things been recently? I'm sorry to hear that it has been getting worse. It must be a very difficult time for you.

(Continued)

Exploration of memory difficulties	Have there been any problems with your short-term memory? By that I mean are there times in which you misplace things? Have there been times in which you forget whether or not you have had a meal?	What about your memories for things in the past? Can you still remember things that happened years ago?	
Exploration of orientation and visuo-spatial dysfunction	Have there been any occasions in which you muddle up the day and dates?	Are you still able to recognize your loved ones? What about distant relatives that you hardly ever meet?	
Exploration of language, communication and recognition difficulties	Have there been times in which you have difficulties with finding the right words in a conversation?	Are there times in which you seem to have great difficulties with understanding a normal conversation?	Can you find the right words to name objects?
Exploration of functioning	Do you need additional help with any of the following recently? • Dressing • Washing • Toileting • Ambulation	Do you need additional help with any of the following? • Finances • Shopping • Food preparation • Transportation	
Risk assessment	Have there recently been any other concerns that you have?	Have you ever gotten lost when you were out of the house?	Have you been aggressive verbally or physically at home?
MMSE: Assess for orientation	Before we begin, can I check whether you have any visual or hearing impairment? Can you see and hear me clearly?	Do you know where we are at the moment? What level are we on? Which part of the county is this? What is the greater country that we are in?	Do you know what time it is? Do you know what year this is? Can you tell me what season, month and the day and date today?
MMSE: Assess for registration	I would like you to remember three objects, which I will ask you to repeat immediately and again in 5 minutes.	The three objects I would like you to remember are 'apple, table and penny'.	Can you repeat the three objects that I have told you?
Assess for attention and calculation	Can I trouble you to spell the word 'world' for me?	Can you please spell the word 'world' backwards for me?	(If the patient is unable to spell, assessment could be done using calculation/numbers instead)

(Continued)

| MMSE: Assess for recall, naming, repetition, comprehension | Can you tell me the three objects that I asked you to remember earlier? | Can you name these objects for me? *(Show the patient a pen and a watch.)* | Can you please repeat this phrase: 'No ifs, ands or buts'. Please listen to my instructions and follow my instructions. I would like you to take this piece of paper with your right hand, fold it in half and place it on the floor. |
| MMSE: Assess for reading, writing and copying | *(Write 'Close your eyes' on a piece of paper)* Can you please read this sentence and do what it says? | Can you help me to write a complete sentence that has a subject and a verb? | *(Draw two intersecting pentagons)* Can you please help me to copy this figure? |

Common pitfalls

a. Failure to demonstrate empathy when the patient vocalized how much his memory difficulties have been troubling him.
b. Failure to cover the range and depth of the task – there is a need to perform two separate tasks: (1) Taking a history to assess for cognitive impairment and (2) performing a cognitive examination.

Quick recall: Mild cognitive impairments (MCI)*

- The conversion rate from normal ageing to mild cognitive impairment is around 15%. The conversion rate from MCI to dementia is around 5%–10% per year.
- The pathology involves atrophy of the hippocampus, beta-amyloid deposition, depression and vascular atherosclerotic changes.
- Clinical features: MMSE is usually between 24 and 30. There might be subjective complaint of memory loss, with objective evidence of cognitive impairment. There is a noted decline from a previously normal level of function. There is preserved basic ADL. There should be no underlying medical or surgical conditions causing reversible dementia. The cognitive impairments are usually not severe enough to meet the diagnostic criteria for dementia.
- There are commonly two types of mild cognitive impairment: the amnesic type and the non-amnesic type.
- The amnesic type is the most common form and manifests as preclinical manifestation of AD. Patients present with impaired performance on delayed recall. There is objective evidence of impairment of short-term memory, but

---

* Adapted from B.K. Puri, A. Hall and R. Ho (2014). *Revision Notes in Psychiatry*. London, UK: CRC Press, pp. 692–693.

general cognitive functions are normal. There is no substantial interference with work, usual social activities or other activities of daily living. This particular form has a higher chance of conversion to dementia compared with non-amnestic type.

- The non-amnestic MCI may involve multiple cognitive domains (such as executive function) rather than purely amnesia. This type of MCI manifests as localized impairment of other cognitive domains rather than memory. Non-amnestic MCI may develop into non-Alzheimer's dementias.

- With regard to treatment, cognitive rehabilitation is an option. It is essential to encourage individuals to engage in regular physical exercises and to maintain a healthy lifestyle. Underlying vascular risk factors such as hypertension and hyperlipidaemia should be treated. In the event that there is underlying depression, treatment is crucial.

- It is recommended that there is yearly follow-up on instrumental ADL and cognition.

STATION 65: MILD COGNITIVE IMPAIRMENT (PAIRED STATION B: EXPLANATION)

Information to candidates

Name of patient: Norman

Norman is a 75-year-old male who has been having increasing difficulties with his memory over the past 6 months. He has been misplacing things and at times he gets confused and lost in a conversation. He decided to check in with his GP last week, who has referred him over to your specialized service for further assessment and management. You saw the patient, Norman, 1 week ago and assessed him to have mild cognitive impairment. His wife is here today and wishes to speak to you.

Task

Please speak to her and explain the diagnosis. Please also discuss with her your treatment plans for Norman. You should also address all her concerns and expectations.

Outline of station

You are the wife of Norman. You understand that the psychiatrist has seen him and diagnosed him accordingly. You wish to know more about the assessment and the clinical diagnosis. When you're being told that your husband has mild cognitive impairment, you need to ask the candidate whether this is similar to dementia. You are concerned as to whether your husband can live independently now that he has been diagnosed with mild cognitive impairment. In addition, you want to know more about the course and the prognosis of having such a diagnosis. You wonder whether your husband would benefit from the usage of anti-dementia drugs. You also wish to know how else you can help him and fully support him, now that he has mild cognitive impairment. You want to know the relevant risk factors that might predispose someone to developing dementia.

CASC construct table

The CASC construct table is formatted such that candidates will be able to cover adequately both the range and the depth of the assessment required in this station.

Starting off: 'Hello, I am Dr Melvyn, one of the psychiatrists from the mental health unit. I understand that you have some concerns about your husband, Norman. Can we have a chat about it?'			
Clarification of assessment and diagnosis	We spoke to your husband last week, and we understand that he has been having memory difficulties for quite a while. It must be a difficult time for you.	We have performed some clinical assessment and memory testing, and the scores show that he is likely to be having mild cognitive impairment.	Have you heard about mild cognitive impairment before? Thanks for sharing with me your understanding about mild cognitive impairment.
Explanation of rationale for diagnosis of mild cognitive impairment	Mild cognitive impairment is different from dementia.	For individuals who have mild cognitive impairments, they usually have mild cognitive deficits, short of that usually observed and described for dementia. They might have poor performance on memory testing.	However, very often, individuals with mild cognitive impairment are usually able to function independently at home and handle their everyday activities. Do you have any questions about his diagnosis?
Explain course and prognosis	For individuals who age normally, around 15% of them might eventually get mild cognitive impairment.	The average conversion rate from mild cognitive impairment to dementia is around 5%–10% per year.	
Explain pharmacological treatment	Based on the local guidelines, there are unfortunately no medications that have been recommended for treatment of this disorder.	If your husband has other underlying medical issues, such as hypertension, it might be ideal for him to be on medications to ensure that his underlying medical conditions are well controlled.	Control of his underlying medical conditions is essential as they are risk factors that increase the chances of him eventually developing dementia.

(Continued)

Explain non-pharmacological treatments	I'm sorry to inform you that there are currently no medications that are indicated for the treatment of this condition.	Apart from medications, lifestyle modifications could help prevent your husband from eventually developing dementia.	We recommend that he partakes in regular exercises and keeps himself physically and mentally active. It is also essential that he eats a healthy diet.
Address any other concerns	I know that I have shared quite a lot of information today. Can I offer you a leaflet from the Royal College about mild cognitive impairment for you to better understand your husband's condition?	Do you have any other concerns at the moment? Thanks for your question. There are many factors that might predispose one to develop dementia.	Common risk factors include being elderly, having a lower education level, previous history of depression and being female in gender.

Common pitfalls

a. Failure to address all the concerns of the relatives
b. Failure to establish rapport and gradually disseminate information/being too quick to give information.

Quick recall: Mild cognitive impairment*

- The conversion rate from normal ageing to mild cognitive impairment is around 15%. The conversion rate from MCI to dementia is around 5%–10% per year.
- There are commonly two types of mild cognitive impairment: the amnesic type and the non-amnesic type.
- The amnesic type is the most common form and manifests as preclinical manifestation of AD. Patients present with impaired performance on delayed recall. There is objective evidence of impairment of short-term memory, but general cognitive functions are normal. There is no substantial interference with work, usual social activities or other activities of daily living. This particular form has a higher chance of conversion to dementia compared with non-amnesic type.
- The non-amnesic MCI may involve multiple cognitive domains (such as executive function) rather than purely amnesia. This type of MCI manifests as localized impairment of other cognitive domains rather than memory. Non-amnesic MCI may develop into non-Alzheimer's dementia.
- With regard to treatment, cognitive rehabilitation is an option. It is essential to encourage individuals to engage in regular physical exercises and to maintain a healthy lifestyle. Underlying vascular risk factors such as hypertension

---

* Adapted from B.K. Puri, A. Hall and R. Ho (2014). *Revision Notes in Psychiatry*. London, UK: CRC Press, pp. 692–694.

and hyperlipidaemia should be treated. In the event that there is underlying depression, treatment is crucial.

- Please refer to the table below for the classification of the risk and the protective factors of dementia.

Modifiable risk factors	Non-modifiable risk factors	Protective factors
• History of diabetes • Physical inactivity, repetitive head injury and smoking • Psychiatry history of depressive disorder • Vascular: hyperlipidaemia, stroke	• Demographics: advanced age and late retirement • Genetics: APP E4 on chromosome 19, abnormalities in chromosome 1, 14 and 21, family history of dementia • Intelligence: low intelligence and limited education • History of MCI	• Bilingualism • Cognitive engagement and late retirement • Fish intake (more than once a week) • High level of education (longer than 15 years) • High level of physical activities (more than three times a week) • Usage of non-steroidal anti-inflammatory drugs (NSAIDs) and statin

STATION 66: DELIRIUM (PAIRED STATION A: HISTORY TAKING)

Information to candidates

Name of patient: Mr Jones

Mr Jones is a 75-year-old male who has been admitted to the medical ward for altered mental state. According to the history given by the family, it was noted that he had been having high fever for the past 4 days. He was noted to be confused as well. The medical team is still doing the routine blood work as well as scans for him. The medical team has referred him to psychiatry as they are concerned that there might be a potential underlying psychiatric cause. Sarah, the daughter of Mr Jones, is here and is keen to speak and give further information about her father.

Task

Please speak to her with the aim of obtaining more information to come to a possible diagnosis of the condition that Mr Jones is having.

Outline of station

You are Sarah, the daughter of Mr Jones. You are the main caregiver of both your father and mother. You noted that over the past 4 days, your father has been spiking a high temperature of 40°C. In addition, you noted that he has been very confused most of the time. He is not able to tell the time and recognize your mother or yourself. At times, he seemed to react and respond to visual stimuli. His gout acted out around 1 week ago, and you have brought him to the local GP, who has given him new painkillers in addition to his routine gout medications. You are very concerned about his current condition. Prior to this, he did not have a history of any memory issues.

CASC construct table

The CASC construct table is formatted such that candidates will be able to cover adequately both the range and the depth of the assessment required in this station.

Starting off: 'Hello, I am Dr Melvyn, one of the psychiatrists from the mental health unit. I understand that your father has been admitted to the medical unit. I'd like to ask you some information that might be helpful for the team in terms of managing his condition. Would that be alright for you?'			
Clarification of presenting complaint	Can you tell me more about what has happened? How long has this been?	Are there times in the day in which you noticed that he is less confused? Is he aware of his surroundings? Can he still recognize his caregivers? Does he know roughly what time of the day it is when you ask him?	Apart from the confusion you have mentioned, does he seem to be more sensitive to environmental changes? (Or) Is he more inattentive and quieter than usual?
Exploration of possible underlying aetiologies	Does your father have any underlying chronic medical conditions that I need to know of?	Over the past week, has he been seen by his GP? Can you tell me more about why he needed to see the GP?	Has the GP offered him new medications? Do you know what medications he is currently on? Have there been problems such as constipation? Does he complain of pain on urination? Have you noticed an increase in his frequency of urination? Has he complained of foul-smelling urine?
Explore comorbid psychiatric symptoms	Over the past 2 weeks, what would you say his mood has been like? Does he still have interest in things he used to enjoy prior to the onset of these confusion episodes?	Have there been any problems with his sleep or his appetite?	Have you noticed that he seemed to be troubled and responding to things that were not there (such as visual stimuli or auditory stimuli)? Does he seem to be more suspicious than usual?

(Continued)

Assess for risk	Have you noticed that he is more agitated recently?	Has he done anything to harm himself or others around him?	
Assess for underlying memory impairments	Prior to the onset of this confusion, what would you say his memory is like? Does he have any problems with his short-term memory? Does he seem to forget where he has placed things? What about his long-term memory? Have there been any issues?	Does he get confused with the day and dates of a week? Are there times in which he cannot recognize your relatives or loved ones? Does he have problems finding the right words to speak at times?	Is he able to function independently in his everyday activities such as grooming and dressing? Is he able to manage his finances? Have there been any episodes in which he has wandered out of the house and got lost? Has he been involved in anything dangerous?

Common pitfalls

    a. Failure to cover the range and depth of information required for the station

    b. Failure to determine whether there is any underlying cognitive issues

Quick recall: Delirium*

1. Overview of *Diagnostic and Statistical Manual of Mental Disorders* (DSM) diagnostic criteria for delirium due to general medical condition.
    a. Disturbance of consciousness (such as reduced clarity of awareness of the environment) and with reduced ability to focus, sustain or shift attention.
    b. A change in the cognition (such as memory deficit, disorientation, language disturbances) or the development of a perceptual disturbance that is not better accounted for by a pre-existing, established or evolving dementia.
    c. The disturbance develops over a short period (usually hours to days) and tends to fluctuate during the course of the day.
    d. There is evidence from history, physical examination or laboratory finding that the disturbance is caused by the direct physiological consequences of a general medical condition.
2. Differentiating between dementia and delirium:
    a. The onset of delirium tends to be rapid.
    b. The duration of delirium tends to last from hours to weeks.
    c. There are changes and fluctuating consciousness.
    d. There is more impaired recent and immediate memory.

---

* Adapted from B.K. Puri, A. Hall and R. Ho (2014). *Revision Notes in Psychiatry*. London, UK: CRC Press, p. 690.

e. In dementia, there is the presence of word-finding difficulties, but in delirium, the speech is incoherent.

f. There is frequent disruption in sleep (such as day–night reversal in delirium).

g. Presence of disorganized thoughts in delirium.

h. In delirium, there is the presence of either hypervigilance or reduced vigilance.

STATION 67: DELIRIUM (PAIRED STATION B: MANAGEMENT)

Information to candidates

Name of patient: Mr Jones

Mr Jones is a 75-year-old male who has been admitted to the medical ward for altered mental state. According to the history given by the family, it was noted that he had been having high fever for the past 4 days. He was noted to be confused as well. The medical team is still doing the routine blood work as well as scans for him. The medical team has referred him to psychiatry as they are concerned that there might be a potential underlying psychiatric cause. Sarah, the daughter of Mr Jones, is here and is keen to speak and give further information about her father. In the previous station, you assessed Mr Jones and came to a possible diagnosis. The ward team and consultant are here, and they are expecting some updates from you.

Task

Please speak to the team's consultant, sharing more about the likely diagnosis as well as the possible management options.

Outline of station

You are Dr Ian, and you have heard from this newly admitted patient. You wish to find out from your trainee more about the presenting complaints and his current working differential diagnosis. In addition, you hope the trainee can substantiate his claims for his proposed differential diagnosis. You will question the trainee about the necessary investigations that should be conducted. You wish to know more about the potential treatment for the patient as well. You expect the trainee to provide more information about how the patient could be managed in the current ward.

CASC construct table

The CASC construct table is formatted such that candidates will be able to cover adequately both the range and the depth of the assessment required in this station.

Starting off: 'Hello, I am Melvyn. Can I discuss the case that I have just seen with yourself and the team?'

Formulation of case	Mr Jones is a 75-year-old gentleman who has been admitted to the inpatient unit and referred to psychiatry for acute changes in behaviour associated with a high temperature. I have spoken to him and also his daughter.	He does not have any psychiatric history and no known family psychiatric history. He has no known past chronic medical illnesses. However, he has recently been seen by his GP.	He is currently staying with his wife and his daughter, who are his main caregivers.
Explain diagnosis and aetiology	Upon interviewing the patient, I note that he has features suggestive of a likely ongoing delirium episode. He was very inattentive throughout the conversation and was confused and not orientated to time, place and person. He reports of visual hallucinations as well.	I have checked the nursing charts, and I have noted that he has sleep–wake disturbances as well. The observations I have noted are consistent with the collaborative history that his daughter has provided me.	With this in mind, my differential diagnosis is that of delirium. I cannot exclude the possibility of an underlying dementing process. With regard to the potential causes of delirium, there are likely many causes to be considered. It might be due to an underlying infection, constipation, dehydration, pain or due to drugs.
Explain investigations	I would like to contact the GP to get more information about his recent assessment. I would also like to know what medication the GP might have started him on as well.	I understand that the medical team has ordered some basic blood work. I would like to check for any abnormalities in the bloods obtained. If a urine analysis has not been ordered, I would like to request it as well.	Ideally, I would like to request some imaging studies if they have not been done as well.
Explain management plans – pharmacological	I suggest that the patient would be best managed in a medical ward.	If the diagnosis is indeed delirium, medications could be started to treat the underlying cause (such as infection).	In the event that he does have disturbing behaviours, I would not recommend that the team commence him immediately on psychotropic medications. Non-pharmacological measures should be tried first.

(Continued)

| Explain management plans – non-pharmacological | It is essential to optimize the environment and nursing care for the patient. It would be advisable for the patient to have a consistent nurse caring for his needs. | The nurse could help to provide regular re-orientation to the environment, which would be helpful for the patient. | Only in circumstances that non-pharmacological measures, fail, should psychotropic medications be considered. Usually antipsychotics like haloperidol could be considered. However, I would monitor him very closely for side effects such as extrapyramidal side effects. His vital signs should also be monitered. I will also do an electrocardiogram (EKG) and check for any prolonged QTc. |
| Explain prognosis | The prognosis is very much dependent on the underlying aetiological causes of the delirium process. | Usually, with adequate treatment, the delirium will clear up in around 2–3 weeks. | Do you have other questions for me? |

Common pitfalls

a. Failure to cover the range and depth of information required for the station
b. Failure to determine whether there is any underlying cognitive issues

Quick recall: Delirium management*

Treatment:

- The primary goal of treating should be to establish the underlying cause of delirium and to treat the underlying cause accordingly.
- The other important goal of treatment is the provision of physical, sensory and environmental support.
- With regard to pharmacotherapy, medications would be helpful in the event that the patient has challenging psychotic behaviours or has insomnia. The most commonly used medication is haloperidol.
- Atypical antipsychotics could also be used for delirium management.

---

* Adapted from B.K. Puri, A. Hall and R. Ho (2014). *Revision Notes in Psychiatry*. London, UK: CRC Press, p. 690.

- For insomnia, hypnotics that are short- or intermediate-acting should be considered.
- With regard to non-pharmacological treatment, it is always essential to provide a supportive and calm environment for the patient. It is essential for 1:1 nursing at homes, to avoid patients getting into serious situations that might result in them having accidents. It is also crucial to note that patients with delirium should not be sensory deprived, and they should also not be placed in an environment that is too stimulating. It would be helpful for them to have their family members at their bedside and would also be helpful for them to have regular re-orientation to the environment by having a calendar and a clock in the ward.

STATION 68: ELDERLY MANIA (PAIRED STATION A: HISTORY TAKING)

Information to candidates

Name of patient: Mr Stephen

Mr Stephen is a 65-year-old male who has been brought in to the emergency services today by his son. Over the past 2 weeks, his son noted that his father had been having increasingly strange behaviours. He was more irritable in his mood and was not sleeping well. Despite the lack of sleep, he has still been capable of helping out with the family business. Three days ago, his son found out from his mother that his father had withdrawn £400,000 from his account to invest in a new piece of property. His son is very concerned about this sudden change in behaviour. Your colleague in the emergency services has done some basic blood tests for him, which were all normal. An imaging study has been done, and it was normal as well.

Task

Please speak to Mr Stephen and take a history with the aim of coming to a diagnosis. Please also do a mental state examination.

Outline of station

You are Mr Stephan, and you are unsure why you have been brought in to the emergency services. You feel perfectly well, and you have already refused to see the medical doctor. You turn irritable when being told that you need to see the psychiatrist. You tell the psychiatrist that there is absolutely nothing wrong with you. You insist that the psychiatrist complete his evaluation quickly, as you have a lot of plans. You withdrew £400,000 from your bank account 3 days ago. You invested in a new property and have plans to distribute the rest of the money to the local charity service. You have not been sleeping well, but it does not concern you as your energy levels are superb. You shared that the royal family has granted you special rights, and you cannot be involuntarily admitted. You hear the royal family speaking to you at times. You do not have any thoughts of harming yourself or others.

CASC construct table

The CASC construct table is formatted such that candidates will be able to cover adequately both the range and the depth of the assessment required in this station.

Starting off: 'Hello, I am Dr Melvyn, one of the psychiatrists from the mental health unit. I understand that your son brought you in today. Can we have a chat?'				
Eliciting core manic symptoms	How have you been feeling in terms of your mood? If I were to ask you to rate your mood on a scale from 1 to 10, what score would you give your mood now? Have others commented that you have been more irritable recently?	How has your energy level been? How has your sleep been? Are you still as energetic as ever despite the decreased amount of sleep? How has your appetite been?	Are you able to think clearly? Do you feel that there are many thoughts racing through your mind at any moment?	How long have you been feeling this way?
Eliciting grandiose delusional beliefs and challenging beliefs	It seems to me that you feel that you are specially chosen. Can you tell me more?	Are there any special powers or abilities that you have that others do not have? Can you tell me more about it?	Can there be any other explanations for why you are having all these symptoms/all these special abilities? Can it be because you have been unwell?	Do you feel increasingly more self-confident recently?
Eliciting hallucinations in all other modalities, elicit thought disorders and elicit passivity experiences	Auditory hallucinations Do you hear sounds or voices that others do not hear? How many voices can you hear? Are they as clear as our current conversation? What do they say?	Second person auditory hallucinations Do they speak directly to you? Can you give me some examples of what they have been saying to you?	Third person auditory hallucinations Do they refer to you as 'he' or 'she', in the third person? Do they comment on your actions? Do they give you orders or commands as to what to do?	How do you feel when you hear them? Can there be any alternative explanation for these experiences that you have been having? Do you feel that your thoughts are being interfered with by an external force? Do you feel in control of your own actions and emotions?

(Continued)

Risk assessment – risk of excessive spending, intimacy, self-harm and violence	Have you engaged in any activities recently that might be dangerous? By that I mean have you been involved with the police recently?	Have you been spending more money than usual?	Have you been recently involved in • any intimate relationships with others? • any unprotected sexual activity?	Have you been so troubled by all these that you have entertained thoughts of ending your life? Have you gotten into trouble with others around you?
Impact and coping mechanisms	How have you been coping with all these?	Have you made use of any substances, such as alcohol, to help you cope?	What about street drugs?	

Common pitfalls

a. Failure to elicit core manic symptoms from patient/failure to cover the range and depth of the station
b. Failure to perform a complete risk assessment

Quick recall*

Mania in the elderly:

- It has been noted that in most elderly people who are suffering from mania, the age of onset is usually in their young adult life. However, in the elderly population, it has been noted that the onset of first manic episode is actually bimodal distributed, with peaks at 37 and also at 73.
- Mania in the elderly is relatively uncommon and accounts for only around 5% of all the elderly psychiatric admissions.
- Late-onset cases appear to have much less genetic loading than younger-onset cases, with fewer of the former giving a family history of affective disorder. It is also important to consider organic causes for late-onset mania. Secondary mania is that arising in a patient with no previous history of affective disorder, soon after a physical illness, such as cerebral tumour or infection. People with late-onset mania have a greater number of large subcortical hyper-intensities on brain MRI compared with that of controls. It is thought that some cases of late-onset mania are a subtype of secondary mania attributing to changes in the brain's deep white matter.
- In terms of clinical features, they are very much similar to the features in younger adults, but it is thought that the following are more common in the elderly manic patients: (1) slow flight of ideas, (2) speech more circumstantial and less disorganized, (3) more paranoid delusions, (4) less hyperactivity, (5) cognitive impairment, (6) irritable, anger and less euphoria, (7) mixed

---

* Adapted from B.K. Puri, A. Hall and R. Ho (2014). *Revision Notes in Psychiatry.* London, UK: CRC Press, p. 711.

affective states, (8) depression following soon after mania recovers, (9) longer duration and higher frequency of acute episodes and (10) presence of neurological abnormalities, especially in elderly male patients.

STATION 69: ELDERLY MANIA (PAIRED STATION B: MANAGEMENT)

Information to candidates

Name of patient: Mr Stephen

Mr Stephen is a 65-year-old male who has been brought into the emergency services today by his son. Over the past 2 weeks, his son had noted that his father had been having increasingly strange behaviours. He was more irritable in his mood and had not been sleeping well. Despite the lack of sleep, he was still capable of helping out with the family business. Three days ago, his son found out from his mother that his father has withdrawn £400,000 from his account to invest in a new piece of property. His son is very concerned about this sudden change in behaviour. Your colleague in the emergency services has done some basic blood tests for him, which were all normal. An imaging study has been done, and it was normal as well. You saw Mr Stephen in the previous station. His wife is here and wishes to know more about what is wrong with him.

Task

Please speak to Mr Stephen's wife and discuss the most probable diagnosis for Mr Stephen. Please also discuss your management plan with her and address all her concerns and expectations.

Outline of station

You are Mr Stephan's wife, Lydia, and you are very concerned about what has been wrong with your husband. You want to know his diagnosis after the psychiatrist has seen him. If the psychiatrist tells you that he has mania, you appear surprised and want to know why this diagnosis has been given. Given the acute changes in behaviour, you want to know whether this could be an acute confusion state. You want to know what the psychiatrist would recommend in terms of further management: Should he be hospitalized? You appear very concerned about hospitalization, as you know that your husband will not be amenable towards staying in the hospital. If the psychiatrist mentions more about using the Mental Health Act to detain your husband, you appear very concerned. You wish to know whether you can give consent on his behalf. You hope that the psychiatrist will keep you updated throughout the entire hospitalization.

CASC construct table

The CASC construct table is formatted such that candidates will be able to cover adequately both the range and the depth of the assessment required in this station.

Starting off: 'Hello, I am Dr Melvyn, one of the psychiatrists from the mental health unit. Thanks for coming today. I have assessed your husband, and I hope we can have a chat to address all the concerns you have'.

Explanation of diagnosis	I have spoken to your husband to understand more about the circumstances leading to the current admission. I have also performed a mental state examination.	I understand that it has been a difficult time for you over the past week. It seems to me that your husband most likely has mania with psychotic symptoms. Have you heard of mania or bipolar disorder before?	Other possibilities could include an acute confusion state or a drug-induced manic episode. However, these seem to be less likely given that his routine blood screens and drug screen seem to be normal. In addition, the imaging study conducted is normal.
Clarification of diagnosis	It is quite likely that your husband has had a manic episode. This is because he has some symptoms consistent with a manic episode, such as having flights of ideas, being more circumstantial in speech and having more paranoid ideations. Sometimes, when patients are in a manic state, they tend to be more irritable as well.	Can I check with you whether your husband has a previous psychiatric history? Does he have any other chronic medical conditions that we need to know of? (Or) If he has a chronic medical condition, has he been on consistent follow-up with any specific doctors?	Would you mind if we obtain further information from the regular doctor that he has been following up with?
Management	I understand that your family has had difficulties with managing your husband's behaviour over the past week. We would like to recommend a short period of inpatient observation and management.	The aim of inpatient admission is largely for us to continue observation of his mental state and to commence treatment. We are hoping that the inpatient observation will help to minimize the associated risks. It is very likely that your husband will also benefit from the inputs of our multidisciplinary team.	We could try pharmacological treatment using medications like lithium and/or antipsychotics to help stabilize his mood. Unfortunately, if he is not responsive to or even intolerant of this combination, electroconvulsive therapy might be indicated.

(Continued)

Other concerns and expectations	Do you have any other concerns about how we are going to manage your husband? I hear that you have some concerns about him not wanting to be admitted.	Given the acute change in mental state and the risk involved, we could detain him involuntarily under the Mental Health Act. I'm sorry we have to resort to doing this. Unfortunately, if he is detained under the Mental Health Act, it is not possible for relatives to give proxy consent.	I hear that you are very concerned about your husband. Please rest assured that my team and I will keep you updated about his clinical progression during his inpatient stay. Please feel free to contact us and make an appointment to meet us should you have further queries.

Common pitfalls

a. Failure to consider alternative differential diagnosis and explain alternatives conceptualized
b. Failure to explain why it is most likely mania, given the history obtained and the mental state examination done previously
c. Failure to address concerns adequately
d. Failure to explain in detail management plans for elderly mania

Quick recall*

- Management: Acute manic episodes may require treatment in the hospital.
- It is important to rule out underlying medical causes and to order baseline blood tests as well as measure the baseline body weight.
- It is also essential for the psychiatrist to check potential drug interactions from existing medications.
- Treatment could be commenced with either antipsychotics or with lithium or a combination of both in some cases.
- Lithium should be started at 150 mg daily if the elderly person is frail, or 300 mg daily if the elderly person is physically fit. The dose is increased by 150 mg on a weekly basis.
- The maximum daily dose is recommended to be less than 600 mg/day. The blood lithium level is aimed to be between 0.6 and 0.9 mmol/L during acute mania and between 0.4 and 0.6 mmol/L during the maintenance phase of the treatment.

---

* Adapted from B.K. Puri, A. Hall and R. Ho (2014). *Revision Notes in Psychiatry.* London, UK: CRC Press, p. 712.

- The elderly will require monthly monitoring of the blood lithium levels in the initial period and regular monitoring of the thyroid, renal and cardiac status and measurement of the body weight.
- The response rate for lithium has been deemed to be similar for both young and elderly people.
- If the elderly person is not responsive to lithium treatment, or intolerant to the combination, electroconvulsive therapy could be effective for manic or mixed affective states.
- With regard to prognosis, the prognosis is the same as that for bipolar disorder.

Recurrence of the disorder is usual, and hence, mood stabilizers are needed in the longer term.

STATION 70: ATTENTION-DEFICIT HYPERACTIVITY DISORDER (ADHD) HISTORY TAKING

Information to candidates

Name of patient: David

The local general practitioner (GP) has referred David, a 5-year-old boy, to your service for further assessment. He is here today with his mother, Mrs Flowers. It was noted on the referring memo that David has been having a lot of difficulties both at home and in school, and his mother is very concerned.

Task

Please speak to Mrs Flowers, David's mother, to elicit more information about him, looking for features suggestive of a childhood disorder. Please also consider other associated comorbidities and rule them out in your history taking.

Outline of station

The purpose of providing an outline of the station is to allow candidates to be familiar with the structure of the station. This outline could also be helpful when candidates practice for the MRCPsych, joining with their colleagues to act out the station.

Please note that the outlines provided are based on the experiences of the authors. There may be variations in the actual examination.

You are Mrs Flowers, David's mother. He is 5 years old this year and has been having problematic behaviours both in school and at home. Both you and his teacher have noted that he is hyperactive and cannot sit still. He is inattentive most of the time. In addition, you are especially concerned about his impulsive actions. There was an occasion in which he was almost involved in an accident as he dashed across the traffic junction. There are no other abnormal behaviours that you have noted. He has not gotten himself into any major conduct problems, and he is still able to handle the work expected for his academic level. His speech is normal. There is no family history of any psychiatric disorders.

CASC construct table

The CASC construct table is formatted such that candidates will be able to cover adequately both the range and the depth of the assessment required in this station.

Starting off: 'Hello, I am Dr Melvyn, one of the psychiatrists from the mental health unit. I understand that you came to see us today as you have some concerns about your son, David. Would you mind telling me more?'			
Background information	I understand from your GP that you have been having some difficulties with managing David. Can you tell me when this first started?	Would you mind sharing with me the difficulties you have been facing? I'm sorry to be hearing of all these. Are these behaviours limited only to school? Are there other occasions in which you have noticed such behaviours?	In what way do you think David is different from a child typical of his age? Thanks for sharing with me your concerns. I hope to be of help. Can we spend the next few minutes helping me understand more about the difficulties?
Eliciting hyperactivity symptoms	You mentioned that David is always on the go. Can you give me some examples?	Is he able to remain in his seat when he is at school? What happens if you are out with David for a family meal?	Are there times in which he climbs on furniture?
Eliciting inattention symptoms	I understand that one of your other concerns is that he seems to be inattentive. What has his teacher reported of when he is in school?	Have you noticed similar problems when he is at home? Can he concentrate on tasks that you have asked him to do?	Are there times in which you noticed that he seemed quite forgetful and kept misplacing things?
Eliciting impulsiveness symptoms	I am very concerned to hear about what he has done previously (dashing out onto the roads). Is that an isolated incident?	Have there been any other similar episodes that have caused you to be concerned about his safety?	Did his teacher report similar incidents in school? Did his teacher ever mention that he is always having problems waiting for his turn?
Consideration of other comorbidities	I'm sorry to know how tough things have been for you with regard to managing his difficult behaviours. Does anyone in the family have any previous psychiatric history?	Apart from the symptoms that you have reported, have you noticed any unusual movements that David has? Does he happen to have any language problems? Is he able to play with the other children? Is he able to reciprocate when you show your affection towards him?	Can you tell me more about his school performance? Has he got himself into any conduct problems in school or with the police? How has his mood been? Is he still able to enjoy doing the things he used to enjoy doing? Thanks for sharing with me. I am hopeful our team can help your son, David, with his condition.

Common pitfalls

a. Failure to ask sufficient questions to cover the range and depth of the information required to make a diagnosis of ADHD or hyperkinetic disorder

b. Failure to ask questions about and exclude other possible comorbid conditions

Quick recall*

- 'ADHD' is an American term. In the United Kingdom, it is often known as hyperkinetic disorder.
- In the United Kingdom, 1.7% of school-aged children suffer from hyperkinetic disorder, based on the *International Statistical Classification of Diseases and Related Health Problems,* 10th revision (*ICD-10*) criteria, which are more stringent and require both hyperactivity and inattention to be present.
- Male-to-female gender ratio has been estimated to be 3:1.
- The peak age of onset is around 3–8 years of age.
- The clinical features include persistent pattern of inattention, hyperactivity and impulsivity across two different settings, which result in significant functional impairments. The behaviours are maladaptive and inconsistent with the developmental level.
- The onset of symptoms is usually before the age of 7 years.

Symptoms of inattention include the following:

- Starts tasks or activities but not being able to follow through and finish.
- Organization of tasks or activities being impaired.
- Loses things necessary for tasks and activities such as school assignments or stationary.
- Instructions are not being followed.
- Distraction by external stimuli.
- Other features include careless mistakes and forgetfulness in daily activities.

Symptoms of hyperactivity and impulsivity include the following:

- Waiting in lines or awaiting turns in games causing frustration.
- On the move most of the time, such as running and climbing.
- Restlessness and jitteriness.
- Squirms on the seat.
- Talks excessively without appropriate response to social constraints.
- Fidgets with hands and feet.
- Answers are blurted out before questions.
- Interruption of other people's conversations.
- Loud noise in playing (hyperactivity).

---

* Adapted from B.K. Puri, A. Hall and R. Ho (2014). *Revision Notes in Psychiatry.* London, UK: CRC Press, p. 630.

The *Diagnostic and Statistical Manual of Mental Disorders,* 5th edition (*DSM-5*) classifies ADHD into three individual subtypes:

- Inattentive type: at least six symptoms of inattention but not hyperactivity and impulsivity symptoms for 6 months
- Hyperactivity type: at least 6 symptoms of hyperactivity and impulsivity symptoms for 6 months
- Combined type: at least 6 symptoms of both inattention and hyperactivity/impulsivity for 6 months

STATION 71: ADHD MANAGEMENT

Information to candidates

Name of patient: David

The local GP has referred David, a 5-year-old boy, to your service for further assessment. He is here today with his mother, Mrs Flowers. It was noted on the referring memo that David has been having a lot of difficulties both at home and in school, and his mother is very concerned. You have spoken to the mother, obtained a school report and have done some psychometric testing for David. It has been established that David has a diagnosis of ADHD. His mother has booked another appointment today as she has some concerns about the diagnosis. She wants to have more information about the medications that might be started. As David is her oldest child, she is very concerned that the rest of her children will get ADHD as well.

Task

Please speak to Mrs Flowers, David's mother, and explain the diagnosis and address all her concerns and expectations.

Outline of station

You are Mrs Flowers, David's mother. You heard that the team has diagnosed David with ADHD. You have only heard about ADHD from the media. You want the doctor to explain to you in a simple manner what ADHD really is. You are curious about the condition and wish to know more. You wonder whether you are responsible for David having ADHD. You would like to know what are the other causes of ADHD. You understand that treatment is available. If the doctor proposes some medication, you appeared to be very concerned and want to know the exact side effects. You have concerns about the major side effects of growth suppression. As you have other children, you wonder what is the likelihood of them having ADHD. You also wonder whether there are blood tests that could confirm the diagnosis. You have heard in the news that a special diet might be helpful. You are curious as to whether you could try some sort of special diet as well for David.

CASC construct table

The CASC construct table is formatted such that candidates will be able to cover adequately both the range and the depth of the assessment required in this station.

Starting off: 'Hello, I am Dr Melvyn, one of the psychiatrists from the mental health unit. I understand that you came to see us today as you have some concerns about your son, David. Would you mind telling me more?'			
Explanation of diagnosis	Thanks for coming today. I understand that you have some concerns about the diagnosis we have made for David.	Yes, you're right in saying that the team has diagnosed him with ADHD. Have you heard about ADHD before?/What is your understanding of ADHD?	'ADHD' is a terminology commonly used in the United States. In the United Kingdom, the disorder is termed 'hyperkinetic disorder'.
Clarification of symptoms and underlying aetiology	Children diagnosed with this condition tend to have three groups of symptoms, which are hyperactivity, inattention and impulsiveness.	Unfortunately, there is no specific blood test or brain imaging that would guide us towards the diagnosis. We have diagnosed David with ADHD based on the history you have provided us with, as well as the collaborative history we have obtained from the school. In addition, we have administered the Conner scale for David, and he was in the abnormal range on the scale.	Hyperkinetic disorder is a common disorder in the United Kingdom, affecting 1.7% of all school-going children. It tends to be more common in males compared with females. With regard to your concerns about the causation of the disorder, there are multiple factors that may be responsible. If there is a family history of the disorder, there is a twofold increment in the risk of the child having the disorder. Disturbances in the normal brain chemicals, as well as infections or problems during pregnancy, might predispose individuals towards ADHD as well.
Explain management (pharmacological)	I'm sorry to inform you that David has ADHD. I am hopeful that our team can help him with his condition. There are medications that are available to help him. The most commonly used medication is methylphenidate, a stimulant. Have you heard about it before?	Like all medications, methylphenidate does have its side effects. Prior to commencement of the medications, we need to do some baseline blood tests as well as a heart tracing. We will commence the lowest dose and adjust the medication in accordance to his response to the medication.	Methylphenidate works by normalizing the amounts of certain chemicals in the brain. It helps to make the child calmer, more focussed and with increased attention. The most common side effects that you need to take note of include abdominal discomfort, headaches and difficulties with sleeping. The most common long-term side effect is growth suppression, and hence we make it a point to measure his height and weight during each clinic review.
Explain management (non-pharmacological)	Apart from medications, there are also other non-pharmacological methods that we could use to help David.	It is of importance that you are referred to educational programs for you to learn more about ADHD, its management and coping strategies.	We can also refer David to see a psychologist to be engaged in behaviour therapy. Environmental modifications such as placing the child in the front row of the class may help to reduce distractions.
Address concerns	I know that we have discussed quite a lot today. Do you have any questions for me?	Existing research has not proven that a special diet will be helpful for children.	As hyperkinetic disorder is a heritable condition, there is an increased chance that your other children might develop the disorder.

Common pitfalls

a. Failure to explain ADHD in a concise manner
b. Failure to address the mother's concerns about stimulants and explain the most common side effects
c. Failure to address the effects of the child's ADHD on other children

Quick recall*

Aetiology

- ADHD is a heritable disorder. It has been proven that siblings of ADHD children most likely have twice the risk of ADHD compared with that of the general population.
- Biological parents of children with the disorder have a higher risk for ADHD than adoptive parents.
- It has been noted that genes related to the dopaminergic functions are implicated (such as the dopamine receptor D4 gene, the dopamine transporter gene, alpha 2A gene, the norepinephrine transporter gene and the catechol-o-methyltransferase (COMT) gene).
- It has been noted that September is the peak month for births of children with ADHD with or without comorbid learning disorders.
- Early infection, inflammation, toxins and trauma could cause circulatory, metabolic and physical brain damage and lead to ADHD in adulthood.
- Psychosocial adversity is associated with ADHD in childhood.
- A dysfunction in the peripheral noradrenaline could lead to negative feedback to the locus coeruleus, which leads to the reduction of noradrenaline in the central nervous system.

Rating scales and cognitive assessment

- Corner's rating scale is a diagnostic scale for ADHD using the *DSM-5* criteria. This scale includes measures of behaviour described by parents and teachers. The behaviour scale includes the following: (a) ADHD symptoms, (b) anxiety, (c) cognitive problems, (d) oppositional behaviour, (e) perfectionism and (f) social problems.
- It is crucial to arrange direct school observation by a member of the Child and Adolescent Mental Health Service (CAMHS).
- Psychometric testing such as intelligence quotient (IQ) assessment or academic assessment is essential if there is evidence of learning disability.

Commonly associated medical conditions

- Speech or language impairment is present in 50% of children with ADHD.
- Oppositional defiant disorder (40% of children would meet the diagnostic criteria, but at least 75% of children with ADHD show behavioural symptoms of aggression).

---

* Adapted from B.K. Puri, A. Hall and R. Ho (2014). *Revision Notes in Psychiatry*. London, UK: CRC Press, p. 630.

- Conduct disorder is present in approximately 30%–50% of children.
- Anxiety disorders are present in 25% of children.
- Tic disorder is present in 11% of children.
- The other common associated condition is substance abuse.

Treatment

- Prior to the initiation of medication, the psychiatrist needs to look out for the following:
  - Look out for exercise syncope, undue breathlessness and other cardiovascular symptoms in the history.
  - Perform a full physical examination including measurement of heart rate and blood pressure and examination of the cardiovascular system.
  - Measurement of baseline height and weight.
  - Ordering an electrocardiogram if there is a history of cardiac disease.
- The most commonly used drug is a stimulant, which includes methylphenidate.
- The stimulant inhibits the dopamine reuptake and causes direct release of dopamine.
- Stimulants are indicted for ADHD without comorbidity or ADHD with comorbid conduct disorder.
- The beneficial effect of methylphenidate is that it helps to improve attention span and hyperactivity for a certain number of hours.
- With regard to dosing: Regular Ritalin requires 5–10 mg three times daily (TID). Could consider modified release preparations that allow for single-day dosing and promote adherence.
- The common side effects include reduction in appetite, gastric discomfort, insomnia, headache, elevation of blood pressure, tics and irritability.
- The most serious and rare side effect includes liver impairment, leucopenia and sudden cardiac death.
- Continuous monitoring for height and weight (every 6 months), cardiovascular status (every 3 months), seizure, tics, psychotic symptoms, anxiety symptoms and drug diversion is required.
- It is essential to note that there is a risk of misuse in patients with history of stimulant misuse.
- It is appropriate to continue treatment for as long as it is effective with regular review of clinical need, benefits and side effects.
- If stimulants are contraindicated, then non-stimulants could be considered. Examples of non-stimulants include atomoxetine, imipramine, bupropion and clonidine.
- The indications for non-stimulants include (a) inability to tolerate side effects associated with the usage of stimulant, (b) unsatisfactory response to two types of stimulants, (c) history of stimulant usage and (d) presence of comorbid conditions that will make the usage of stimulant contraindicated.
- Apart from pharmacological treatment, non-pharmacological treatment is indicated as well. Parent training and education programs could be considered. Parents could be offered referral to educational programmes to learn more about ADHD, the management and the coping strategies. Individual or

group-based parent training could be useful for children and adolescents suffering from ADHD. Academic remediation is indicated for the child as well.

- Behaviour treatment is indicated as well. It is essential to provide the child with positive reinforcement (for example, reward system and praises to promote positive behaviour). It is also of importance to teach them time-out skills that include planned ignoring to reduced negative behaviour. Environmental modifications could be implemented, such as placing the child in the front row of the class, to reduce the amount of distraction.
- Prior research has demonstrated that the combination of behaviour therapy and medication may be better than medication alone.

Prognosis

- ADHD symptoms tend to persist at the age of 30 years in one-quarter of the ADHD children. Most patients do not require medications when they get older. However, it will be appropriate to continue medications and treatment in adults whose ADHD symptoms remain disabling for them.
- It has been noted that although the symptoms of hyperactivity often improve as the child grows older, the inattentive symptoms tend to remain disabling.
- Remission of the symptoms is unlikely prior to the age of 12 years. When remission does occur, it usually takes place between the ages of 12 to 20 years. Hyperactivity is usually the first symptom to remit. Distractibility is the last symptom to remit.

The following are predictors for the persistence of ADHD symptoms into adulthood:

- Presence of family history of ADHD
- Psychosocial adversity
- Comorbid conduct disorder
- Comorbid depressive disorder
- Comorbid anxiety disorder
- Of importance, approximately 20% of children with ADHD do develop antisocial personality disorder in adulthood. Fifteen per cent develop substance misuse in adulthood.

STATION 72: CONDUCT DISORDER – HISTORY TAKING

Information to candidates

Name of patient: Samson

The school counsellor has requested an early appointment for Samson, a 14-year-old male, with the child psychiatrist. Samson has been physically threatening his peers in school and has been recently involved in a theft as well. The school feels that he would benefit from further assessment and management. His mother, Mrs Thomas, has been informed of the referral and is here with her son today.

Task

Please speak to Mrs Thomas, Samson's mother, and take a history to arrive at an appropriate diagnosis. Please obtain other relevant personal history from his mother as well.

Outline of station

You are Mrs Thomas, Samson's mother, and you have heard about his increasingly difficult behaviour in school. You're very concerned to learn that your son has been involved in a recent theft case in school. You hope this is not because he is mixing with bad company. You have noted that since he was young, he has been cruel towards animals. When he was in junior school, you received feedback from his teachers, who said that he was physically aggressive and had been threatening to harm his peers. Now that he is in high school, you understand that he has been frequently missing school as well. You hope that this is not because you are struggling to make ends meet and cannot provide your son with quality time and care, given that you need to work long hours. Your husband is currently in prison, following a grievous crime that he committed 3 years ago. You hope that the psychiatrist can help your son with regard to his behaviour issues, as you hope that he will not end up in a similar state as your husband.

CASC construct table

The CASC construct table is formatted such that candidates will be able to cover adequately both the range and the depth of the assessment required in this station.

Starting off: 'Hello, I am Dr Melvyn, one of the psychiatrists from the mental health unit. I understand that the school counsellor has some concerns for your son, Samson, and hence have arranged this appointment. Can we have a chat about your concerns?'			
Clarification of history	Thank you for being here today. I understand that this must be a difficult time for you. Can you share with me more about your concerns pertaining to Samson?	How long have you noted Samson to be having these difficult behaviours for? (Or) Do you remember when all these difficult behaviours first started?	Would you say that in the past 12 months, Samson has violated rules, been aggressive, been destructive or been deceitful? Or in the past 6 months, has he violated any rules, been aggressive, been destructive or been deceitful?
Specific symptoms (towards adults)	Has he been having frequent arguments with adults/yourself? Does he defy set rules or any other specific requests set by adults/yourself?	Has he stayed out after dark against your prohibition?	

(Continued)

Specific symptoms (towards other people)	How has he been around other people? Have you noticed that he has been annoying them intentionally? Does he tend to blame others for his own mistakes?	Has he gotten into any fights with others? If he has, has he used any weapons to harm the others? Has he exhibited any cruelty towards others or even to animals?	Do you know if he has forced others into sexual activities?
Specific symptoms (towards objects or properties)	Has there been any occasion in which he has deliberately destroyed properties?	My understanding is that he has been recently involved in a theft. Can you tell me more about it? Has he been involved in any other crimes previously?	Has there been any time in which he has run away from home?
Eliciting predisposing risk factors	Can I check whether there is a family history of any psychiatric-related disorder? Can you tell me more about your husband? Do you know if he had conduct problems whilst he was in school? Has he been involved in any crimes?	Is there a history of substance usage in the family (such as alcohol)? How are the finances in the family?	Were there any problems with Samson when he was growing up? Was there anyone who was harsh to him or resorted to using severe physical and verbal punishment to deal with his difficult behaviours?
Ruling out comorbidity	How has Samson's mood been in the past month or so? Have you realized that he is losing interest in things he used to enjoy? Would you say that Samson has been more anxious lately?	Can Samson focus on tasks that you assign him to do? Is he always on the go (hyperactive)? Does he have any learning difficulties? How is his current academic performance?	Are you aware whether Samson is using any alcohol or street drugs at the moment?

Common pitfalls

a. Failure to cover the range and depth required for the station
b. Failure to elicit predisposing risk factors that would contribute towards the child developing conduct disorder
c. Failure to rule out comorbidities

Quick recall*

- Conduct disorder has been diagnosed in approximately 4% of children, based on the Isle of Wight study.
- The prevalence is usually higher in socially deprived inner city areas and larger families. The male-to-female gender ratio for conduct disorder is 3:1.
- The age of onset of conduct disorder begins earlier in boys (10–12 years) compared with girls (14–16 years). The comorbidity of ADHD and aggressive behaviour is associated with early onset of conduct disorder.
- Aetiology: (a) Genetics factors: Conduct disorder is associated with inheritance of antisocial trait from patents that have demonstrated conduct disorder. (b) Parental predisposing factors include the failure to set rules and monitor, presence of harsh, punitive parenting with severe physical and verbal aggression, parental psychopathology, having a parent (father) with antisocial personality disorder and alcohol dependence, maternal depression, repeated physical and sexual abuse, rejection from parents and low income.
- The protective factors against conduct disorder include (1) economic stability in family, (2) family commitment to normal societal value, (3) being of female gender, (4) good coping strategies, (5) high IQ, (6) positive social interaction, (7) pre-pubertal anxiety such as separation anxiety, (8) resilience, (9) stable social organization in the community and (10) warm supportive family.
- Criteria for diagnosis of conduct disorder: Based on the *ICD-10*, there is a repetitive and persistent pattern of behaviour in which either the basic rights of others or major age-appropriate societal norms are violated. The minimum duration of symptoms lasts for at least 6 months.
- Individual symptoms: The child often displays severe temper tantrums, being angry and spiteful and often telling lies and breaking promises. To adults, there is normally frequent argument, refusing adult's requests or defying rules and staying out after dark even after parental prohibition (onset earlier than age 13 years). Regarding behaviour towards other people, the child might annoy them deliberately, blaming them for his mistakes and initiating fights with the others, using weapons to harm the others and exhibiting physical cruelty (also to animals), confronting victims during a crime or forcing another person into sexual activity and frequently bullying the others. Towards objects or properties, the child might deliberately destroy properties, set fire, steal objects of value within the home or outside and breaking into someone's house.
- The *ICD-10* criteria classify conduct disorder into mild, moderate and severe. The *ICD-10* criteria recommend specifying the age of onset as childhood onset (younger than 10 years) and adolescent onset (older than 10 years). Substance abuse is not a diagnostic criterion for conduct disorder.
- The *DSM-5* criteria suggests the following with regard to conduct disorder: Conduct disorder involves the repetitive and persistent pattern of behaviours in which the basic rights of others or major age-appropriate societal norms or rules are violated, as manifested by the presence of three or more of the

---

* Adapted from B.K. Puri, A. Hall and R. Ho (2014). *Revision Notes in Psychiatry.* London, UK: CRC Press, p. 635.

following: aggression, destruction, deceitfulness, serious violation of rules) in the past 12 months, with at least one criteria being met in the past 6 months.

- The common comorbidities for conduct disorder include ADHD (50% of children with conduct disorder), mood disorders (5%–30% of the patients) and anxiety disorder (30% of children with anxiety disorder also suffer from conduct disorder).
- With regard to pharmacological treatment for aggression and behavioural problems: antipsychotics such as risperidone, olanzapine and haloperidol can reduce the physical aggression and assault. For depression and impulsivity, selective serotonin reuptake inhibitors (SSRIs) can help to reduce impulsivity, irritability and depression. For conduct disorder associated with ADHD, stimulants can help reduce behavioural problems associated with hyperactivity and improve attention.
- The multimodal treatment is an indicated treatment option for conduct disorder. The National Institute for Health and Care Excellence (NICE) guidelines recommend group-based parent training and education programmes. Individual-based parent training or education programmes are recommended if there are particular difficulties in engaging with the parents or the family's needs are too complex.
- Individual psychotherapy is indicated, such as problem-solving therapy, impulse control, anger management and social skills training.
- With regard to prognosis, approximately 40% of young people with conduct disorder will develop dissocial personality disorder in adulthood. Borderline IQ, mental retardation and family history of dissocial personality disorder are predictive factors. Approximately 35%–75% of patients have comorbid ADHD, and the presence of ADHD predicts a worse outcome for boys with conduct disorder. Callous emotional trait predicts a more severe and persistent course of conduct disorder.

STATION 73: AUTISM – HISTORY TAKING

Information to candidates

Name of patient: Mrs Young

Mrs Young has been having some concerns about her 4-year-old son, Jonathan. She feels that his language abilities are limited and not on par with the rest of the normal children of his age. In addition, she noticed that her child is not able to reciprocate her affection at times and has very minimal eye contact, even towards the rest of the family members. Her local GP has recommended that she seek help from a child psychiatrist for Jonathan, and she is here today to share her concerns.

Task

Please speak to Mrs Young and elicit more history to come to a possible diagnosis. Please also take other necessary personal and developmental history that might be pertinent towards formulation of the eventual diagnosis.

Outline of station

You are Mrs Young, and Jonathan is your only child. Prior to his turning 3 years old, you noted that he had delayed language abilities. You have also noticed that

Jonathan has abnormal reciprocal social interaction. He has poor eye contact and is not able to play with the rest of the children in the playgroup. He is not able to show his affection towards you. He does not usually play with his toys in the usual way, like how the other children play. He tends to be preoccupied with parts of the toys instead. Thus far, you have not noticed any other additional problems, such as any sleeping or eating disturbances or aggression or any self-injurious behaviour.

CASC construct table

The CASC construct table is formatted such that candidates will be able to cover adequately both the range and the depth of the assessment required in this station.

Starting off: 'Hello, I am Dr Melvyn, one of the psychiatrists from the mental health unit. I understand that your local GP has arranged for you to see us as you have some concerns about your child, Jonathan. Can we have a chat about this?'			
Clarification of the history and onset of symptoms	I'm sorry to hear about the difficulties that you have been facing with Jonathan. I'm hoping to understand the situation better, so that we can help your child.	Can you tell me approximately how old Jonathan was when you first noticed these behavioural changes? (Or) Did you first notice these behavioural difficulties when Jonathan was younger than 3 years old?	Since then, how have things progressed?
Presence of abnormal reciprocal social interactions	Is Jonathan able to make eye contact with you or your family members when you speak to him?	Is he able to reciprocate your affections when you give him a hug?	Is he able to make friends with other children? Is he able to share toys and play together with other children?
Presence of abnormal communication	Can you tell me more about his language abilities? Do you know what his language difficulties are?	Is he able to initiate and sustain a normal conversation with you? Does he tend to make use of or say the same phrase repetitively?	Have you noticed whether he tends to repeat spoken words others have said? Does he keep repeating what he has just said?
Presence of restricted, stereotyped and repetitive behaviour	Have you noticed anything odd when Jonathan is allowed to play by himself? Does he seem to be preoccupied with parts of certain toys?	Does he play with his toys in the same way that other children play? Is he able to have imaginative play? Can you tell me more about what his interests are? Does he only have particular interests? Does he tend to do anything repeatedly/follow particular rituals?	Do you think he is able to adapt to changes in the environment? Have you noticed whether Jonathan has any other characteristic body movements (such as hand flapping, body rocking)? Is he sensitive to touch?

(Continued)

Other psychiatric comorbid	How has his mood been? Is he still able to keep up with his interests? How have his sleep and appetite been?	Are there any specific things that Jonathan is afraid of?	Has there been any aggressive behaviour? Has there been any self-injurious behaviour?
Developmental history	Can you tell me more about your pregnancy? Were there any complications prior to, during or after the pregnancy and delivery?	I would like to enquire more about his developmental milestones. Do you remember when he first started to smile, turn over, crawl, sit and walk?	Are there any other developmental issues I need to know of?

Common pitfalls

a. Failure to cover the range and depth of the information required to confirm the diagnosis of autistic disorder
b. Failure to elicit information about developmental history

Although this is a history-taking station, it is important to demonstrate empathy towards the parent, who may be distressed, worried and anxious.

Quick recall*

- The prevalence of autism has been estimated to be 7–28/10,000 individuals.
- The male-to-female ratio has been estimated to be 4:1.
- *ICD-10* diagnostic criteria and clinical characteristics: (a) Presence of abnormal development that is manifested before the age of 3 years, including abnormal selective or reciprocal social interaction and abnormal functional or symbolic play. Children with autism are often attached to odd objects and have a relative lack of creativity and fantasy in thoughts. (b) Abnormal reciprocal social interactions that include failure in eye gaze and body language, failure in development of peer relationships, lack of socio-emotional reciprocity and lack of spontaneous sharing with other people. (c) Abnormal communication that includes the lack of development of spoken language, lack of social imitative play and failure to initiate or sustain conversational language. Their languages are frequently associated with pronoun reversals. (d) Restricted, stereotyped and repetitive behaviour includes preoccupation with stereotyped interest, compulsive adherence to rituals, motor mannerisms and preoccupation with parts of objects or non-functional elements of play materials. There might be

---

* Adapted from B.K. Puri, A. Hall and R. Ho (2014). *Revision Notes in Psychiatry*. London, UK: CRC Press, p. 635.

other nonspecific problems such as phobias, sleeping and eating disturbances, temper tantrums, self-directed aggression and self-injury.

- To make the diagnosis, there might be the absence of other causes of pervasive developmental disorders, socio-emotional problems and schizophrenia-like symptoms.
- The common psychiatric comorbidity is learning disability, academic learning problems in literacy or numeracy, ADHD (50%), obsessive–compulsive disorder (10%), tics syndrome, anxiety disorders, depression (irritability or social withdrawal), temper tantrums, oppositional defiant disorder and self-injurious behaviour.

Psychological treatment includes the following:

- Applied behavioural analysis: Operant conditioning helps to develop special social, communication and behavioural skills by reinforcing positive behaviour. The triggers for problematic behaviours are analysed.
- Intensive behavioural intervention: The design, implementation and evaluation of environmental modifications that aim to produce meaningful changes in behaviour.
- Sensory integration therapy: Techniques such as brushing of the skin or swinging to stimulate vestibular response will help to reduce the hypersensitivity to stimuli.
- Facilitated communication: Training in reading and writing.

Pharmacological treatment

- Risperidone: helps with the reduction in the repetition and aggression and helps to improve behaviour
- Fluoxetine: reduces the levels of ritualistic behaviour and improves mood and anxiety
- Anticonvulsants: reduction of self-injurious behaviours
- Naltrexone: reduction of self-injurious behaviours
- Atomoxetine: reduces inattention, hyperactivity and aggression

Prognosis

- Within the first 3 years of life, approximately 70% of children with this condition do not achieve normal development.
- There is a chance that inappropriate sexual behaviour may emerge in adolescence and early adulthood.
- Most children with this condition do show improvement in social relations and communication. However, their rituals and repetitive behaviour may not improve over time.
- The condition in itself predisposes to lifelong disability.

NICE guidance recommendations

- The NICE guidelines recommend patients with autism to be treated by a multidisciplinary team that includes a paediatrician and/or a child psychiatrist, speech therapist, clinical or educational psychologist and occupational therapist.

- Autistic children often do well in a well-structured educational setting with experienced teachers and educational psychologists.
- Behaviour therapy establishes underlying reasons for disruptive behaviour and provides alternative and more socially acceptable ways of indicating needs. Behaviour therapy also aims at reducing behavioural problems such as temper tantrums, feeling and toilet problems, aggression, rituals and obsessions.
- Social skills training helps the child to understand the beliefs and emotions of others based on theory of mind, teaching a child to mind-read by first helping a child understand his own thoughts or feelings and thus eventually be able to deduce actions of other people.
- Speech therapist: can help the child to facilitate communication and the parents to understand echolalic speech and consider an alternative mode of communication.
- Occupational therapist: can assess the child's behaviour from the sensory processing and self-regulation perspectives and help the child to develop more adaptive ways to self-regulate.
- Parent education and support are provided for parents and family members about childhood autism, referring them to community resources for further support.

STATION 74: EARLY-ONSET PSYCHOSIS (PAIRED STATION A: HISTORY TAKING)

Information to candidates

Name of patient: Paula

The local GP has referred Paula, a 17-year-old student, as her parents feel that she has not been her usual self. They are very worried that there might be something wrong with her mental health, as her grades have been declining, and she is also reluctant to go to school.

Task

Please speak to Paula in this station, and elicit a history to come to a possible diagnosis. Please perform a relevant mental state examination.

Outline of station

You are Paula, and you went to the GP with your parents last week. You were told that you need to see a child psychiatrist. For the past 2 months, you have not been going to school as you feel that your friends are all talking about you behind your back. Despite you feeling this way, you have not confronted them about this matter. Your grades have declined as well. You do not hear voices and do not have any other strange experiences. You have tried cannabis once (which your parents are not aware of) when your close friends asked you to try. You have no thoughts of self-harm or suicide.

CASC construct table

The CASC construct table is formatted such that candidates will be able to cover adequately both the range and the depth of the assessment required in this station.

Starting off: 'Hello, I am Dr Melvyn, one of the psychiatrists from the mental health unit. I understand that your local GP has arranged for you to see me. Can we have a chat?'			
Eliciting core delusion and other delusional beliefs	I understand that there have been some difficulties at school. Can you tell me more? I'm sorry to hear that you have been feeling this way. It must have been a very difficult time for you.	How do you know that your friends are talking about you? Could there be any other alternative explanations for the way they behave?	Do you feel that other people out there are trying to harm you in any other way? Do you feel that you have some special powers or abilities? Do you feel that certain things have a special meaning for you?
Hallucinations	Auditory hallucinations Do you hear sounds or voices that others do not hear? How many voices can you hear? Are they as clear as our current conversation? What do they say?	Second person auditory hallucinations Do they speak directly to you? Can you give me some examples of what they have been saying to you? Third person auditory hallucinations Do they refer to you as 'he' or 'she', in the third person? Do they comment on your actions? Do they give you orders or commands as to what to do?	How do you feel when you hear them? Could there be any alternative explanation for these experiences that you have been having?
Thought disorders	Thought interference Do you feel that your thoughts are being interfered with? Who do you think is doing this? Thought insertion Do you have thoughts in your head that you feel are not your own? Where do you think these thoughts come from?	Thought broadcasting Do you feel that your thoughts are being broadcasted, such that others would know what you are thinking?	Thought withdrawal Do you feel that your thoughts are being taken away from your head by some external force?

(Continued)

209

Passivity experiences	Do you feel in control of your own actions and emotions?	Do you feel that someone or something is trying to control you? Who or what do you think this could be?	
Impact on mood and coping	Has this affected your mood in any way? Are you still interested in things you used to enjoy?	I understand that this must be a difficult time for you. How have you been coping?	Have you made use of any substances, such as alcohol, to help you cope? What about street drugs?
Risk assessment	Are you feeling so troubled that you have entertained thoughts of ending your life?	What plans have you made?	Have you made any plans to approach those who have been speaking about you?

Common pitfalls

a. Failure to explore other delusional beliefs
b. Failure to cover the range and the depth of the task required for the station
c. Failure to perform a comprehensive risk assessment (risk assessment needs to take into account risk towards oneself as well as risk towards others)

Quick recall*

- Prodrome of schizophrenia refers to a range of subjective experiences before the onset of schizophrenia.

There might be the presence of attenuated positive symptoms such as the following:

- Unusual perception.
- Odd beliefs.
- Vague and circumstantial speech.
- Preoccupation with religion, occult and philosophy.
- Suspiciousness.
- Pre-psychotic anxiety.
- Praecox feeling refers to a subjective sense by the clinician that the patient is odd. The patient is usually concrete, woolly, exhibiting mild formal thought disorder or socially blamed or reporting perceptual disturbances.

There might be the presence of negative symptoms such as the following:

- Blunted affect
- Amotivation
- Isolation and social withdrawal

---

* Adapted from B.K. Puri, A. Hall and R. Ho (2014). *Revision Notes in Psychiatry*. London, UK: CRC Press, p. 370.

- There might be the presence of cognitive symptoms such as the following:
  - Deterioration in academic, work and social functioning and self-care
  - Reduced attention and concentration
- There may be general symptoms such as the following:
  - Sleep disturbances, usually with initial insomnia
  - Irritability
  - Depressed mood
  - Poor hygiene

STATION 75: EARLY-ONSET PSYCHOSIS (PAIRED STATION B: MANAGEMENT)

Information to candidates

Name of patient: Paula

The local GP has referred Paula, as her parents feel that she has not been her usual self. They are very worried that there might be something wrong with her mental health, as her grades have been declining, and she is also reluctant to go to school. You assessed her in the previous station and performed a mental state examination.

Task

Please speak to Dr Cullen and discuss the differential diagnosis and your management plans for the patient.

Outline of station

You are Dr Cullen, the child psychiatrist on call. You understand that your core trainee has just seen Paula. You need to know more about the case and are keen to hear from the core trainee regarding his formulation of the case. You need the trainee to tell you what possible differentials he is considering, and his management plans in accordance with the differentials that he has suggested. You need the trainee to tell you specifically how he would manage the patient in the acute setting, as well as in the long term.

CASC construct table

The CASC construct table is formatted such that candidates will be able to cover adequately both the range and the depth of the assessment required in this station.

Starting off: 'Hello, I am Melvyn, the on-call trainee. I have seen Paula and have performed a mental state examination of the patient. Can I present my assessment and my management plans to you?'

Summary of psychiatric formulation	I have spoken to Paula, a 17-year-old student. She has been isolating herself from school for the past 2 months, as she has been having paranoid ideations towards her fellow classmates. These ideations are of delusional intensity. She does not have any other first-rank symptoms.	She does not have any significant medical or psychiatric history that I have taken note of. She does not have any family history of any psychiatric disorder.	With regard to her mental state, she appears neat and groomed. She maintains some eye contact during the interview. Her mood is not overtly low, and her affect is appropriate. She is relevant throughout the interview. She denies any hallucinations, but she does have paranoid delusions. She denies harbouring any suicidal or homicidal ideations.
Explain differential diagnosis	Can I go on to discuss the possible differential diagnosis that I have considered?	I like to consider the possibility of her having first-episode psychosis.	My other differentials that I would like to consider and exclude are that of substance-induced psychosis as well as depression with psychotic symptoms.
Explain general management (pharmacological)	With regard to management, the necessary blood work should be done to exclude an underlying organic aetiology. In addition, a toxicology screen would be essential to exclude the possibility of this being drug-induced psychosis.	Once we have ascertained that this is indeed first-episode psychosis, based on the NICE guidelines, we could commence her on a low dose of antipsychotics. My preference would be to commence her on an atypical antipsychotic, as it is associated with lesser side effects.	An example of an antipsychotic that I would consider will be that of risperidone. I will adjust the dose of the medications in accordance to how she responds to the initiation of the medication.
Explain management (non-pharmacological)	Apart from medications, I would like to suggest other alternatives to help Paula and her family. Providing education to Paula and her family about her condition and reinforcing compliance to medications will be essential.	In addition, the family needs to be educated about the relapse indicators, so that they can bring her back for an admission if need be. At times, psychological therapy such as cognitive behavioural therapy (CBT) might be beneficial. I will closely monitor Paula's condition and will refer her to a psychologist when she is more settled in her mental state.	If there are highly expressed emotions within the family, I will recommend family therapy for the family as well.

(Continued)

Address consultant's concerns	I hope that I have adequately discussed how best we can help Paula. Are there any questions you have for me? I would like to manage Paula as an outpatient for now, as there are no risk factors that I was able to elicit. She would benefit from engagement with the early psychosis intervention team.	If she is not compliant with her medications, I would like to consider getting her more support in the community. This might involve having a community nurse doing home visitation. If she is still not compliant, I might consider speaking to the patient and the family about the commencement of a depot medication.	I am hoping she will respond to the antipsychotic we are intending to start. Should she not respond to adequate trials of both typical and atypical antipsychotics, clozapine might be an option.

Common pitfalls

a. Failure to cover the range and depth needed for the station (explain both pharmacological and non-pharmacological treatments needed).
b. Failure to discuss more about getting the first-episode psychosis team involved.
c. Failure to address adequately the concerns raised by the consultant about outpatient monitoring, administration of a depot and commencement of clozapine. It is essential to know the NICE guidelines about schizophrenia treatment to explain treatment options in this station.

Quick recall*

Recommended interventions

- There is a need for careful observation.
- It is necessary to consider other differential diagnoses, including that of organic diagnosis.
- It is necessary to exclude other common comorbidities such as substance abuse.
- It is essential to strive towards minimization of the risk of relapse.
- The aim is to eliminate the exposure to cannabis and psycho-stimulants through psycho-education and appropriate stress management and maintenance antipsychotic treatment.
- It is essential to discuss in advance treatment options such as antipsychotics and CBT.

NICE guidelines

In the United Kingdom, the NICE issued guidelines in June 2002 with respect to the prescription of atypical antipsychotics for patients with schizophrenia. They are as follows:

- The atypical antipsychotics should be considered when deciding on first-line treatment of newly diagnosed schizophrenia.

---

* Adapted from B.K. Puri, A. Hall and R. Ho (2014). *Revision Notes in Psychiatry.* London, UK: CRC Press, p. 370.

- An atypical antipsychotic is considered the treatment of choice for managing an acute schizophrenic episode when discussion with the individual is not possible.
- An atypical antipsychotic should be considered for an individual who is suffering from unacceptable side effects with a conventional antipsychotic.
- An atypical antipsychotic should be considered for an individual in relapse whose symptoms were previously inadequately controlled.
- Changing to an atypical antipsychotic is not necessary if a conventional antipsychotic controls symptoms adequately, and the individual does not suffer from unacceptable side effects.
- Clozapine should be introduced if schizophrenia is inadequately controlled despite the sequential use of two or more antipsychotics (one of which should be an atypical antipsychotic) each for at least 6–8 weeks.
- The conversion to schizophrenia has been estimated to be around 35%. Approximately, 70% of individuals diagnosed with schizophrenia achieve full remission within 3–4 months.
- Eighty per cent achieve stable remission within the course of 1 year.

STATION 76: CHILDHOOD SEXUAL ABUSE

Information to candidates

Name of patient: Annie

You are the on-call core trainee and have been called to see a 15-year-old girl in the accident and emergency department, as she has overdosed on 50 paracetamol tablets. The medics have done basic blood work for her and have started her on medical management for her overdose. During the psychiatric clinical interview, the girl, Annie, showed you a paper with the word 'rape' on it when you asked her what was her stressor recently. She also pointed out a man in the waiting area (who you know was her stepfather) when you asked who was involved.

Task

Please discuss the information you have obtained with the consultant on call. Please discuss with the consultant how you wish to manage this case.

Outline of station

The questions asked in the CASC Grid will cover the outline of this station.

CASC construct table

The CASC construct table is formatted such that candidates will be able to cover adequately both the range and the depth of the assessment required in this station.

Starting off: 'Hello, I am Melvyn, the on-call trainee. I have a patient in the emergency room, and I would like to discuss this case with you. Can I proceed?'		
Summary of the case	I have spoken to Annie, a 15-year-old girl, who has been admitted to the emergency department following an overdose on 50 paracetamol tablets.	During the clinical interview, she was not willing and forthcoming about the circumstances that led her to overdose. She eventually showed me a paper with the word 'rape' on it and pointed to her stepfather in the waiting area when I asked who was involved.	In view of the seriousness of the allegations, I had to terminate the interview at that point, so as to avoid contamination of the information obtained from the child. I have asked a nurse to be with her for now, whilst I discuss this case with you.
Explain limitations	I am not able to obtain more information about the allegation, in view of my concerns about the possible contamination of the evidence. However, I have obtained sufficient information to evaluate her current suicide risk.	In addition, in view of the seriousness of the allegations, I have informed Annie, the child involved, that there is a need for me to break confidentiality of the information.	I have clearly explained to her that I needed to share this information with my colleagues to ascertain the nature of the facts involved.
Acute management	Annie would require continued medical management given that she has just overdosed on a large number of pills. I would like to offer her admission to the inpatient child medical ward or the child psychiatric unit for further observation and monitoring.	It is clear to me that she is still distressed by the circumstances that she has been in. I will inform my nurses to place her on suicide caution and ideally, also recommend one-to-one nursing for her. I want to make an urgent referral to the social worker. In addition, I would like to inform the child protection officer from the relevant agencies and the police as well.	I have to inform her mother, as her mother has parental responsibility over Annie. I would like to briefly explain to her the current situation and advise her that a period of inpatient observation is essential in order for us to find out more about the allegation. I need to inform her mother that we need to restrict the access that her stepfather has with regard to visitation. In view of the circumstances involved, there is need for me to ascertain from the mother whether there are other vulnerable individuals currently at home and advise her accordingly.

(Continued)

Intermediate and long-term management	I hope that the on-call consultant can discuss with the lead consultant in charge of child abuse cases, and a formal interview be conducted with the child.	In the intermediate short term, the social worker or the police can offer an emergency protection order or a police protection order to ensure that the child is placed in a place of safety. If the allegations are subsequently ascertained to be true, they could help with facilitating an alternative accommodation for the child. In the event that the parents do not agree, a care order can be issued.	I would like to recommend that the child be engaged with a counsellor for counselling services to deal with the emotional issues that have arisen due to the abuse. Other modalities of psychological therapy might also be helpful for the child.

Common pitfalls

a. Failure to explain why the interview needs to be stopped once information pertaining to the sexual abuse has been shared
b. Failure to explain in depth the recommended acute, intermediate and long-term management plans

Quick recall*

- In the United Kingdom, 7% of children were rated as experiencing serious physical abuse, and 6% had serious emotional maltreatment.
- 3/1000 children are on the official child protection register for the ages between 0 and 18 years.
- Ten per cent of children have been victims of sexual abuse.
- The male-to-female ratio is approximately 1:2.5.
- Each year, 3% of children up to the age of 13 years are brought to the attention of professional agencies because of suspected abuse.
- There are four common types of abuse: physical abuse, sexual abuse, emotion abuse and neglect.
- The assessment should include all of the following:
  - Evaluate and validate the claim of abuse from the child's perspective.
  - Assess the impact of abuse on the physical and emotional condition.
  - Look for further evidence to support the claim of abuse and consistency in the child's accounts.
  - Assess cognitive and language competence of the child.
  - Identify emotional and behavioural disturbances in the child such as conduct disorder and truancy.

---

* Adapted from B.K. Puri, A. Hall and R. Ho (2014). *Revision Notes in Psychiatry.* London, UK: CRC Press, p. 653.

- Recognize the emotional, physical and therapeutic needs of a child.
- Seek the child's view on staying in a safe and protective environment (such as staying in a shelter).
- Assess family dynamics, family members involved and parental psychopathology.
- For young children, special techniques of interviewing such as drawing and using anatomically correct dolls may facilitate disclosure of sensitive information from the child's perspective.
- It is important not to ask leading questions as they could suggest certain answers.
- Psychiatrists should use age-appropriate language and ask one question at a time.
- After the initial assessment, a further interview may be videotaped with parental consent and permission from the child. This will avoid the child mentioning the traumatic experience repeatedly to different professionals.
- Address the dilemma whether the other family members shall be involved in the assessment of the child. Psychiatrists should always seek the child's view on this issue.
- Physical examination is key and should be carried out by an appropriately experienced paediatrician or gynaecologist.
- If abuse is indeed confirmed, the psychiatrist needs to assess the child to determine the effects of abuse, safety issues and recommend further treatment.

Management

- The safety of the child is the most important, and the psychiatrist needs to discuss with the paediatrician and the social worker to notify the authorities accordingly and to remove the child from danger.
- Recognize the physical and emotional consequences of abuse. It might lead to anxiety, guilt, psychiatric comorbidity secondary to sexual abuse, fears about disclosure and regression to an earlier developmental stage.
- It is always essential to evaluate the continuing risk to the child and the siblings.
- It is necessary to evaluate the therapeutic needs of the child and parents.
- Individual psychotherapy may help the child to overcome the symptoms of post-traumatic stress disorder and poor self-esteem.
- Family therapy may be useful to restore the roles and boundaries in family.

STATION 77: BULLYING AND OVERDOSE

Information to candidates

Name of patient: Amelia Smith

You are the core trainee on call, and you have been asked to see Amelia Smith, a 15-year-old girl, who has been brought into the accident and emergency department following a massive overdose on her mother's psychiatric medications. Her mother shared with the medical team that her daughter has been experiencing some difficulties at school. She is extremely distressed with her daughter's condition. The medical team has done the necessary blood work and stabilized her condition. You have been asked to further evaluate Amelia.

Task

Please speak to Amelia to identify her reasons for her overdose and to perform an appropriate suicide risk assessment.

Outline of station

You are Amelia, a 15-year-old girl who has just overdosed on all your mother's psychiatric medications. You come from a single-parent family, and your new school has been too much for you to handle. Because of your size, your peers in your new school have been calling you nasty names. There was an occasion in which they tried to lay hands on you after you argued with them. You have contemplated overdosing on medications for the past 2 weeks and decided to go ahead today, as you feel that life is no longer worth living, and you are too distressed by your experience in school. There is no one with whom you can share your problems, not even your mother, as she is busy working to make ends meet. You're willing to share the circumstances with the doctor, but you do not feel that sharing with the psychiatrist would help matters at school.

CASC construct table

The CASC construct table is formatted such that candidates will be able to cover adequately both the range and the depth of the assessment required in this station.

Starting off: 'Hello, I am Dr Melvyn, one of the psychiatrists from the mental health unit. I have some information about why you have been admitted to the hospital. Can we have a chat about it?'			
Exploration of current attempts	I understand from the medical doctor that you have been admitted to the hospital following an overdose. I am sorry to hear that. It seems that things have been difficult for you. Can you take me through what has happened today? How long have you been thinking about overdosing? Where did you get those tablets? Did you write any last notes or letters to your loved ones before consuming all the tablets?	Can you tell me where you were when you took all those medications? Was there anyone with you? (Or) If you were at home, did you take steps to ensure that no one would discover you? Did you take all the medications at once? Did you take the medications with any other substances? What was running through your mind when you took those tablets? Did you have thoughts of ending it all? How dangerous did you think taking that amount of medications would be? How did you feel after taking all the medications? How were you discovered? Who brought you to the hospital?	Now that you are in hospital, do you regret that your overdose attempt was not successful? (Or) Are you remorseful about what you have done?
Exploration of underlying stressors	I understand that it has been a very difficult time for you. Can you share with me more about what has been bothering you?	(Or) Can you tell me about what sort of things you have been bothered by? How have things been at home, in school or at work?	Do you have any relationship issues?

(Continued)

In-depth exploration of core stressors	I'm sorry to hear about the issues that have been troubling you. Can you tell me more about it?	What have they done towards you? Have they called you names? Have they been physical against you? Have they done other things to cause you emotional hurt, such as spreading rumours about you?	How long has this been going on for you? Did you manage to share with anyone more about this?
Other psychiatric comorbid	Has this affected your mood in any way? Are you still interested in things you used to enjoy?	How have you been sleeping and eating?	Are you frequently bothered by flashbacks of the events that happened? Are you bothered by nightmares in your sleep? Do you avoid school? Would you say that you have been feeling more on edge recently?
Risk assessment and coping mechanisms	Are you feeling so troubled that you have entertained thoughts of ending your life? What plans have you made?	I understand that this must be a difficult time for you. How have you been coping?	Have you made use of any substances, such as alcohol, to help you cope? What about street drugs?

Common pitfalls

a. Failure to perform a comprehensive suicide risk assessment
b. Forgetting to ask about emotional bullying apart from verbal and physical bullying

Quick recall*

- The rate of attempted suicide is noted to be around 8%–9% of individuals in Western countries.
- The rate of suicidal ideations is 15%–20%.
- Suicide is common amongst young people at an age between 14 and 16 years.
- The male-to-female ratio for self-harm is 1:6.
- The male-to-female ratio for suicide is 4:1.
- Suicide is the third most common cause of death for young people after accident and homicide.
- Self-harm is the most common cause of admission to a general hospital.

---

* Adapted from B.K. Puri, A. Hall and R. Ho (2014). *Revision Notes in Psychiatry*. London, UK: CRC Press, p. 370.

Aetiology

- Due to the presence of underlying psychiatric disorders such as depression, psychosis, substance abuse, conduct disorder, isolation, low self-esteem and physical illness.
- For girls, self-harm is strongly predicted by depressive disorder. For boys, self-harm is strongly predicted by previous suicide attempts.

The increase in adolescence suicide is likely due to the following:

- Factors influencing reporting (copycat suicide as a result of media coverage, the fostering of illusions and ideals through Internet suicide groups and pop culture).
- Factors influencing the incidence of psychiatric problems (problems with identity formation, depression, substance abuse and teenage pregnancy).
- Social factors (such as bullying, the impact of unemployment for older adolescents, living away from home, migration, parental separation and divorce).

Common self-harm and suicide methods:

- Self-harm: Cutting and scratching are common impulsive gestures. Cutting often has a dysphoric effect.
- Suicide: Self-poisoning is a common method used by British adolescents.

Management of self-harm and suicide (NICE guidelines)
It is important to offer physical treatment with adequate anaesthesia. There should not be any delays in terms of psychosocial assessment. It is mandatory to explain the care process. For those who repeatedly self-poison, one should not offer minimization advice on self-poisoning because there is no safe limit. For those who self-injure repeatedly, it is essential to teach self-management strategies on superficial injuries, harm minimization techniques and alternative coping strategies.

Management of suicidal adolescent
It is essential to consider inpatient treatment after balancing the benefits against loss of family support. It is necessary to involve the young person in the admission process. Electroconvulsive therapy (ECT) may be used in adolescents with very severe depression and suicidal behaviour not responding to other treatments.

- With regard to prognosis, for those who self-harm, approximately 10% of them will repeat in 1 year. The risk of repetition is higher especially in older male adolescents, those with a history of suicide attempts, those with persistent suicidal ideations, psychotic symptoms, substance misuse and use of methods other than overdose or self-laceration.
- For suicide, 4% of girls and 11% of boys will kill themselves in 5 years after the first episode of suicide attempt.

STATION 78: ENURESIS

Information to candidates

Name of patient: Joseph

Joseph is a 7-year-old male who has just started school. Sarah, Joseph's mother, has recently received feedback from his teachers that his academic performance in school is poor. Sarah has noted that over the past month, there were many nights during which Joseph wet his bed. She is increasingly concerned about this. She has brought Joseph for an evaluation by the local GP, who has referred him to see you.

Task

Please speak to Sarah, Joseph's mother, and elicit more history about the current presenting problem, with the aim of establishing and arriving at a diagnosis.

Outline of station

You are Sarah, Joseph's mother, and you are quite concerned about your son's condition. He has just recently started school, and you have already received feedback from his teachers that his performance in school is poor. You are trying your best to tutor him at home but to no avail. You cannot afford to hire a private tutor for Joseph. In addition, you noticed that over the past month, there were many nights during which Joseph wet the bed. You are very concerned about this and have decided to seek help from your local GP. Your local GP feels that there might be an underlying mental health issue and hence has referred you to see the child psychiatrist.

CASC construct table

The CASC construct table is formatted such that candidates will be able to cover adequately both the range and the depth of the assessment required in this station.

Starting off: 'Hello, I am Dr Melvyn, one of the psychiatrists from the mental health unit. I received some information from your GP about Joseph. I understand you have some concerns. Can we have a chat about it?'			
History of current presenting problem	Can you tell me more about your concerns? Thanks for sharing with me. I understand that it must be a difficult time for you as a parent.	Can you tell me roughly when you first noticed that Joseph has been wetting his bed? How has this problem progressed over the past month or so?	How often has Joseph been wetting his bed in the past week or so?
Clarifying history of enuresis	With regard to your current concern, can I check with you whether this is the first time such a problem has occurred? Has he had similar issues in the past?	So it seems like it has just started over the past month and has been progressively increasing in frequency. Is he able to stay dry in the day? Have you received any feedback from his teachers regarding this?	Does Joseph have other problems, such as him having difficulties with bowel movement? What do you do if you find out that Joseph has wet the bed? How do you usually react? How does he feel about you finding out? What does he say?

(Continued)

Identification of stressors	Do you have other worries for Joseph? Can you tell me more?	Apart from the concern about schoolwork and his poor performance in school, is there anything else you think might be bothering Joseph?	How have things been at home? Have there been any recent changes in the home environment? How is his relationship with yourself and the rest of the family?
Identification of other comorbid psychiatric conditions	Over the past 2 weeks or so, how do you think Joseph's mood has been? Is he still able to keep up with things that he used to enjoy? Does he seem to be more anxious than usual?	How has his sleep been? How has his appetite been?	Are there problems with him going to school? Does he refuse to go school? Has Joseph been seen by a psychiatrist before?
Developmental history	Can you tell me more about his development? Was the pregnancy normal? Was the delivery normal?	Were there any issues in the early years? Did the doctors pick up any developmental delays?	Have you noted that he used to be achieving his milestones much slower than the other children? Were there any previous issues with potty training?
Rule out medical comorbid	I understand that the GP has seen him before referring him to our service. Do you know if blood tests as well as urine analysis were done?	Does Joseph have any underlying chronic medical conditions that I need to know of? (If he does have) Can I know the medications that he is on at the moment? Have there been any changes to his medications recently?	Has Joseph been complaining of any difficulties with urination? Have you noticed that he needs to go to the toilet frequently? Does his urine smell foul? (If there is an underlying history of seizure) Can I know when he has had his last fit? What kind of fits does he usually have? Does he lose consciousness?

Common pitfalls

a. Failure to cover the range and depth of the station (there is a need to take a developmental history and exclude other possible medical comorbidities in this station)

Quick recall*

- In accordance with *ICD-10*, nonorganic enuresis is characterized by the involuntary voiding of urine, by day and/or by night, which is abnormal in relation to the individual's mental age and which is not a consequence of a lack of bladder control resulting from any neurological disorder, epilepsy or a structural urinary tract abnormality.

---

* Adapted from B.K. Puri, A. Hall and R. Ho (2014). *Revision Notes in Psychiatry*. London, UK: CRC Press, p. 642.

- The minimum duration of enuresis is 3 months. It is usually not diagnosed before the age of 5 years and may be subdivided into (1) primary: urinary continence never achieved and (2) secondary: urinary continence has been achieved in the past.
- The *DSM-5* criteria are similar to *ICD-10* and further subdivide enuresis into (1) nocturnal only: passage of urine only during night time sleep, (2) diurnal only: passage of urine during waking and (3) nocturnal and diurnal: a combination of both subtypes.
- The prevalence of nonorganic enuresis at different ages has been found to be 7 years – 6.7% in boys and 3.3% in girls, 9–10 years – 2.9% in boys and 2.2% in girls and 14 years – 1.1% in boys and 0.5% in girls.
- At the age of 5 years, the male-to-female ratio is the same. However, it reaches approximately 2:1 in teenage years.
- The following possible cause of this underlying condition has been proposed:
  - Genetics: Approximately 70% of children have at least one first-degree relative with late attainment of continence.
  - Stressful environment and life events, which might result in a doubling of the normal frequency.
  - Delayed in toilet training.
  - Developmental delay.
  - Abnormalities of bladder structure: Children diagnosed with this condition usually have a different shape of bladder baseplate as well as a reduction in functional bladder volume.

Management

- A full assessment that includes a physical assessment is essential. It is necessary to exclude a physical cause.
- Urinary microscopy and microbiological analysis should be ordered and sent for analysis.
- Urodynamic studies should be considered if the patient is older than 15 years of age.
- There should be a period of observation. Measures such as fluid restriction could be taken.
- Star charts could be used. The relapse rate has been noted to be approximately 40%.
- Pad and buzzer could be used; in older children, a pants alarm. The relapse rate has been approximately 40%.
- If pharmacological treatment is needed, low-dose tricyclic antidepressants could be initiated. However, it is noted that there are side effects, and there is a high rate of relapse on discontinuation. Nasal desmopressin could be recommended but should not be continued for more than 3 months without stopping for a week.
- Exercises are helpful to increase the functional capacity of the bladder.
- Habit training can be done.
- With regard to prognosis, the course is generally good.

STATION 79: ELECTIVE MUTISM

Information to candidates

Name of patient: Shane

The local GP has referred Shane to your service for further assessment. She has just started school in the past month, and the teachers have reported that she has been refusing to speak in school. She is noted to be totally mute and does not answer anyone in school. This behaviour of Shane is strange as she is able to communicate without any issues at home. You have assessed Shane, and she is also reluctant to speak to you. Her mother, Mrs Parker, is here and hopes to find out more from you.

Task

Please speak to Mrs Parker and explain the current assessment as well as your management. Please address all her concerns and expectations.

Outline of station

You are Mrs Parker, the mother of Shane. You have received feedback from the teachers informing you that Shane has been totally mute at school. You are quite surprised by this, as she is able to communicate normally at home. You have asked her why she is mute at school, but she becomes teary and refuses to say anything. You are quite concerned as to whether there is anything wrong with her. You have sought help from your GP, who has recommended that she sees a child psychiatrist. You understand from the assessment conducted by the child psychiatrist that she was mute throughout the interview as well. You are anxious and wish to understand what is wrong with your child and how the psychiatrist can help you with her sudden change in behaviour.

CASC construct table

The CASC construct table is formatted such that candidates will be able to cover adequately both the range and the depth of the assessment required in this station.

Starting off: 'Hello, I am Dr Melvyn, one of the psychiatrists from the mental health unit. I received some information from your GP about Shane and have assessed her. I understand you have some concerns. Can we have a chat about it?'			
Explain assessment and information needed	Thanks for sharing with me your concerns. The information you shared with me with regard to the onset of the behavioural changes is essential in helping us to formulate the diagnosis.	In addition to the information you have provided, we might also need additional information from your GP, as well as from the school. Would that be fine with you? At times, we also request a formal school report. Is that fine with you?	Do you know if any educational psychologist has seen Shane in the school? If an educational psychologist has done so, we would like to obtain some information from her regarding her assessment of Shane. In addition, I would like to find out whether there have been any other problems at school. Do you know whether she has been bullied at school? How have things been at home? Have there been any changes in the home environment? How does she communicate at home?

(Continued)

Obtain developmental history	I have seen Shane in my clinic previously, but she is not willing to share much. I hope you can share with me more about her development in her younger years to help me understand Shane better.	Can I ask whether there were any problems whilst you were having Shane? Were there any problems with the delivery and thereafter?	Can I check whether Shane met all her developmental milestones? Did any doctor inform you that Shane is developing slower as compared to normal children? Did Shane ever have any serious childhood infection that required prolonged hospitalization? Does Shane have any chronic medical issues that I need to know of? Is she on any chronic medications?
Discuss possible differential diagnosis	Once we have gathered more information from the school, and taking into account the information you have shared with us, we will have a better idea of the likely underlying condition causing this.	For now, it seems that what Shane is having is what is known as elective mutism. Have you heard of this before?	The other conditions I would like to consider might be those of emotional disorders and natural shyness.
Explain investigations	We would like to suggest further investigations to determine the exact cause of the condition. As a baseline, we need to conduct a physical and neurological examination.	Psychometric testing must be beneficial. As the problems are confined to the school environment, assessment by an educational psychologist will be essential. We would like to suggest conducting a school visit to observe her interaction in the school setting.	We will also consider referring her for further speech and language assessment to determine whether she has underlying speech or language problems accounting for her not speaking in school.
Explain treatment	The modality of treatment depends on the exact cause of her problems. If she is selectively not speaking only in the school setting, we might need the psychologist to make use of behavioural methods to address this issue. In behavioural therapy, positive behaviours such as talking are being rewarded in the school setting, and this will reinforce the positive behaviour.	If there are underlying speech or hearing abnormalities, appropriate interventions can be conducted, such as speech therapy.	
Explain prognosis	The prognosis for the condition is usually good.		

Common pitfalls

a. Failure to explain that more information needs to be obtained prior to the formulation of a diagnosis

Quick recall*

- Elective mutism usually occurs in early childhood with a peak age of around 6–10 years.
- There is no noted difference in the gender ratio.
- The prevalence is usually around 0.8 per 1000 children.
- The common causes include (1) overprotection by family members, especially mother, (2) distant father figure and (3) trauma.
- According to the *ICD-10*, it is characterized by a marked, emotionally determined selectivity in speaking, such that the child demonstrates language competence in some situations but fails to speak in other situations. The duration of symptoms needs to last for 4 weeks.
- This condition tends to be associated with personality factors such as (1) social anxiety, (2) withdrawal, (3) sensitivity and (4) resistance.
- The common management approaches include (1) exclusion of any underlying speech abnormalities, (2) behavioural approaches, (3) play therapy, (4) art therapy and (5) family therapy.
- With regard to prognosis: In the long term, the prognosis is good, unless there are other conditions that are also present.
- Poor prognosis is usually associated with having the presence of the disorder for longer than 12 months.

---

* Adapted from B.K. Puri, A. Hall and R. Ho (2014). *Revision Notes in Psychiatry*. London, UK: CRC Press, p. 639.

STATION 80: LEARNING DISABILITY WITH CHALLENGING BEHAVIOUR: HISTORY TAKING

Information to candidates

Name of patient: David

David has severe learning disability and has been staying in a residential home for the past 2 years. The manager of the home, Mr Thomas, called the outpatient clinic, urgently requesting an appointment to see you, the learning disability service psychiatrist, as soon as possible. In view of the urgency of the referral, an appointment was made to see you. Mr Thomas mentioned during the clinic consultation that David has seemed like a changed person for the past 2 weeks. His nursing staff in the home is finding it tremendously difficult to cope with his challenging behaviours. Mr Thomas hopes that you can help him with his current situation, as he has not previously noted David to have such abnormal behaviours since he has been with them.

Task

Please speak to Mr Thomas with the aim of getting more history and to identify a likely cause for the changes in behaviour. Please make use of the available time to explain to Mr Thomas the most likely reasons for the drastic changes in behaviour.

Outline of station

The purpose of providing an outline of the station is to allow candidates to be familiar with the structure of the station. This outline could also be helpful when candidates practice for the MRCPsych, joining with their colleagues to act out the station.

Please note that the outlines provided are based on the experiences of the authors. There may be variations in the actual examination.

You are Mr Thomas, the manager of the home. David has been a resident in the home for the past 2 years. Your staff has noticed a dramatic change in David's behaviour over the past 2 weeks. At times David seems to be very irritable, and at times he refuses his meals as well as his medications. He has been refusing to participate in the usual activities that he used to enjoy. Your staff has been finding it a struggle to help

David with his behaviour and have related this to you. You are at your wit's end, and hence you need to arrange an appointment with the psychiatrist as soon as possible, as you hope that some medications will help fix the problem. You do know that David has a history of seizures and has seen the neurologist recently and was continued on the same dose of the medications for his seizures. He has been complaining recently of pain during urination. There have not been other complaints. There have not been any other changes to the schedule of activities at the nursing home.

CASC construct table

The CASC construct table is formatted such that candidates will be able to cover adequately both the range and the depth of the assessment required in this station.

Starting off: 'Hello, I am Dr Melvyn, one of the psychiatrists from the mental health unit. I understand that you have requested for us to see David as early as possible, as there have been increasing difficulties managing him in the nursing home. Can you tell me more about this?'			
Clarification of the history of presenting symptoms	I'm sorry to hear that it has been a difficult and challenging time for you and your staff. I would like to try to understand the situation better, so that we can help David.	Can you tell me when these changes in David's behaviour began? How was David before these all began? Can you tell me more about his difficult behaviours? What does he do? Are there times in which he is aggressive?	When David has these challenging behaviours, how do your nurses handle him? Does he require any additional doses of medications to calm him down? Has something like this happened before?
Consider and exclude mood disorders and psychosis	Can you tell me how has David's mood been? Does he seem to be very irritable or tearful at times? Is he still able to enjoy things he used to enjoy doing?	How has his sleep been? How has his appetite been?	Are there times in which he seems preoccupied? Are there times in which he seems to be responding to voices or some other external stimuli? How has he been getting on with the rest of the residents in the home?
Consider and exclude medical disorders	Can you share with me whether he has other underlying medical conditions that I need to know of? (Or) Is he on any long-term medications that I need to know of? Have there been any recent changes in his medications?	Has he been ill recently? Can you tell me more about his recent illness? Did he seek any medical help for his recent illness?	

(Continued)

Consider and exclude changes in the environment	Can you share with me whether there have been any changes in your home environment?	Have there been any new nursing staff in your home? Have there been any new residents in the home?	Do you know whether David's parents have visited him recently? Have they provided any inputs about his behaviour?
Psycho-education about reasons for behavioural change	Thanks for sharing with me your concerns. I have a better understanding of the problem. It seems to me that there might be a variety of reasons as to why David has a change in behaviour.	I am concerned that there have been some changes in the environment that he is placed in. In addition, I am concerned that there are changes in the doses of the medications that he has been using for his epilepsy condition.	I need to discuss David's case with my consultant to see how best we can help you. Do you have any other questions for me?

Common pitfalls

a. Failure to explore the possibility of other physical conditions causing the changes in behaviour.
b. Failure to explore the possibility of changes in the environment resulting in behavioural changes.

Quick recall*

- The *International Statistical Classification of Diseases and Related Health Problems,* 10th revision (*ICD-10*) classification of mental disability
- Mild mental retardation: The intelligence quotient (IQ) is in the range of 50–69; 85% of all have learning disability. There is delayed understanding and usage of language. There are possible difficulties in gaining independence. Work is possible in practical occupations. Any noted behavioural, social and emotional difficulties are similar to the normal.
- Moderate mental retardation: The intelligence quotient is in the range of 35–49. It accounts for 10% of all learning disability. There are varying profiles of abilities. Language usage and development can be variable. It is often associated with epilepsy and neurological and other disabilities. There is a delay in achievement of self-care. Simple practical work is possible. Independent living is rarely achieved.
- Severe mental retardation: The intelligence quotient is in the range of 20–34. It accounts for 3% of all learning disability. There are more marked impairments, and achievements tend to be at the lower end.

---

* Adapted from B.K. Puri, A. Hall and R. Ho (2014). *Revision Notes in Psychiatry.* London, UK: CRC Press, p. 663.

- Profound mental retardation: Intelligence quotient can be difficult to measure but is usually less than 20. It accounts for 2% of all learning disability. There are severe limitations in ability to understand and comply with requests or instructions. Individuals usually are capable of little or no self-care. There is severe mobility restriction and basic or simple tasks may be acquired.
- The *Diagnostic and Statistical Manual of Mental Disorders,* 5th edition (*DSM-5*) adopts similar classification. For mild mental retardation, the individual is still able to maintain age-appropriate personal care. For moderate mental retardation, an extended period of teaching and time is needed to teach the patient to become independent. For severe mental retardation, they may require full support for basic activities of daily living. For profound mental retardation, they are dependent on other people for daily living.
- The usual onset age is prior to the age of 18 years.
- The prevalence of learning disability, defined as having an intelligence quotient of less than 70, has been around 3.7%, which is higher than what would be expected based on a normal distribution of IQ scores.
- The prevalence of self-injurious behaviours amongst people with learning disability is between 20%–50%. The peak age of self-harm is between 15 and 20 years and is much higher in males.

Severely challenging behaviour

1. The intensity and the frequency of certain behaviour would place the patient at an increased risk.
2. This would also imply that there will be restrictions with regard to the individual's usage of common community resources.

Medications

1. Mood stabilizer: Carbamazepine is usually considered to be useful in the treatment of episodic destructive behaviour. Valproate could be used to reduce aggression as well. Lithium is helpful to reduce aggression and self-injurious behaviour.
2. Beta-adrenergic receptor antagonists: Propranolol can help to reduce the explosive rages.
3. Behavioural therapy: It can help to shape social behaviours and reduce destructive behaviour.
4. Opiate antagonist: Naltrexone is used for those individuals with self-injury.

STATION 81: DEMENTIA IN DOWN'S SYNDROME – HISTORY

Information to candidates

Name of patient: Joseph

The local general practitioner (GP) has referred Joseph to the learning disability service. His brother, Thomas, previously brought him for an assessment with their local GP, as Thomas has been very concerned about Joseph's declining memory and his need for more assistance in his daily activities. Joseph has been previously diagnosed with mild learning disability and has been able to work previously in a sheltered workshop up until 1 year ago.

Task

Please speak to Thomas, the brother of Joseph, to obtain further history to arrive at a diagnosis. Please also perform an appropriate risk assessment based on the history and the diagnosis you are suspecting.

Outline of station

You are Thomas, the brother of Joseph. Joseph was diagnosed with mild learning disability at the age of 8 years. He is capable of independent living and previously even managed to sustain a job at the local handicraft workshop, up until last year. He was dismissed from his job due to his poor work performance. Over the past year, you have been noticing that Joseph is no longer his usual self. He has been having progressive difficulties with his short-term memory. His long-term memory is still intact. At times, he does seem to be confused about the day and the dates as well. He is having more difficulty finding the right words to say at the right time. He also requires more assistance in terms of daily living, especially in the area of finances. You are also particularly concerned about the risks involved when he is alone at home. There was an occasion during which he actually forgot to switch off the gas. You are hoping that by speaking to the psychiatrist today, you can gain some clue as to what is going wrong for Joseph.

CASC construct table

The CASC construct table is formatted such that candidates will be able to cover adequately both the range and the depth of the assessment required in this station.

Starting off: 'Hello, I am Dr Melvyn, one of the psychiatrists from the mental health unit. I understand that the GP has referred your brother to see us soon, as you have some concerns. Can we have a chat about it?'			
Clarification about the presenting complaint	I understand that you have brought your brother to see the GP in view of your concerns about his memory difficulties. Can you tell me more?	Can you tell me when these memory difficulties first started? (Or) How long have there been difficulties with his memory?	How have things been recently? I'm sorry to hear that things have been worsening. It must be a very difficult time for you.
Exploration of memory difficulties	Have there been any problems with his short-term memory? By that I mean are there times in which he misplaces things? Have there been times in which he forgets his meal?	What about his memories of things in the past? Can he still remember things that have happened years ago?	Would you say that his memory is progressively getting worse, since the time in which it first started?

(Continued)

Exploration of orientation and visuo-spatial dysfunction	Does he seem to muddle up the day and the dates in a week?	Have there been times in which you noticed that he seemed to be very confused?	Is he able to recognize loved ones? What about distant relatives that he hardly meets?
Exploration of language, communication and recognition difficulties	Have there been times in which he has difficulties finding the right words in a conversation?	Are there times in which he seems to have great difficulties with understanding a normal conversation?	Is he able to recognize and identify everyday objects? Can he find the right words to name those objects?
Exploration of functioning	Is he still able to manage himself? Can you tell me more about the difficulties that he has been having?	Does he require additional help with any of the following? • Finances • Shopping • Food preparation • Transportation	Does he need additional help with any of the following? • Dressing • Washing • Toileting • Ambulation
Assessment of other psychiatric disorders	How has his mood been recently? Is he still able to enjoy the things that he used to enjoy?	How has his sleep been? How has his appetite been?	Have you noticed whether he has any abnormal behaviour?
Risk assessment	Have there been any other concerns with regard to his behaviour of late?	Has he been aggressive verbally or physical at home? Has he accidentally hurt himself recently?	Has he wandered out of the house previously? Has he done anything dangerous at home recently? Thanks for sharing with me your concerns.

Common pitfalls

a. Failure to cover the range and depth of the information necessary to make a diagnosis of dementia
b. Failure to cover a comprehensive risk assessment

Quick recall*

- Down's syndrome is the most common cytogenic cause of learning disability.
- It accounts for 30% of all children with mental retardation. The prevalence is estimated to be 1 in 800 live births if the mother is younger than the age of 30 years, and 1 in 80 if the mother is older than 40 years old.
- Approximately 94% of the cases are caused by meiotic non-disjunction, or the trisomy 21 (47 chromosomes); 5% of the cases are caused by translocation,

---

* Adapted from B.K. Puri, A. Hall and R. Ho (2014). *Revision Notes in Psychiatry*. London, UK: CRC Press, p. 663.

which refers to a fusion between chromosomes 21 and 14 (46 chromosomes); 1% of the cases are caused by mosaicism, which refers to the non-disjunction that occurs after fertilization in any cell division.

- Screening for Down's syndrome: Maternal serum markers at 16 weeks of gestation showed raised human chorionic gonadotropin (HCG), lowered alpha-foetoprotein and lowered unconjugated estriol.
- Intelligence: The IQ of people with Down's syndrome is between 40 and 55. IQ of less than 50 is present in approximately 85% of the cases. Verbal processing skills are usually better than auditory processing skills. Social skills are more advanced than intellectual skills.
- Growth: People with Down's syndrome have stunted growth, with an average height of 141 cm in females and 151 cm in men.
- Behavioural features: They tend to be passive and affable. They might be obsessional and stubborn. Twenty-five per cent of them have associated hyperkinetic disorder.
- It should be noted that these individuals are particularly predisposed to a higher risk of developing Alzheimer's disease. The incidence for those between 50 and 59 years old is around 36%–40% and for those between 60 and 69 years old is 55%. Over the age of 40 years, there is a high incidence of neurofibrillary tangles and plaques with an increase in P300 latency.
- There might also be associated hearing loss in 50% of people with Down's syndrome.
- The immune system might be affected as well (with impairments), and thus, they are at an increased risk of developing diabetes mellitus.
- They tend to have low thyroid levels as well.
- The common associated psychiatric conditions include obsessive–compulsive disorder, depression, autism, bipolar disorder, psychosis and sleep apnoea.
- The average life expectancy of people with Down's syndrome is between 58 and 66 years.
- The most common cause of death is chest infection.

STATION 82: DEPRESSION IN LEARNING DISABILITY

Information to candidates

Name of patient: Mr Brian Smith

The local GP has referred Mr Brian Smith, a man previously diagnosed with mild learning disability, to your specialist outpatient service. His family members have noticed that over the past month, he has been increasingly withdrawn and low in mood.

Task

Please speak to Mr Smith and elicit features of depression. Please also perform an appropriate risk assessment.

Outline of station

You are Mr Brian Smith, and your family has asked to come to see the psychiatrist. Over the past month, you have been having low mood. You used to be able to work in the nearby store, owned by your family, doing simple chores, but over the past month you find yourself having no energy for work at all. You find it tough to go to sleep at night, and you have not much appetite as well. You have lost a significant amount of weight over the past month. You do not have any suicidal ideations.

CASC construct table

The CASC construct table is formatted such that candidates will be able to cover adequately both the range and the depth of the assessment required in this station.

Starting off: 'Hello, I am Dr Melvyn, one of the psychiatrists from the mental health unit. I understand that the GP has referred you to see us today. Can we have a chat?'			
History of presenting complaint	I understand that you have been having some difficulties lately. Can you please tell me more?	I'm sorry to hear about all these. How long have you been troubled by these difficulties?	(Or) Do you know when all these difficulties first started? Do you feel that things are worsening?
Core clinical features of depression	How has your mood been recently?	You mentioned that your mood has not been good. Have you been more emotional and been crying more recently? If I were to ask you to rate your mood on a scale from 1 to 10, where 1 is low and 10 is happy, what number would you give your mood?	What are your hobbies? Have you been able to enjoy things you used to enjoy? Do you find that you have lost interest in things you previously liked to do?
Biological symptoms of depression	How has your energy been? Do you feel that you don't have the energy even to do everything things?	How has your sleep been? Do you wake up earlier in the morning?	How has your appetite been? Do you find that you have lost a lot of weight recently?
Other depressive features	Can you watch a television program?	How confident do you feel in yourself? Do you feel that you're as good as others?	Do you feel that you have done something wrong? Do you blame yourself for anything? I understand that this has been a very stressful time for you. Have you had any unusual experiences when stressed? Such as hearing voices?

(Continued)

Risk assessment	Do you feel that life is no longer worth living? Do you feel that you are better off dead?	Have you had thoughts of ending your life? Have you made any plans?	Thanks for sharing and for speaking to me.

Common pitfalls

a. Failure to communicate effectively and to tailor questions in accordance with the intelligence level of the individual

Quick recall*

Depressive disorder

- This could be easily missed during a clinical interview.
- It is important to consider the biological symptoms, such as lack of interest, changes in the activity level and changes in the appetite. The changes in the biological symptoms are more pertinent and will guide the diagnosis.
- Negative cognitions and suicide ideation are typically rare.
- Antidepressants are helpful for depression or with anxiety disorder. They can also be used to help with self-injurious behaviours. They are helpful if there are any associated obsessions and compulsions as well.
- The common antidepressants used are fluoxetine, paroxetine and sertraline.

Other psychiatric conditions associated with learning disabilities include the following:

Schizophrenia

- People with learning disability tend to have higher prevalence of schizophrenia (around 3%).
- The prevalence of schizophrenia is inversely related to the IQ score.
- Schizophrenia cannot be accurately diagnosed if the IQ is much less than 45.

Bipolar disorder

- Mania should always be differentiated from other causes of overactivity.
- For those with cyclical disorders, individualized recording schedules would be very useful.

Anxiety disorder

- Individuals with learning disabilities may present just with somatic complaints. Facial expression and physiological signs are usually more reliable in the diagnosis.
- Phobia could manifest simply as the absolute avoidance of the feared situation.

---

* Adapted from B.K. Puri, A. Hall and R. Ho (2014). *Revision Notes in Psychiatry*. London, UK: CRC Press, p. 674.

Discovery Library

Tel. 01752 439111

- For post-traumatic stress disorder (PTSD), the individual might have sudden and unexplainable changes in arousal, avoidance of certain activities, fear and the presence of pre-existing evidence of trauma.

  Attention deficit and hyperactivity

- Individuals with learning disabilities might present with attention deficits and hyperactivity.

STATION 83: TEMPORAL LOBE EPILEPSY

Information to candidates

Name of patient: Mr Johnson

The local GP has referred Mr Johnson to the emergency department. In the memo, it is stated that Mr Johnson is a 25-year-old male with a history of mild learning disability. He has been recently seen by the psychiatrist and has been started on an antidepressant known as dothiepin for his sleep and also for his mood symptoms. Since the commencement of the antidepressant, it was stated that his family has noted that Mr Johnson does behave out of the norm at times. There were times during a conversation in which he actually lost consciousness. This had never happened before. The GP is concerned and hence has urgently referred him to the emergency services for further evaluation. Mr Johnson is here with you in the emergency, with his elder brother, Thompson.

Task

Please speak to his elder brother, Thompson, to understand more about what has been happening. Please elicit more information to arrive at a possible diagnosis.

Outline of station

You are Thompson, the brother of Mr Johnson. Over the last month, you have noticed on multiple occasions that your brother does not seem the same as before. You know that your brother saw the psychiatrist 1 month ago and was started on an antidepressant for his sleep and mood symptoms. Over the course of the last month, you've noticed that he blanks out at times during a normal conversation. It starts off usually with him appearing dazed and being unresponsive to commands, and he will then lose consciousness for the next 5 minutes or so. Thereafter, he usually complains of feeling confused and sleepy. You are very concerned about the reasons accounting for this change in behaviour. Your brother does not have any other medical history of note, but there is a family history of seizure.

CASC construct table

The CASC construct table is formatted such that candidates will be able to cover adequately both the range and the depth of the assessment required in this station.

Starting off: 'Hello, I am Dr Melvyn, one of the psychiatrists from the mental health unit. I understand that the GP has referred your brother to see us today. Can we have a chat for us to understand more about his condition?'

Presenting complaint	I understand how difficult it must be for you, given your worries for your brother. I am hoping to be able to understand more from you so as to better help your brother with his condition.	Can you tell me the changes that you have noticed? When did this first begin? (Or) How long have there been these changes in behaviour?	How frequently have you been noticing such changes? Have these changes in behaviour been progressively worsening?
Pre-ictal	Can you tell me what usually happens before your brother has an episode of this abnormal behaviour?	Does he seem to stare blankly into space? Did he mention any unusual experience (visual disturbance, etc.) or sensation (epigastric) prior to the onset of the episodes?	Does he seem to be totally unresponsive to external commands? Are there any abnormal involuntary movements (e.g., uprolling of eyes, grimacing) that you have observed prior to the onset of those episodes?
Ictal phase	Can you tell me what happens then? Do you know roughly how long these episodes last?	Does he lose consciousness during those episodes?	Apart from losing consciousness, does he have any other abnormal movements during those episodes? Has he ever lost continence during these episodes?
Post-ictal phase	Can you tell me more about what happens after each episode?	Does he appear to be confused or sleepy?	Does he remember what happened during the episode itself? Does he complain of any headache?
Medical history	I understand that your brother has a history of learning disability and has just been in recent contact with his psychiatrist. Do you know whether he has been on chronic medications from the psychiatrist? Have there been any recent changes in his medications that you are aware of?	Does your brother have any underlying medical conditions that I need to know of? Is he on any other chronic medications? Does he use any other substances such as alcohol or any other drugs?	Can I check whether there is a family history of seizure? Thanks for sharing with me the above information.

Common pitfalls

a. Failure to cover the range and depth of the information required for this station

Quick recall*

- Based on the International League Against Epilepsy classification, epilepsy can be classified into partial seizures (seizures which begin locally), generalized seizures (bilaterally symmetrical without lead onset) and unclassified epileptic seizure (inadequate or incomplete data).
- The special clinical features associated with epilepsy include aura (rising epigastric sensations, déjà vu and olfactory or auditory hallucinations), autonomic signs (change in skin colour, temperature and palpitations), absence seizure (motor arrest and motionless state) and amnesia (amnesia of the entire seizure).
- The frequency of partial seizure according to neuroanatomical areas is as follows: temporal lobe epilepsy 75%, frontal lobe epilepsy 15%, parietal lobe epilepsy 5% and occipital lobe epilepsy 5%.
- Temporal lobe epilepsy: (1) predisposing factors include the presence of birth injury and infantile febrile convulsions; (2) aura might be complex and varied, presenting as lip smacking, forced thinking, visual hallucinations and tinnitus; (3) behaviour can include the presence of hyper-emotionality and hypo-sexuality.
- The other variant is frontal lobe epilepsy. It is essential to know some of the clinical features and manifestations of frontal lobe epilepsy.
- Frontal lobe epilepsy: (1) non-specific cephalic aura; (2) motor automatisms: fencing posture, aversive eye and head movement, speech arrest and bizarre vocalization (such as singing), with a duration of usually less than 5 minutes; (3) bilaterally coordinated limb movements (such as clapping); (4) contralateral clonic Jacksonian march when supplementary motor area is involved; (5) brief, frequent, dramatic, nocturnal seizures with immediate recovery. This particular form of epilepsy is often diagnosed as hysterical. Prolactin levels remain the same after frontal lobe epilepsy. Frontal lobe epilepsy is usually associated with phonation (such as speech during seizure).
- Investigation: Electroencephalogram (EEG) is normal during and after the seizure. Video telemetry further examines the very stereotyped (and thus likely epileptic) or the very non-stereotyped (and probably non-epileptic) nature of the seizure.
- Serum prolactin is another marker of a seizure activity. Serum prolactin should be taken within 20 minutes after the seizure. For a generalized seizure,

---

* Adapted from B.K. Puri, A. Hall and R. Ho (2014). *Revision Notes in Psychiatry*. London, UK: CRC Press, p. 494.

the level is around 1000. For a partial seizure, the levels are around 500. For pseudo-seizure, the levels are 0.

- Treatment: If the child is being admitted as an inpatient, regular nursing monitoring will be required. Titration of existing psychotropic medications, or switching the class of medications, can be considered.

STATION 84: LEARNING DISABILITY – STERILIZATION

Information to candidates

Name of patient: Mr John Smith

Dorothy is the mother of John Smith, a 30-year-old male who has been previously diagnosed with mild learning disability. He has been staying at a residential home, in view of the fact that Dorothy needs to work long hours to make the ends meet. Recently, Dorothy has learnt that John has had a relationship with another female member at the residential home, and the girl is currently 4 months pregnant. Dorothy has requested for an early appointment to see you as she has quite a few concerns.

Task

Please speak to Dorothy, the mother of John Smith, and address all her concerns and expectations.

Outline of station

You are Dorothy, the mother of John Smith. John was diagnosed with mild learning disability at a young age. You had a hard time raising him, coupled with the fact that your husband left home as he could not accept the fact that John has learning disability. You learnt about John having a girlfriend only 2 months ago. You are now very surprised to know that the girl is actually 4 months pregnant. You are very concerned that in view of John and his girlfriend's intellectual disabilities, the child will be removed from them by the social services. In addition, you are also doubtful whether they could parent the child. You are very worried that you might end up being the one who will have to parent the child. You are also very worried that your grandchild might have a learning disability. You wonder why individuals with learning disabilities are not sterilized. You appear extremely distressed throughout the interview.

CASC construct table

The CASC construct table is formatted such that candidates will be able to cover adequately both the range and the depth of the assessment required in this station.

Starting off: 'Hello, I am Dr Melvyn, one of the psychiatrists from the mental health unit. I understand that you have some concerns about John, your son. Can we have a chat about it?'		
History of presenting complaint	I have some understanding of what has happened. Can you share with me more what your concerns are?	I understand how difficult this must be for you. Thanks for sharing with me.	Do you know when your son first met his current girlfriend? Do you know roughly how many months into the pregnancy his girlfriend is?
Parenting of child	I understand that John has underlying mild learning disabilities. Do you recall when it was first diagnosed? Did the doctors tell you he had learning disabilities? How has he been coping ever since? Is he able to doing things independently? (Or) Does he need assistance even for very simple daily tasks? Is he currently working? If so, how is his work performance?	Do you know more about John's girlfriend? Do you know what extent of learning disabilities she has? Are you aware of how independent she is? Does she require assistance even in daily activities? Is she currently working? I hear that you have some concerns about the social services taking away your grandchild. Am I right in saying so? My understanding is that the social workers will not automatically take away the child. Usually, when the child is born, they will conduct a series of parenting assessment to determine whether your son and his girlfriend are capable of taking care of the child. There are also several programmes that your son and his girlfriend can attend during the pregnancy, to help them prepare for taking care of the baby. After birth, social services can also provide further training.	Very often, only in exceptional cases in which both parents do not have the capacity would the child be taken away for alternative care arrangements. I understand your concerns about them imposing upon you to take care of your grandson. I'm sorry to hear how difficult it was previously when you had John. Let me reassure you that the social worker would make the best arrangement in this circumstance.
Sterilization	Thanks for bringing up this issue regarding sterilization for David and his girlfriend.	Even though David and his girlfriend have mild learning disabilities, it does not necessarily mean that they cannot have children. They do have the same rights as any other human being. Moreover, sterilization is an irreversible surgical procedure and requires the consent of your son.	Only in exceptional circumstances, when there is a lack of capacity for both individuals, would a court be involved. And the decision would have to be in the best medical interest for your son.

(Continued)

| Possibility of child having learning disabilities | I hear your concerns about your grandchild having learning disabilities as well. Before I address that, can I check with you how John was diagnosed with learning disability? Is there anyone in the family with a history of learning disability, apart from John? | There are a variety of causes for learning disabilities. Inheritance in itself plays a role, but there are also many other factors in place. | Are you aware whether his girlfriend has gone for any antenatal checks? The underlying reason why this needs to be done is to facilitate the early recognition of abnormalities. |

Common pitfalls

a. Failure to cover the range and depth of the information required for this station

Quick recall*

Adapted from *Oxford Handbook of Clinical Psychiatry*:

- According to societal norms, it might be tough to acknowledge the fact that individuals diagnosed with learning disabilities can have normal sexual desires as well.
- There have been reports of many individuals with mild learning disabilities who are capable of being successful parents. In addition, studies have shown that they are also capable of being successful as parents. Most of them can provide their child with a nurturing environment with some support from the community at large.
- In this station, it is essential to understand the concerns of the mother, which accounts for the reasons as to why she is keen for sterilization of her child.
- Having a child with learning disability is something major for every family. Very often, depression sets in for the carers or the parents. The protective factors against depression might include having a good relationship with their parents, as well as having more support from relatives and friends.
- In this situation, it might be recommended for there to be early genetic testing to determine whether the child has learning disabilities. This might alleviate blame on the parents as well as the carer.
- It is essential to acknowledge that there is a tremendous burden of care on the carers. Hence, it is essential that carers are provided with access to high-quality and appropriate primary healthcare. In addition, they should be given advice and access to the appropriate resources for help.

---

* Adapted from B. K. Puri, A. Hall & R. Ho (2014). *Revision Notes in Psychiatry*. London: CRC Press, p. 494.

STATION 85: LEARNING DISABILITY – ABUSE

Information to candidates

Name of patient: Mr Charlie Brown

You have been tasked to speak to the key worker for Mr Charlie Brown, a 25-year-old male who has a history of moderate learning disability. The key worker has requested for an early consultation as he is concerned that Charlie has been increasingly withdrawn in the day centre. He used to have interest and was still able to participate in the daily activities in the day centre until 2 weeks ago.

Task

Please speak to Mr Brown's key worker to assess for the potential causes leading to his current presentation. Please obtain enough information to come to a diagnosis.

Outline of station

You are the key worker of Mr Charlie Brown. You are very concerned about the acute behavioural changes that you have noted over the past 2 weeks. You noticed that Mr Brown has been increasingly withdrawn over the past 2 weeks. This took place immediately after he went back home during the weekend with his parents. When he returned, you noticed some bruising over his bilateral arms. Charlie is not able to tell you the reasons as to why he has the bruises. You have contacted his parents to find out more information, in response to which they claimed he might have hurt himself accidentally. Charlie does have an underlying medical condition (that of epilepsy), but he has not had a seizure for the past year. Due to his degree of learning disability, he is only able to gesture to indicate his needs. Over the past 2 weeks, he has been more withdrawn and does not even gesture to indicate his needs.

CASC construct table

The CASC construct table is formatted such that candidates will be able to cover adequately both the range and the depth of the assessment required in this station.

Starting off: 'Hello, I am Dr Melvyn, one of the psychiatrists from the mental health unit. I understand that you have some concerns about Charlie, one of your residents in your home. Can we have a chat about it?'			
History of presenting complaint	I understand that you have some concerns about how Charlie has been. Can you tell me more about it?	I'm sorry to learn that. Can you kindly let me know when this first started? (Or) How long has Charlie has had these changes in behaviour?	Do you feel that the changes in behaviour are progressively worsening? (Or) Have there been further changes in his behaviour since you first noticed it?

(Continued)

Exploration of social circumstances	You mentioned that the changes first started after the outing that Charlie had with his parents. Can you share with me more about his relationship with his family?	How often is he allowed to head home and spend time with his family? Does his family visit him at the home he is currently living in?	You mentioned that you noticed some bruises the last time Charlie came back from home leave. Have you asked him about it? Have you asked his parents about the bruises?
Exploration of comorbid psychiatric symptoms	I am concerned to hear that Charlie has been more withdrawn recently. Can you tell me more? Is Charlie no longer able to enjoy activities he used to enjoy?	How has his mood been over the past 2 weeks? Have your workers in the home noticed any change in his sleep? Does Charlie seem to be having a poor appetite?	Apart from being withdrawn, are there any other abnormal behaviours that your staff has noticed? Is he more aggressive and violent in the residential home? Also, does he seem more easily startled recently?
Establishment of baseline communication and skills	In order for me to understand the problem better, I would like to know more about what Charlie was like before all this happened. My understanding is that Charlie has moderate learning disability. Am I right?	Can you tell me how Charlie usually communicates his needs? Is he able to say any words? Does he use only gestures? What activities of daily living can Charlie perform independently?	How does Charlie interact with the rest of the residents of the home? Does Charlie have any issues with any of the residents?
Exclude medical causes	Can I check whether Charlie has any underlying medical conditions that I need to know of? If so, is he on long-term chronic medications?	You mentioned that he does have epilepsy. Do you know when was the last time he had a fit? Have his medications for his epilepsy been adjusted recently?	Thanks for sharing with me. Do you have other concerns you wish to share?

Common pitfalls

a. Failure to cover the range and depth of the information required for this station

STATION 86: ALCOHOL DEPENDENCE – HISTORY TAKING (PAIRED A)

Information to candidates

Name of patient: Samuel

The local general practitioner (GP) has referred Samuel to your service. His recent blood tests done with the local GP have shown that he has a deranged liver function test. His local GP has written you a memo asking you to help evaluate his condition, as he understands that Samuel has been a chronic drinker for years.

Task

Please speak to Samuel and elicit a history to come to a diagnosis of alcohol dependence.

Outline of station

The purpose of providing an outline of the station is to allow candidates to be familiar with the structure of the station. This outline could also be helpful when candidates practice for the MRCPsych, joining with their colleagues to act out the station.

Please note that the outlines provided are based on the experiences of the authors. There may be variations in the actual examination.

You are Samuel, and you have been referred by your local GP to see the psychiatrist. You are ambivalent about attending today's appointment, but you are quite concerned to learn recently that your liver is not working well. Your local GP has told you that it might be due to the alcohol that you have been using over the years. You started drinking when you were a teenager and previously used only beer. Recently, due to stressors from work and from your relationships, you have been using more alcohol to cope. You are beginning to find that you need more to get the same effect and you need to drink to avoid having bad withdrawals. You are here to see whether the psychiatrist can help you with this drinking problem.

CASC construct table

The CASC construct table is formatted such that candidates will be able to cover adequately both the range and the depth of the assessment required in this station.

Starting off: 'Hello, I am Dr Melvyn, one of the psychiatrists from the mental health unit. I understand that your GP has referred you to our service, as he has shared some concerns about your recent liver function test. Can we have a chat?'			
History of presenting complaint	Can I understand more about what your GP has told you? Did he inform you of the possible reasons for the changes found in your blood test?	Can you share with me more about your usual drinking habits? Can you tell me when you first started to drink? What did you start drinking?	How have things changed since the time you first started drinking? Can you take me through a typical day and tell me more about your drinking patterns?
Compulsive drinking, tolerance and withdrawals	Do you find it difficult at times to control the amount of alcohol you use? How long have you been feeling this way?	Do you find that you need to drink much more to feel similar effects from alcohol you have previously consumed?	Have you missed a drink before? What would happen if you missed a drink? Do you get bad tremors if you do not drink? Have there been any episodes in which you lose consciousness or went into a fit? When was the last time this happened? Were there times in which you missed your drink and had unusual experiences?
Primacy, relief drinking, reinstatement, stereotype	Would you say that alcohol has been a priority for you? Is it far more important to get a drink compared with other commitments that you have in life?	Do you start drinking the first thing in the morning? With whom do you usually drink?	Have you tried to stop drinking previously? What happened when you attempted to stop drinking?
Complications	How has your alcohol problem affected you? How has it affected your physical health? Blackouts, fits, gastric, liver dysfunction, memory impairment, sexual dysfunction, etc.	Apart from it affecting your physical health, has it affected your work?	Has your drinking problem affected your relationships? Have you gotten into any trouble with the law because of your drinking habits?

(Continued)

| Current mental state | I understand that you have some concerns about your health and also your drinking habits. Can I check how your mood has been recently? What about your interest? Are you able to enjoy the things you used to enjoy? | How has your sleep been recently? What about your appetite? | Sometimes, when people are under stress, they do report of having unusual experiences. Have you had any unusual experiences recently? Have you been feeling recently that life is not worth living or that life is meaningless? |
| Insight and readiness for change | Do you feel that you might have a problem with alcohol? What makes you feel so? | How do you want us to help you with your alcohol problem? Any thoughts of quitting alcohol drinking? | Do you have any questions for me? |

Common pitfalls

a. Failure to cover the range and depth of the information required for this station
b. Failure to assess the complications that might have arisen from his current drinking habits
c. Failure to assess for insight and readiness for change

It is important to be familiar with Prochaska and DiClemente's stages of change.

Quick recall*

The *International Statistical Classification of Diseases and Related Health Problems,* 10th revision (*ICD-10*) criteria for alcohol dependence state the following:

- There must be three or more of the following manifestations, which should have occurred together for at least 1 month. If the manifestations persist for less than 1 month, they should have occurred together repeatedly within a 1-year period:
- There must be a strong desire or sense of compulsion to consume alcohol.
- There must be impaired capacity to control drinking in terms of its onset, termination or levels of use. Alcohol is thus often being taken in larger amounts or over a longer period than intended.
- There is persistent desire to or unsuccessful efforts to attempt to reduce or control alcohol usage.

---

* Adapted from B.K. Puri, A. Hall and R. Ho (2014). *Revision Notes in Psychiatry.* London, UK: CRC Press, p. 522.

- There must be the presence of a physiological withdrawal state characterized by feeling shaky, restless or excessively perspiring.
- There is a need for significantly increased amounts of alcohol to achieve intoxication or the desired effect or a markedly diminished effect with continued use of the same amount of alcohol.
- Important alternative pleasures or interests are being given up or reduced because of drinking or a great deal of time is being spent in activities necessary to obtain, take or recover from the effects of alcohol.
- There must be persistent alcohol use despite clear evidence of harmful consequences even though the person is actually aware of the nature and the extent of the harm.
- Specific course specifier includes currently abstinent (early, partial and full remission), currently abstinent but in a protected environment, currently on supervised maintenance or replacement regiment, currently abstinent but receiving treatment with aversive or blocking agent, currently using the substance with or without psychotic features, continuous use and episodic usage.

STATION 87: ALCOHOL DEPENDENCE – DISCUSSION (PAIRED STATION B)

Information to candidates

Name of patient: Samuel

The patient, who has been previously assessed, has been admitted to the medical ward, as he sustained a fall whilst he was out drinking. The medical team has completed their work-up for his condition, but they are hoping that the psychiatrist can review him before he is allowed home. His wife, Sarah, is here and wants to find out more about his condition.

Task

Please speak to Sarah, the wife of Samuel, and address all her concerns and expectations.

Outline of station

You are Sarah, the wife of Samuel. You are aware that he has been admitted to the hospital following a fall whilst he was intoxicated last night. You are very worried about the complications of his long-term alcohol dependence. You wish to know more about how best the addiction team here can help him with his condition. You wish to know whether there are medications and talking therapies that might be effective for him.

CASC construct table

The CASC construct table is formatted such that candidates will be able to cover adequately both the range and the depth of the assessment required in this station.

Starting off: 'Hello, I am Dr Melvyn, one of the psychiatrists from the mental health unit. I understand that you have some concerns about your husband, Mr Samuel. Can we have a chat about this?'			
Updates about current condition	I'm sorry to inform you that your husband has been admitted to the medical ward following a fall whilst he was intoxicated with alcohol.	Since he has been admitted, our medical team has worked him up, and he is stable at the moment. I would like to reassure you that they have called me to speak to your husband and you, as we understand you have some concerns about his condition.	Can you share with me more about your concerns? Can you share with me how long you have realized that your husband has a problem with alcohol?
Explanation of the complications associated with alcohol dependence	Thanks for sharing your concerns. I understand that it must be a very difficult time for you. Are you aware of the complications that might arise from long-term alcohol usage?	There are several complications that might arise as a result of long-term alcohol usage. It might cause physical health problems. Alcohol is acted upon by the liver, and very often the liver might be affected. The acute withdrawal of alcohol might also precipitate seizures or fits in some individuals.	In addition, patients with chronic alcohol dependence are also at risk for the development of other comorbid psychiatric conditions, such as depression and anxiety. Sometimes, patients with chronic alcoholism might also get into trouble with the law (such as due to drunk driving). In the long run, there is a concern that the chronic usage of alcohol might induce what is commonly known as alcoholic dementia.
Management approach	Thanks for coming down today. I hope to discuss with you several options that we could adopt to help your husband with this condition. Your continued support will determine the success of the treatment program.	There are programs such as alcohol detoxification programs that your husband might benefit from.	I would like to discuss with you some medications, talking therapies and other help that I feel might benefit your husband. Is it alright for me to move on to share this information with you?

(Continued)

Pharmacology management	In terms of medications, there are several options. If your husband is agreeable to a detoxification program, we will start him on a tapering dose of hypnotics to help him with the withdrawal symptoms.	There are other medications that have been licensed for use. There are anti-craving medications.	In addition, there are medications that would help him to maintain abstinence.
Psychological management	Apart from medications, there are other forms of therapy that might benefit him.	We could refer him to the psychologist for a talking therapy such as cognitive behavioural therapy.	At times, brief intervention such as FRAMES (Feedback, responsibility, Advice, Menu, Empathy and Self-efficacy) can also be utilized to help patients with their symptoms.
Social management	We need your continued support to help your husband be abstinent from alcohol.	In addition, we can link him up with support groups such as Alcoholics Anonymous.	
Prognosis	The good prognostic factors for the condition include having an insight into the condition.	In addition, a close network of support from family and friends promises a better prognosis.	I understand that I have shared quite a lot of information today. Can I leave you with some leaflets about what we have discussed today?

Common pitfalls

a. Failure to cover the range and depth of the information required for this station
b. Failure to discuss alternative medications apart from recommending detoxification program
c. Failure to discuss social factors such as family and GP support

Quick recall*

- For screening purposes for the outpatient, the CAGE questionnaire is commonly used. Positive answers to two or more of the four questions are indicative of problem drinking. The CAGE questionnaire includes the following:
  - Have you felt that you should cut down your drinking?
  - Have people annoyed you by speaking about your drinking?

---

* Adapted from B.K. Puri, A. Hall and R. Ho (2014). *Revision Notes in Psychiatry*. London, UK: CRC Press, p. 521.

- Have you felt guilty about your drinking?
- Have you ever needed a drink the first thing in the morning as an eye-opener?
- For patients who are in alcohol withdrawal, clinical assessment tools such as the Clinical Institute Withdrawal Assessment (CIWA) scale should be utilized in addition to conventional history taking.
- The CIWA scale is a validated 10-item scale to help to quantify the severity of the alcohol withdrawal and to monitor patients throughout the detoxification period.
- When alcohol dependence is suspected or diagnosed, it will be essential to carry out a full physical examination, as multiple bodily systems might be affected due to the long-term chronic usage of alcohol.
- In terms of investigations, blood tests, in particular, liver function tests, need to be done.
- National Institute for Health and Care Excellence (NICE) guidance on the management setting in acute alcohol withdrawal: It is important to offer admission to hospital if the person is at risk of alcohol withdrawal seizures or delirium tremens and if the patient is younger than 16 years old and in acute alcohol withdrawal. There should be consideration for admission to hospital for vulnerable people who are frail and who have cognitive impairments or multiple comorbidities.
- The score of the CIWA scale could be used as a reference to determine treatment setting. If the score of the CIWA scale is less than 10, the patient should be suitable for home treatment. However, if the score of the CIWA scale is more than 15, the patient is suitable for community or hospital treatment.
- NICE guidance on the treatment for acute alcohol withdrawal: Benzodiazepine should be considered to offer. Both diazepam and chlordiazepoxide have UK marketing authorization for the management of acute alcohol withdrawal symptoms. The alternatives to benzodiazepines include carbamazepine, which could be used in the management of alcohol-related withdrawal symptoms, but it does not have UK marketing rights. Clomethiazole can be used in the management of alcohol-related withdrawal symptoms for patients who are determined to discontinue drinking and in the inpatient setting, as it could lead to fatal respiratory depression when combined with alcohol in patients with cirrhosis. It does have UK marketing rights.
- It is essential to take into account the state of hydration as well as the nutrition of the patient. Prior to the administration of thiamine, a glucose load should be avoided as it could worsen the underlying thiamine deficiencies.
- NICE guidelines on the prevention of Wernicke's encephalopathy: (a) Thiamine should always be given to people who are at high risk of developing or with suspected Wernicke's encephalopathy, (b) indications for prophylactic oral thiamine include malnourishment, decompensated liver disease and acute withdrawal, (c) indications for prophylactic parental thiamine include malnourishment or decompensated liver disease, attendance at the emergency department and suspected Wernicke's

encephalopathy. Parental thiamine should be given for a minimum of 5 days and followed by oral thiamine.

- Prior to the commencement of pharmacological and psychological treatment to maintain abstinence, it is essential first to access the patient's readiness to change. Motivational interviewing can at times help to move the patient from the pre-contemplation stage to the contemplation stage.

Pharmacological treatments:

Disulfiram	This is an aversive agent, and the prescribing doctor has to ensure that the patient has not consumed any alcohol for at least 1 day prior to the commencement of the medication. Patients should be well motivated and be aware of the risks associated with the taking of alcohol with this agent. Efficacy depends on compliance with taking the aversive agent. It inhibits the ALDH2, thus leading to acetaldehyde accumulation after drinking alcohol and hence resulting in unpleasant side effects.
Acamprosate	This medication, in combination with counselling, may also be helpful towards maintaining abstinence. It should be initiated as soon as possible, and it should be maintained if a relapse occurs. The patient is allowed to have only one relapse whilst they are taking the medication. If there is more than one relapse, the psychiatrist should advise the patient to stop the medication. It is a *gamma*-Aminobutyric acid (GABA) agonist and glutamate antagonist. It inactivates the N-methyl-D-aspartate (NMDA) receptors and prevents the influx of calcium. This will reverse the GABA and the glutamate imbalance when abstaining from alcohol and reduce the long-lasting neuronal hyper-excitability.
Naltrexone	It is currently not licensed for usage in the United Kingdom for the treatment of alcohol dependence due to the risk of mortality after overdose and potential withdrawal. It is only used in people who are in abstinence and who are highly motivated. It functions as an opioid antagonist. Alcohol thus would become less rewarding when opioid receptors are blocked, and the individual does not experience any of the euphoric effects.

Psychological treatments:

Alcoholics Anonymous (AA): This is a self-help group which some alcoholics would find to be useful. It supports the families of alcoholics and also the teenage children of alcoholics. It offers largely a 12-step approach program, which emphasizes that addiction damages the whole person and group therapy allows peer pressure to overcome the denial and resistance common in people addicted to alcohol or other substances. The AA group usually meets two or three times per week. The strongest predictor of AA group attendance is the severity of alcohol-related problems.

The 12 steps are as follows:

- Having to admit being powerless over alcohol
- Believing that a greater power can help to restore the person back to sanity
- Agreeing to seek help from God
- Admitting to God their respective wrongs
- Asking God to remove their shortcomings
- Searching for moral inventory

- Making a list of the people who were harmed
- Direct amends to the victims
- Continuing to take personal inventory
- Seeking help through prayer and mediation
- Eventually arriving at a spiritual awakening

Other psychological therapies include the following:

- Brief intervention known as FRAMES, which stands for feedback about drinking, responsibility enforcement, advice to change, menu of alternatives, empathetic style and self-efficacy.
- Cognitive behaviour models appear to be particularly effective in relapse prevention. Such therapies include cue exposure, relapse prevention, contingency management, social skills and assertiveness training.

Prognostic factors

- Good prognostic factors include good insight, strong motivation and good social and family support.
- Relapse can be triggered by emotional stress, interpersonal conflict and social pressures.

STATION 88: EFFECTS OF ALCOHOL ON MOOD

Information to candidates

Name of patient: Mr Roger Smith

Mr Roger Smith has been referred by his local GP to your service. You note that the referral memo states that the patient has a long-standing history of alcohol consumption. He has been referred to your service today as the patient has been having 1 month's worth of low mood with fleeting suicidal ideations.

Task

Please speak to Mr Smith and obtain a brief history of his drinking habits and the impact of his habits on his mood.

Outline of station

You are Mr Smith and have visited your GP, as you have been feeling low for the past month, with reduction in interest to do things you used to enjoy. Your work performance has deteriorated, and there have been relationship issues with your wife as well. You have difficulties with sleep, and your appetite is poor. In view of your stressors, you have been coping by increasing your alcohol intake. You thought that alcohol could help you get over this difficult period. There were several occasions in which you had fleeting thoughts of hurting yourself, but you did not succumb to that. You are desperate for help and hope that the psychiatrist can help you.

CASC construct table

The CASC construct table is formatted such that candidates will be able to cover adequately both the range and the depth of the assessment required in this station.

Starting off: 'Hello, I am Dr Melvyn, one of the psychiatrists from the mental health unit. I understand that your GP has referred you to our service. Can we have a chat?'			
History of presenting complaint	I understand from the memo from my colleague that you have been feeling low in your mood and have been using alcohol to help you cope. Before we explore more about your mood, can I get a general understanding of your drinking habits?	Can you share with me more about your usual drinking habits? Can you tell me when you first started to drink? What did you start drinking?	How have things changed since the time you first started drinking? Can you take me through a typical day and tell me more about your drinking patterns?
Compulsive drinking, tolerance and withdrawals	Do you find it difficult at times to control the amount of alcohol you use? How long have you been feeling this way for?	Do you find that you need to drink much more to feel similar effects from alcohol that you have previously consumed?	Have you missed a drink before? What would happen if you miss a drink? Do you get bad tremors if you do not drink? Have there been any episodes in which you lost consciousness or went into a fit? When was the last time this happened? Were there times in which you missed your drink and had unusual experiences?
Primacy, relief drinking, reinstatement, stereotype	Would you say that alcohol has been a priority for you? Is it far more important to get a drink compared with other commitments that you have in life?	Do you start drinking the first thing in the morning? With whom do you usually drink?	Have you tried to stop drinking previously? What happened when you attempted to stop drinking?
Complications	How has your alcohol problem affected you?	Apart from it affecting your physical health, has it affected your work?	Has your drinking problem affected your relationships? Have you got into any trouble with the law because of your drinking habits?

(Continued)

Assessment of depressive symptoms	Thanks for sharing with me your drinking history and habits. I would like to understand more about your mood. Can I check how your mood has been recently? Does your mood vary across the day? What about your interest? Are you able to enjoy the things you used to enjoy?	How has your sleep been recently? What about your appetite? How has your energy levels been? Are you still able to keep up with your routine daily chores? Have you made mistakes at work recently? How do you find your attention and concentration to be like?	Sometimes, when people are under stress, they do report having unusual experiences. Have you had any unusual experiences recently? Have you had experiences in which you feel extremely guilty?
Risk assessment	Are there times in which you find that life no longer has a meaning for you?	Have you felt that life is not worth living?	Do you have any plans to do anything to end your life?

Common pitfalls

a. Failure to cover the range and depth of the information required for this station
b. There are two parts to the task, and hence candidates must allocate sufficient time for both tasks
c. It is crucial to perform a risk assessment in a patient who is depressed, and this should not be neglected

Quick recall*

- It has been noted that chronic heavy drinking can produce severe, usually transient depressive symptoms, which generally clear up if drinking is stopped. If symptoms persist with abstinence, antidepressants should be considered and commenced.
- The suicide rate has been estimated to be at least 50 times higher in those who drink compared with that of the general population.
- Approximately one-fourth to one-third of completed suicides happen to those who drink, and up to four-fifths of those who kill themselves have been drinking prior.
- Other psychiatric conditions closely associated with alcohol include alcoholic dementia, pathological jealousy, personality disorder, neurotic disorder, and sleep disturbances as well as psychosexual disorders.

---

* Adapted from B.K. Puri, A. Hall and R. Ho (2014). *Revision Notes in Psychiatry*. London, UK: CRC Press, p. 518.

- Alcoholic dementia: It has been demonstrated that those who have abused alcohol for some years commonly suffer from mild-to-moderate cognitive impairments, which may improve with stopping the usage of alcohol. Women, who are more prone to suffer physical complications of alcohol abuse earlier than men, also do develop cognitive impairments much earlier.
- Pathological jealousy: Previous research has demonstrated its correlation with that of alcoholism.
- Personality disorder: Personality disorders could be a predisposing factor towards alcohol abuse; but alcohol abuse in itself could lead individuals to engage in antisocial activities as well. Hence, the correlation between the onset of the disorder and the timing of onset of the alcoholism does matter. Two types of alcoholism have been described by Cloninger (1987). Type 1 is generally less severe and occurs in men and women of adult onset (older than 25 years), independent, anxious, rigid and those whose biological parents may have a mild adult-onset alcohol problem. Type 1 drinkers have a greater ability to abstain from alcohol. Type 2 is generally severe and usually of early onset (less than 25 years of age). It usually occurs in men who are socially detached and confident and whose biological fathers often have teenage-onset alcoholism and criminality. This particular type has been proposed by some to be due to underlying sociopathic personality disorder.
- Neurotic disorders: The disorder in itself may predispose individuals towards alcoholism, as patients might make use of alcohol to self-medicate. Generalized anxiety disorder, anxiety disorders such as panic attack, phobic disorders and post-traumatic stress disorders may precede alcoholism.
- Sleep disturbances: Alcohol can decrease sleep latency and also reduce the duration of rapid eye movement (REM) sleep. It could potentially lead to more fragmentation in sleep and result in longer episodes of awakening.
- Psychosexual disorders: Extensive alcohol intake has been associated with psychosexual disorders. It can lead to erectile impotence as well as delayed ejaculation. Chronic heavy drinking can lead to loss of sexual drive, reduction in the sizes of the testes and penis, loss of body hair as well as gynaecomastia.

STATION 89: SOCIAL AND LEGAL IMPLICATIONS OF ALCOHOL

Information to candidates

Name of patient: Roger

Roger has been referred to your addiction clinic by his GP. In the referral memo, it was stated that Roger has a long-standing history of alcohol usage. Due to his alcohol usage, he has been facing some difficulties in his relationships, in his work and also with the police. He is keen to seek further help.

Task

Please speak to Roger and explore his current level of alcohol consumption. Please also assess his social and legal problems associated with his current long-standing history of alcohol usage.

Outline of station

You are Roger and have been referred by your GP to the local addiction services to get some help for your alcohol problem. You have been a chronic drinker and need to drink daily, or else you have several withdrawal side effects. Because of your chronic drinking habits, you have gotten into fights, and the police have been involved. There was an occasion in which you were also caught for drunk driving. In addition, you are not performing well in your work, and your company has dismissed you. You are having problems with your finances. Also, things are not working out well for your relationship. You have been having frequent fights with your wife, who is not agreeable to your drinking habits. You are keen to seek help.

CASC construct table

The CASC construct table is formatted such that candidates will be able to cover adequately both the range and the depth of the assessment required in this station.

Starting off: 'Hello, I am Dr Melvyn, one of the psychiatrists from the mental health unit. I understand that your GP has referred you to our service. Can we have a chat?'			
Current usage of alcohol	I understand from the memo from my colleague that you have been having several problems as a result of your long-term drinking. Before we explore more about your problems, can I get a general understanding of your drinking habits?	Can you share with me more about your usual drinking habits? Can you tell me when you first started to drink? What did you start drinking?	How have things changed since the time you first started drinking? Can you take me through a typical day and tell me more about your drinking patterns?
Work-related complications	Do you have any problems with regard to work due to your current problems with drinking?	Have there been days you were late for work? How often has this occurred? Have you missed days at work due to your problems with drinking?	Have you been less attentive and been making mistakes at work due to your current drinking habits?
Relationship-related complications	Do you have any problems with regard to your relationships due to your current problems with drinking?	Have you been having arguments and fights with your partner recently?	Has there been a time in which you have been physically abusive towards your partner?

(Continued)

Forensic complications	Have you gotten involved with the police due to your problems with drinking?	Have you been involved in any drunk-driving offenses?	Have you been drunk, and have you been involved in fights when you were drunk? Are there any outstanding charges against you at the moment?
Financial complications	Can you tell me whether you are having financial difficulties due to your current drinking habits?	Can you tell me how you have been financing your alcohol habits?	Have you borrowed money to finance your drinking habits?
Social complications	How has drinking affected your social life?		

Common pitfalls

a. Failure to cover the range and depth of the information required for this station

Quick recall*

- Abuse of alcohol has been found to be associated with other addictive behaviours, such as gambling and the usage of other illegal substances.
- Social complications of alcohol abuse and dependence include (1) family breakdown, (2) crime, (3) road traffic accidents and trauma and (4) economic harm.
- Approximately one-third of problem drinkers tend to cite their marital relationship as one of their problems. One-third of those undergoing divorce highlighted alcohol as a contributory factor, and three-fourths of wives being abused acknowledge the fact that their husbands are chronic drinkers.
- Children of alcoholics are at risk as well, as they tend to suffer from neglect and poverty as well as being subjected to physical violence.
- Legal complications: Alcohol abuse has been known to be strongly associated with crime, particularly against persons and also against properties. Half of those who commit homicide have been drinking at the time of the offence. Half of the rapists convicted were drinking at the time of the offence as well.
- Approximately one-fifth of all the deaths on the roads result from drunk driving.
- One-third of accidents at home are due to drowning following the consumption of alcohol.

---

* Adapted from B.K. Puri, A. Hall and R. Ho (2014). *Revision Notes in Psychiatry*. London, UK: CRC Press, p. 519.

STATION 90: OPIOID DEPENDENCE – HISTORY TAKING

Information to candidates

Name of patient: Mr Aaron

You have been tasked to speak to Mr Aaron, who has been referred to the dual addictions service by his GP. The GP has written in the memo that Mr Aaron has a history of opioid dependence.

Task

Please speak to Mr Aaron to elicit a history of opiate dependence.

Outline of station

You are Mr Aaron and have been referred by your GP to see the drug and addiction service. You were at your GP 2 days ago as there was an infection around the site in which you have been injecting heroin. You have been using heroin since you were a teenager but have escalated over the past 2 years in view of work-related stress and relationship difficulties. You have not used any other drugs. You do use alcohol on an occasional basis. You use heroin via both the intranasal route and the intravenous route. You used to share needles but have not done so recently as you are aware that there is a chance you might acquire an infection such as human immunodeficiency virus (HIV). You cannot afford to stop using heroin as you will experience significant withdrawal symptoms. You do not have any other features of any other psychiatric disorder. You feel that you need some help after the GP counselled you about the risk associated with continued usage of the drug.

CASC construct table

The CASC construct table is formatted such that candidates will be able to cover adequately both the range and the depth of the assessment required in this station.

Starting off: 'Hello, I am Dr Melvyn, one of the psychiatrists from the mental health unit. I understand that your GP has referred you to our service. Can we have a chat?'			
History of presenting complaint	I understand from your GP that you have been using heroin. Can you tell me more about your usage of heroin? Apart from heroin, are there other drugs that you have been using? Do you use alcohol as well? How often and how much do you use?	Can you tell me when you first started using heroin? How much heroin did you use when you first started? How do you use the heroin?	Currently, how much heroin do you use on a typical day? Can you take me through a typical day to help me understand your drug usage? How do you use the heroin? Do you inject the heroin? Have you shared needles before? How much do you spend on drugs on a daily basis?

(Continued)

Dependence symptoms	Do you feel that recently you've needed to use more and more heroin to achieve the same effects?	Are we you finding it tougher to control the amount of heroin that you are using?	Are there times in which you find yourself having cravings when you missed a dose?
Dependence symptoms	Can you tell me more about what happens if you miss a dose or stop using heroin?	Do you experience any withdrawal symptoms? Can you tell me more about the symptoms that you have been experiencing? Have you ever had a seizure or fit if you miss a dose?	The typical withdrawal symptoms include • Muscular aches • Stomach cramps • Nauseated feeling • Yawning • Rhinorrhoea
Complications	I understand that you have been using heroin intravenously. Have there been any complications from where you have been injecting? Have you had infections such as an abscess?	Have you ever needed to be admitted to the hospital due to an infection? Has anyone done any tests for your underlying liver condition? Do you know if you have any specific liver conditions?	How has your drug usage affected you? Has it affected your work? Has it affected your relationships? Has it affected you in terms of your finances? Have you gotten into trouble with the law?
Comorbid psychiatric disorders	How has your mood been recently? Do you find yourself being able to enjoy things that you used to be able to enjoy?	How have you been coping with your sleep and appetite? How is your attention and concentration?	Have you ever had any unusual experiences, such as listening to voices or seeing things that are not there? Have you ever felt that life is not worth living?
Insight and motivation	Do you think you could have a mental health problem?	What do you want to do about your current problem?	What kind of help do you want from us with regard to your problem? How motivated are you for a change?

Common pitfalls

a. Failure to cover the range and depth of the information required for this station

Quick recall*

- Drugs derived from opium poppies are known as opiates. Synthetically derived opiates are known as opioids.

---

* Adapted from B.K. Puri, A. Hall and R. Ho (2014). *Revision Notes in Psychiatry*. London, UK: CRC Press, pp. 535–539.

- Heroin is produced from morphine, which is derived from the sap of the opium poppy. It may be smoked or chased by heating on tinfoil and inhaling the sublimate. It is also injected intravenously and, much less commonly, subcutaneously. Street heroin is usually 30%–60% pure and 0.25–0.75 g is a common daily consumption for addicts.
- Most heroin users are aged between 20 and 30 years. The steepest increase has occurred in those aged 16–24 years.
- The male-to-female ratio is 2:1.
- The stimulation of opiate receptors produces analgesia, euphoria, miosis, hypotension, bradycardia and respiratory depression.
- Euphoria is initially intense and is related in part to the method of administration. Thus, methods delivering a large bolus quickly to the central nervous system (CNS) are associated with a greater initial rush. Intravenous and inhalational techniques of heroin fulfil these conditions; oral and subcutaneous methods do not. Dependence may arise within weeks of regular use.
- The *Diagnostic and Statistical Manual of Mental Disorders,* 5th edition (*DSM-5*) proposes the following opioid-induced disorders: major neurocognitive disorder, amnestic disorder, psychotic disorder, depressive or bipolar disorder, anxiety disorder, sexual dysfunction or sleep disorder.
- Effects of opioid withdrawal: During opioid withdrawal, there is an excessive release of noradrenaline, which results in rhinorrhoea or sneezing, lacrimation, muscle cramps or aches, abdominal cramps, nausea or vomiting, diarrhoea, pupillary dilatation, piloerection, recurrent chills, tachycardia, hypertension yawning and restless sleep. The *ICD-10* criteria require the presence of any three of the aforementioned symptoms. The *DSM-5* criteria are similar to the *ICD-10*. Opioid withdrawal is seldom associated with withdrawal fits.
- Opioid withdrawal usually begins within 4–12 hours of last heroin use. Peak intensity is at around 48 hours, and the main symptoms disappear within a week of abstinence. Although it is unpleasant, opiate withdrawal is not generally dangerous (with the exceptions including that of pregnancy, when abortion may result from acute withdrawal).

Harmful effects include the following:

Drugs	Overdose can be caused by the uncertain concentration of street drugs or due to reduced tolerance, following a period of abstinence.
Intoxications	Intoxication might lead to accidents.
Inhalation	Commonly worsens or causes lung conditions such as asthma. There are increased rates of pneumonia and tuberculosis in those who are HIV positive.

(Continued)

Intravenous usage	Includes transmission of infection through the usage of shared needles. HIV and hepatitis B, C and D are commonly transmitted through this route.
Bacterial infections	Result from the lack of aseptic techniques. The risk is not eliminated by the usage of clean needles since the drug itself is not of pharmaceutical quality.
Skin infection	At injection sites leads to abscess formation and thrombophlebitis.
Blood infection	Most injecting results in transient bacteraemia. This can result in septicaemia and/or bacterial endocarditis, even in those with a previously normal heart valve. Septic emboli can be carried to distant sites. Septic embolism can result in osteomyelitis.
Fungal infection	Systemic fungal infections have been reported, which are difficult to treat.
Vascular complications	Include the obliteration of the lung vascular bed with continued prolonged infection of particular matter. Deep vein thrombosis may develop at the site of femoral administration. Arterial administration can result in occlusion caused by spasm or embolism. The loss of a limb may result.

Management of opiate/opioid dependence

- Help the person to deal with drug-related problems
- Reduce damage occurring during the drug use
- Reduce duration of episodes of drug use
- Reduce the chance of relapse
- Help the person to remain healthy until he or she manages to attain a drug-free state
- Harm minimization: The aims are to stop or reduce the use of contaminated injecting equipment, to prevent the sharing of injecting equipment, to stop or reduce drug use, to stop or reduce unsafe sexual practices, to encourage health consciousness and a more stable lifestyle and to establish and retain contact with the drug services. To achieve these aims, sterile injecting equipment and condoms should be provided, and non-immune individuals should be offered hepatitis B vaccination and substitute oral opiates such as methadone should be given.

NICE recommendations:

- Detoxification should be offered to people who are opioid dependent and have expressed an informed choice to become abstinent after being counselled on the adverse effects of opioid misuse.
- Methadone or buprenorphine should be offered as the first-line treatment in opioid detoxification.

If dependence is not severe, reassurance, support and symptomatic treatment with non-opiate drugs may be sufficient. The following could be considered:

- Clonidine: an alpha-adrenergic antagonist that inhibits noradrenergic overactivity by acting on the presynaptic auto-receptors. It could provide some symptomatic relief in opiate withdrawal, but hypotension could potentially be a problem.
- Lofexidine: It is an alpha 2 agonist, which acts centrally to reduce the sympathetic tone. It is indicated for detoxification within a short period (5–7 days) and also for dependence in young people.
- Propranolol: It can be given for somatic anxiety.
- Thioridazine: It can be used to relieve anxiety in low doses.
- Promethazine: It can be effective for mild withdrawal.
- Benzodiazepine: It can be used to treat anxiety.

Pharmacological treatment:

- Methadone: It is indicated if opioid drugs are taken on a regular basis, and there is convincing evidence of opioid dependence. There needs to be an opportunity to supervise the daily use of methadone for a minimum duration of 3 months. It is contraindicated for individuals with prolonged QTc and those who refuse to be supervised. It is a synthetic opioid that can be taken orally or intravenously. It is a long-acting opioid agonist that allows for once-daily oral prescribing. The dose of 60–100 mg/day is more effective than lower dosages with regard to reducing heroin misuse. The starting dose is 10–30 mg per day and increases by 5–10 mg per week to reach the therapeutic dose. For maintenance, a substitute opiate is prescribed indefinitely in an effort to stabilize the addict's life and reduce the risk of intravenous use. For long-term withdrawal, substitute prescribing takes place over a period of months to years with the long-term aim of opiate abstinence. For rapid withdrawal, withdrawal takes place over a period of weeks by the use of a substitute drug in decreasing doses. For gradual withdrawal, withdrawal takes place over a period of months by the usage of a substitute drug in decreasing doses.
- Buprenorphine: This is a partial mu-opioid agonist and a kappa-opioid antagonist. The titration dosing for induction starts with 2 or 4 mg on the first day. The dose can be increased in 2–4 mg increments to 12–16 mg on the second day. Most people tend to stabilize with a dose of 8–32 mg/day.
- Naltrexone: It is an opioid receptor antagonist. It is indicated for people who prefer an abstinence programme and are fully informed of the risk associated with withdrawal. Naltrexone is most effective in adults who are highly motivated. It cannot be given until all the opioids have been cleared from the body. The initial dose is 25 mg which then increases to a maintenance dose of 50 mg per day. It is particularly helpful if a partner administers it and if used in conjunction with cognitive behavioural therapy.

Psychosocial interventions based on NICE guidance:

- Contingency management: Offering incentive contingent on each drug-negative test, such as giving vouchers that can be exchanged for goods or privileges, that allow the person taking methadone home.

- For people on naltrexone: They have to receive contingency management with behaviour family intervention for the person and a non-drug-misusing family member.
- Psychological methods: Therapeutic outcome is improved if substitute prescribing is combined with various forms of behaviour therapy.
- Motivational interviewing: Motivational interviewing is a cognitive behaviour approach that takes into account the patient's stage of preparedness for change and prompts the patient to consider favourable reasons to change.
- Prognosis: The mortality rate for intravenous drug abusers is 20 times that of their non-drug-using peers. Since the 1980s, the prevalence of HIV infection amongst intravenous drug users has increased to approximately 50%–60% in some groups, and mortality amongst this group has increased further.

STATION 91: SUBSTANCE MISUSE IN PREGNANCY – HISTORY TAKING (PAIRED STATION A)

Information to candidates

Name of patient: Sheena

Sheena is a 31-year-old female known previously to the drug and alcohol services, as she has been using heroin since she was young. She has been maintained on methadone treatment and has been compliant with her methadone treatment thus far. She has missed her menstrual period for the past 2 months and has just discovered that she is pregnant. She has informed her partner about her pregnancy. Her partner is supportive and has recommended that she come by the drug and alcohol services for an evaluation, as he is concerned about her continued usage of methadone whilst she is pregnant. You are the core trainee on call and have been told by your consultant to assess Sheena first.

Task

Please speak to Sheena and elicit a history with regard to her drug usage and also explore more about her social circumstances. Please note that in the next station, you will need to speak to her partner to discuss the relevant management plans.

Outline of station

You are Sheena, a 31-year-old female, and are known to the drug and addiction services. You started using heroin and other drugs (such as crack) when you were a teenager. However, you have stopped using the other drugs and have been dependent on heroin mainly. You realized that you needed some help for your drug issues 2 years ago and have been on constant follow-up with the local drug and addictions service. They have previously started you on methadone. You have been on methadone for a year now and have not gone back to using heroin. Your current pregnancy is unplanned and you feel a little unprepared with regard to the pregnancy. You are willing to share with the core trainee any information that is pertinent to help you with the management of your drug issues during pregnancy.

CASC construct table

The CASC construct table is formatted such that candidates will be able to cover adequately both the range and the depth of the assessment required in this station.

Starting off: 'Hello, I am Dr Melvyn, one of the psychiatrists from the mental health unit. Can we have a chat today to help me understand your problems?'			
Previous history of drug usage and current usage	I understand that you have been seen by our service before. Can you tell me more about it?	You mentioned that you started to see us due to your usage of drugs. Can I clarify what drugs you have been using? Apart from heroin, do you use cannabis, cocaine, amphetamine, methadone, ecstasy, sleeping tablets? Do you also use alcohol?	Thanks for sharing with me. My understanding is that you have been using heroin regularly up till last year, when you were maintained on methadone. Can you tell me how much methadone are you maintained on currently? Can you also share with me more about where you have been getting your methadone?
Explore methods of administration and risky behaviours	In the past, how often did you use heroin? Do you recall when was the last time you have used heroin? How do you use the heroin? Do you smoke it or do you inject it?	If the patient has been injecting: When did you first start injecting? How often do you inject? Have you shared needles previously?	How much heroin do you use on a typical day? How much do you typically spend on your drugs?
Explore withdrawal side effects	Do you find yourself needing more heroin to achieve the same effects as previously? What happens if you miss your dose of heroin?	Have you experienced any side effects or withdrawal symptoms when you are not using heroin?	The typical withdrawal symptoms include the following: - Muscular aches - Stomach cramps - Nauseated feeling - Yawning - Rhinorrhoea
Explore patient's feeling towards current pregnancy	My understanding is that you have realized that you could be pregnant. How do you know?	Is this pregnancy planned or unplanned?	What are your thoughts with regard to having a child?
Explore personal history and social circumstances	Are you currently working? Do you have any current financial difficulties?	With whom do you stay at the moment? How are the relationships at home?	Is there anyone who would help you care for your child at home?

Common pitfalls

a. Failure to cover the range and depth of the information required for this station

Quick recall*

Information for history taking and management

- Substance abuse in pregnancy involves the excessive nontherapeutic use of recreational or prescribed drugs resulting in adverse effects on both the mother and her foetus. Such effects also depend on the trimester of the pregnancy. Anticipated postnatal problems need to be addressed during the antenatal period.
- The basic principle is to consider a substitute (such as methadone) to minimize harm and manage the patient in holistic care with the involvement of an addiction specialist, a neonatologist and an obstetrician. This can take place at any stage of the pregnancy and carries a much lower risk that continuing usage of heroin may lead to withdrawal or overdose as a result of fluctuating opiate level.
- Apart from a clinical history, physical examination needs to be performed to assess the mother's nutritional status and also to look for needle marks and anaemia. Investigations need to be conducted.
- The short-term management includes establishing therapeutic alliance and stabilization of heroin intake by referring the patient to a methadone treatment programme. When the patient reaches the second trimester, the addiction specialist will withdraw the methadone over a period of 4 weeks. The mother needs to undergo regular monitoring by an obstetrician. The drug prevention worker can work with the patient in relapse prevention by motivational interviewing and compliance therapy. The social worker will enhance supports, and the psychologist will offer supportive psychotherapy with a focus on pregnancy issues. The psychiatrist can offer treatment for any comorbid psychiatric disorders.
- The medium-term management includes establishing a delivery plan with input from the other specialists. The psychiatrist will educate the patient on neonatal abstinence syndrome. Both the patient and the newborn will be transferred to the mother and baby unit after delivery. The psychiatrist will monitor her mood and look for signs of other psychiatric disorders. Postnatal education also involves advice on breast-feeding. Methadone is compatible with breast-feeding, and the dose should be less than 20 mg/day.
- For long-term management, the psychiatrist will assess the patient after delivery and decide whether absolute detoxification or harm minimization is more appropriate.

---

* Adapted from B.K. Puri, A. Hall and R. Ho (2014). *Revision Notes in Psychiatry*. London, UK: CRC Press, pp. 565–566.

- *Summary of* Maudsley's Guideline Recommendation of Detoxification of Opiate During Antenatal and Postpartum Period.*
  - First trimester: Minimization of drugs that are harmful in the first trimester, such as benzodiazepines, alcohol and heroin. It is important to optimize nutrition and supplement with folate and iron tablets. Detoxification in the first trimester is not recommend as opiate withdrawal in the first trimester is likely to lead to spontaneous abortion.
  - Second trimester: If detoxification is required, it is best done in the second trimester. Detoxification is safe and abstinence can be achieved in stable cases. The use of methadone is recommended during this antenatal period. Buprenorphine needs more data to support its safety in pregnancy.
  - Third trimester: Increase methadone dose because the metabolism will increase towards the end of pregnancy. Patient should be offered divided dose of methadone to prevent withdrawal. The main objective during the delivery is to minimize withdrawal in the newborn and to ensure assisted breathing for the floppy and sedated newborn. Detoxification is not recommended after 32 weeks because it may lead to preterm delivery and stillbirth.
  - Delivery and postpartum: Antenatal assessment by an anaesthetist is required to handle potential risks. The anaesthetist needs to decide on the analgesic requirements based on the dose of methadone given. Newborns who are born with mother dependent on opiate may develop vomiting and diarrhoea leading to dehydration and poor weight gain. Other signs of neo-natal abstinence syndrome include excessive crying and sucking, hyper-reflexia, increased muscle tone and fever.

STATION 92: SUBSTANCE MISUSE IN PREGNANCY – DISCUSSION (PAIRED STATION B)

Information to candidates

Name of patient: Mr Charlie Brown

Sheena is a 31-year-old female known previously to the drug and alcohol services as she has been using heroin since she was young. She has been maintained on methadone treatment and she has been compliant with her methadone treatment thus far. She has missed a period for the past 2 months and has just discovered that she is currently pregnant. She has informed her partner, Mr Charlie Brown, about her pregnancy. Charlie is supportive and has recommended that she come by the drug and alcohol services for an evaluation, as he is concerned about her continued usage of methadone whilst she is pregnant. You are the core trainee

---

* From B.K. Puri, A. Hall and R. Ho (2014). *Revision Notes in Psychiatry*. London, UK: CRC Press.

on call and have been told by your consultant to assess Sheena first. You have previously spoken to Sheena and now have a better understanding of her drug issues. You are aware that her partner is here and wishes to see you to discuss more about the management of her addiction issues in pregnancy.

Task

Please speak to Charlie and address all his concerns and expectations.

Outline of station

You are Mr Charlie Brown, the partner of Sheena. You know that your partner has abused multiple drugs in the past and has been dependent on heroin for the past few years when you knew her and is currently on methadone treatment. You have some questions to ask the core trainee and hope that your questions can be clarified. You want to know the risks associated with her current pregnancy in view of the fact that she has been on multiple drugs previously. You are concerned about how heroin and methadone might potentially harm the baby. You want to know what might happen to the baby if your partner is still abusing heroin when she is pregnant. You wonder whether it would be safe for the continuation of methadone throughout pregnancy. Also, you wish to know if your partner can breast-feed whilst she is on methadone. Lastly, in view of your partner's drug history, you are concerned that your child might be taken away from you by social services.

CASC construct table

The CASC construct table is formatted such that candidates will be able to cover adequately both the range and the depth of the assessment required in this station.

Starting off: 'Hello, I am Dr Melvyn, one of the psychiatrists from the mental health unit. I understand that you have some concerns about your partner and her usage of drugs. Can we have a chat about this?'			
Explanation of risk associated with drug usage in pregnancy	Can you help me to understand your concerns about your partner and her current pregnancy? I think you have raised a very important issue about your partner's usage of drugs and her being pregnant at the same time. I understand your concerns about the risk associated with her drug use in pregnancy.	My understanding from speaking to your partner just now is that she used several drugs previously, and lately, she has been using heroin before being maintained on methadone.	There is always the inherent risk of drugs causing issues such as stillbirth, premature delivery of the child, as well as some antenatal complications. It might also cause low birth weight. Hence, it is crucial that your partner continues to see us regularly. It is also essential that she follows up and does the necessary antenatal evaluations and checks.

(Continued)

Safety of heroin and methadone in pregnancy	I understand that you are concerned about methadone and its effect on the current pregnancy. Please allow me to share that methadone is relatively safe in pregnancy and will not cause any abnormalities in the child.	However, should your partner continue to use heroin, it might have an impact on your child.	Previous research has shown that the usage of heroin might lead to miscarriage as well as intrauterine-related deaths.
Explanation of neonatal abstinence syndrome	One of the other effects that continued usage of heroin in pregnancy can have is neonatal withdrawal syndrome. Have you heard of this condition before? What's your understanding of this condition? Would it be alright for me to explain more?	In the event that your partner continues to use heroin in pregnancy, your baby might be susceptible towards acquiring neonatal withdrawal syndrome.	In essence, your baby might display some withdrawal symptoms associated with the prior usage of heroin. We would need to monitor your baby for this. In the event that your baby does have clinical signs and symptoms of opioid withdrawal, we might need to treat accordingly.
Explain management in pregnancy	Based on previous research findings, the best time to consider detoxification would be in the second trimester.	Methadone could still be used as a substitute and be continued throughout pregnancy.	However, there needs to be some adjustment of the dosing of methadone when your partner is in her third trimester.
Address concerns about breast-feeding and methadone	I hear your concerns with regard to the suitability of your partner breast-feeding your baby if she is on methadone.	If she is maintained on methadone at a dose of less than 20 mg/day, she can breast-feed your baby.	There are other medications that are contraindicated in breast-feeding, and hence it is essential we continue to follow up on the care of your partner and make the appropriate recommendations.
Address concerns about social services	I hear that you have some concerns about whether your child would be taken away by the social services in view of your partner having a drug history.	I would like to reassure you that your child would not be taken away from you and your partner just because your partner has a drug history.	The social services would consider alternative care arrangements only under special circumstances in which it is deemed that your partner is unable to manage your child. We need your help with advising your partner to come back routinely for her appointments with us.

Common pitfalls

a. Failure to cover the range and depth of the information required for this station

Quick recall*

Information for history taking and management

- Substance abuse in pregnancy involves the excessive nontherapeutic use of recreational or prescribed drugs resulting in adverse effects on both the mother and her foetus. Such effects also depend on the trimester of the pregnancy. Anticipated postnatal problems need to be addressed during the antenatal period.
- The basic principle is to consider a substitute (such as methadone) to minimize harm and manage the patient in holistic care with the involvement of an addiction specialist, a neonatologist and an obstetrician. This can take place at any stage of the pregnancy and carries a much lower risk than continuing usage of heroin that may led to withdrawal or overdose as a result of fluctuating opiate level.
- Apart from a clinical history, physical examination needs to be performed to assess the mother's nutritional status and also to look for needle marks and anaemia. Investigations need to be conducted.
- The short-term management includes establishing therapeutic alliance and stabilization of heroin intake by referring the patient to a methadone treatment programme. When the patient reaches the second trimester, the addiction specialist will withdraw the methadone over a period of 4 weeks. The mother needs to undergo regular monitoring by an obstetrician. The drug prevention worker can work with the patient in relapse prevention by motivational interviewing and compliance therapy. The social worker will enhance supports, and the psychologist will offer supportive psychotherapy with a focus on pregnancy issues. The psychiatrist can offer treatment for any comorbid psychiatric disorders.
- The medium-term management includes establishing a delivery plan with input from the other specialists. The psychiatrist will educate the patient on neonatal abstinence syndrome. Both the patient and the newborn will be transferred to the mother and baby unit after delivery. The psychiatrist will monitor her mood and look for signs of other psychiatric disorders. Postnatal education also involves advice on breast-feeding. Methadone is compatible with breast-feeding, and the dose should be less than 20 mg/day.
- For long-term management, the psychiatrist will assess the patient after delivery and decide whether absolute detoxification or harm minimization is more appropriate.

---

* Adapted from B.K. Puri, A. Hall and R. Ho (2014). *Revision Notes in Psychiatry.* London, UK: CRC Press, pp. 565–566.

- Summary of Maudsley's Guideline Recommendation of Detoxification of Opiate During Antenatal and Postpartum Period.
  - First trimester: Minimization of drugs that are harmful in the first trimester, such as benzodiazepines, alcohol and heroin. It is important to optimize nutrition and supplement with folate and iron tablets. Detoxification in the first trimester is not recommend as opiate withdrawal in the first trimester is likely to lead to spontaneous abortion.
  - Second trimester: If detoxification is required, it is best done in the second trimester. Detoxification is safe and abstinence can be achieved in stable cases. The use of methadone is recommended during this antenatal period. Buprenorphine needs more data to support its safety in pregnancy.
  - Third trimester: Increased methadone dose, because the metabolism will increase towards the end of pregnancy. Patient should be offered a divided dose of methadone to prevent withdrawal. The main objective during the delivery is to minimize withdrawal in the newborn and to ensure assisted breathing for the floppy and sedated new-born. Detoxification is not recommended after 32 weeks because it may lead to preterm delivery and stillbirth.
  - Delivery and postpartum: Antenatal assessment by an anaesthetist is required to handle potential risks. The anaesthetist needs to decide on the analgesic requirements based on the dose of methadone given. Newborns who are born with their mothers dependent on opiate may develop vomiting and diarrhoea leading to dehydration and poor weight gain. Other signs of neo-natal abstinence syndrome include excessive crying and sucking, hyper-reflexia and increased muscle tone and fever.

STATION 93: DELIRIUM TREMENS (DISCUSSION WITH CONSULTANT)

Information to candidates

Name of patient: Mr White

You have been tasked to see Mr White, a 54-year-old man, who has just undergone hip surgery following a fall he sustained whilst intoxicated. His last drink, according to his daughter, was 3 days ago. He was noted to be very distressed and agitated in the ward, and he did vocalize that he was having visual and auditory hallucinations. He has been threatening to leave the ward premises as well, as he does not feel that the environment is safe. Your consultant, Dr Thomson, has heard about this patient and wishes to discuss the case with you.

Task

Please speak to Dr Thomson, your consultant on call, and discuss more about the case with him. Please summarize your findings and discuss a sound management approach for Mr White.

Outline of station

You are Dr Thomson, the on-call consultant, and you have heard about this case, as the nursing manager of the surgery ward has called you. You are aware that your core trainee has assessed the patient and you hope that your core trainee can provide you with a summary of his assessment. You want to discuss with the trainee the differential diagnosis of the case, and the most likely diagnosis given the clinical features. You would like to discuss with the core trainee more about the specific management for the patient as well.

CASC construct table

The CASC construct table is formatted such that candidates will be able to cover adequately both the range and the depth of the assessment required in this station.

Starting off: 'Hello, I am Melvyn, one of the core trainees. Can I discuss a case with you?'			
Brief formulation of current assessment	I have seen Mr White, who is a 54-year-old man referred from the general surgery unit. My understanding is that he has been admitted following a recent fall and has just undergone an operation. I understand that he sustained the fall whilst he was intoxicated with alcohol around 3 days ago.	I have seen the patient, and he is currently confused and not orientated to time, place and person. He does have episodes of agitation, and it is quite hard for the nursing staff to manage him in the ward. He has been reporting both visual and auditory hallucinations.	He seemed to be quite distressed by the visual hallucinations that he is experiencing. He does not find it safe to be in the ward and has been requesting for the team to consider discharging him.
Likely diagnosis and differential diagnosis	Given that he has the presence of altered consciousness and visual and auditory hallucinations, and taking into consideration that his last drink was 3 days ago, the most likely clinical diagnosis at the moment is delirium tremens.	I have obtained a collaborative history from his daughter, who suggests that he is alcohol dependent and that his last drink was around 3 days ago. He previously used a combination of beer and hard liquor.	I would like to consider other differential diagnoses as well. The blood investigations have been done and do not show an infective picture or sepsis at the moment. The acute onset of the current presentation might not be typical for a patient with schizophrenia or other psychotic disorder.

(Continued)

Management – pharmacological	Delirium tremens is considered to be a medical emergency, and he needs immediate and close monitoring in a medical ward. Prior to the commencement of medications, I would like to suggest that there should be more intensive monitoring of his vitals. There should be regular reorientation. He should also be nursed in a quiet room, with familiar nursing staff as well.	We urgently need to replace his thiamine by giving him intravenous thiamine replacement up to 500 mg three times per day. We could consider starting a reducing dose of diazepam, based on his Clinical Institute Withdrawal Assessment of Alcohol Scale (CIWA) withdrawal scores. He should also be monitored closely for withdrawal seizures.	Given his agitated behaviour, antipsychotic medications such as haloperidol could be considered as an adjunctive medication for agitation and aggression.
Management – psychological	We need to educate and explain to the family the symptoms and the medical condition he is having at the moment.	Educate and provide support to the nursing staff to alleviate anxiety. Consistent nursing care and reduction of excessive stimulation may worsen his delirium.	Once he is out of delirium, we need to consider referring him to the addiction service for the counsellor to assess him and to provide motivational interviewing regarding his alcohol issues.

Common pitfalls

a. Failure to cover the range and depth of the information required for this station

It is important to mention non-pharmacological methods before jumping into medications. Consider the approach of a multidisciplinary team. Highlight to the examiner that you are able to weigh the pros and cons of starting antipsychotic medications on a frail elderly patient.

Quick recall*

- In chronic heavy drinkers, a fall in the blood alcohol concentration will lead to withdrawal symptoms, including delirium tremens.

---

* Adapted from B.K. Puri, A. Hall and R. Ho (2014). *Revision Notes in Psychiatry*. London, UL: CRC Press, pp. 516–517..

- The peak onset is within 2 days of abstinence, and it usually lasts for about 5 days.
- There is a prodromal period with anxiety, insomnia, tachycardia, tremor and sweating.
- The onset of delirium is marked by disorientation, fluctuating level of consciousness, intensely fearful affect, hallucinations, misperceptions, tremor, restlessness and autonomic overactivity.
- The hallucinations are often visual and are commonly Lilliputian in nature. Auditory and tactile hallucinations and secondary delusions may also be present.
- There is a mortality rate of about 5% associated mainly with cardiovascular collapse or infection.
- The treatment of delirium tremens is supportive with sedation, fluid and electrolyte replacement and high-potency vitamins (especially thiamine to prevent an unrecognized Wernicke's encephalopathy progressing to Karsakov's psychosis).
- National Institute for Health and Care Excellence (NICE) guidance on the management of delirium tremens or seizures: Oral Ativan should be used as first-line treatment for delirium tremens or seizures. If symptoms persist or there is difficulty with administration of oral medications, one could consider parenteral Ativan, parenteral haloperidol and parenteral olanzapine. The aforementioned medications do not have UK marketing authorization for treating delirium tremens or seizures. Informed consent should be obtained and documented if possible. Phenytoin is not included for the treatment of alcohol withdrawal seizures.

Wernicke's encephalopathy and Korsakov's syndrome

- This is caused by severe deficiency of thiamine, which is usually caused by alcohol abuse in Western countries.
- The important clinical features include ophthalmoplegia, nystagmus, ataxia and clouding of consciousness.
- Ten per cent of patients with Wernicke's encephalopathy have the classical triad including ataxia, ophthalmoplegia and memory disturbances. Peripheral neuropathy may also be present.
- Eighty per cent of untreated Wernicke's could convert to Karsakov's psychosis if untreated.
- Korsakov's syndrome is an alcohol-induced amnesia syndrome that is described as an abnormal state in which memory and learning are affected out of all proportion to other cognitive functions in an otherwise alert and responsive patient. Clinical features include retrograde amnesia, anterograde amnesia, sparing of immediate recall, disorientation in time, inability to recall the temporal sequences of events, confabulation and peripheral neuropathy.

STATION 94: PSYCHOTHERAPY – COGNITIVE BEHAVIOURAL THERAPY (COUNSELLING)

Information to candidates

Name of patient: Mr Johnson

Mr Johnson is a 35-year-old male who has been referred by his general practitioner (GP) to the mental health service, as he has been having low mood with reduction of interest ever since he got dismissed from his workplace. He has been started on an antidepressant. The consultant psychiatrist has recommended for him to also attend a psychotherapy session. The consultant psychiatrist wants you to share more about the specific psychotherapy (cognitive behavioural therapy [CBT]) that he has recommended for the patient.

Task

Please speak to Mr Johnson and counsel him with regard to how cognitive behavioural psychotherapy would work. Please also address all his expectations and concerns.

Outline of station

The purpose of providing an outline of the station is to allow candidates to be familiar with the structure of the station. This outline could also be helpful when candidates practice for the MRCPsych, joining with their colleagues to act out the station.

Please note that the outlines provided are based on the experiences of the authors. There may be variations in the actual examination.

You are Mr Johnson and have been diagnosed with major depressive disorder just 3 weeks ago and commenced on an antidepressant medication. Your mood symptoms came on following a dismissal from your workplace. You understand from the consultant psychiatrist that apart from medications, there are other alternatives such as psychotherapy that might help you with your depressive illness. You wish to know more about the particular psychotherapy offered. You wish to know more about the therapy and how the therapy is structured. You also wish to know the structure of the therapy as well as the expected outcomes, and you wonder whether, if therapy is effective, you could stop antidepressants as you worry about the long-term consumption of antidepressant medications.

CASC construct table

The CASC construct table is formatted such that candidates will be able to cover adequately both the range and the depth of the assessment required in this station.

Starting off: 'Hello, I am Dr Melvyn, one of the psychiatrists from the mental health unit. I understand that you have some questions about the psychotherapy recommended. Can we have a chat about this?'			
Clarifying the nature of the therapy	I understand that the therapy that has been recommended for you is CBT. Have you heard anything about this form of psychotherapy or talking therapy before?	CBT is therapy that is recommended for patients with anxiety as well as depressive disorders.	It focuses on specific issues at present and does not look at past events.
Clarifying the principles of the therapy	In this form of therapy, it is believed that the way we think will in turn affect how we feel and behave. As the name suggest, it is important for you to realize that there are two main principles governing the therapy session.	Cognitive techniques are used during the therapy session. Cognitive restructuring helps you to identify negative thoughts, dysfunctional assumptions and maladaptive core beliefs relating to your underlying problems. It also tests the validity of those thoughts, assumptions and beliefs. The goal is to produce more adaptive and positive alternatives.	Apart from cognitive techniques, specific behavioural techniques are also used. Some of the common techniques include the following: a. Rehearsal: It helps you to anticipate challenges and to develop strategies to overcome difficulties. b. Inclusion of graded assignment on exposure. c. Training oneself to be self-reliant. d. Pleasure and mastery of skills. e. Activity scheduling to increase contact with positive activities and decrease avoidance and withdrawal. f. Diversion or distraction techniques.

(Continued)

| Clarify the structure of the therapy | A total of 12–16 sessions are usually recommended. In the early phase, it is pertinent for the therapist to build on the therapeutic alliance. The client needs to be educated on the model of CBT and the influence of thoughts on behaviour and emotions. Goals are set for the psychotherapy session. Negative automatic thoughts are identified. The therapist makes use of questioning to reveal the self-defeating nature of the client's thought process and identify cognitive triad. | In the middle phase, the therapist asks the patient to keep a dysfunctional thought diary. Through the homework assignment, the therapist can identify cognitive errors and core beliefs. The therapist practices skills for reattribution by reviewing evidence and challenging cognitive errors. Behaviour therapy involves identifying safety behaviours, entering feared situations without safety manoeuvres and applying relaxation techniques, activity scheduling and assertiveness training. The therapist will review progress and offer feedback to the client. | The last stage of therapy involves termination. The therapist helps to identify early symptoms of relapse and predict high-risk situations leading to a relapse. The client is taught coping strategies to overcome negative emotions, interpersonal conflicts and pressure. A plan is formulated for early intervention should relapse take place. The skills and knowledge acquired in therapy are consolidated. |
| Address specific concerns | Do you have any questions thus far? Is there anything else that you are concerned about with regard to the proposed therapy? | Even if there are gains in therapy and you feel better, we would not recommend that you stop your antidepressant immediately. | I know that I have shared a lot of information with you. Please allow me to offer you a brochure on CBT to help you understand more about the therapy. |

Common pitfalls

a. Failure to cover the range and depth of the information required for this station

Quick recall*

- The objectives of CBT are to alleviate symptoms such as anxiety and depression by helping the client to identify and challenge negative cognitions.

* Adapted from B.K. Puri, A. Hall and R. Ho (2014). *Revision Notes in Psychiatry*. London, UK: CRC Press, p. 336.

It helps them develop alternative and flexible schemas. It also helps the client to rehearse new cognitive and behavioural responses in difficult situations.

- Core characteristics of CBT
  - There needs to be engagement and collaboration between the therapist and the client.
  - It focuses on specific issues.
  - Homework is assigned.
  - It is time-limited in nature.
  - It focuses on the here and now.
  - Outcomes can be measured by direct observation, physiological measure, standardized instruments and self-report measures, such the Beck Depression Inventory.
- The indications include the following:
  - Mood disorders such as depressive disorder and bipolar disorder
  - Generalized anxiety disorder, panic disorder and obsessive–compulsive disorder (OCD)
  - Phobia: social phobia and simple phobia
  - Eating disorders
  - Impulse control disorders
  - Schizophrenia (with the main focus being that of targeting delusions and hallucinations, coping enhancement, enhancing adherence to treatment and relapse prevention)
  - Personality disorder
  - Substance abuse
  - Liaison psychiatry
- Cognitive techniques used during therapy:

Cognitive restructuring helps the client to identify negative thoughts, dysfunctional assumptions and maladaptive core beliefs relating to their underlying problems. It also tests the validity of those thoughts, assumptions and beliefs. The goal is to produce more adaptive and positive alternatives. Features of cognitive techniques include the following:

- Identification of negative automatic thoughts
- Identification of dysfunctional or faulty assumption
- Identification of maladaptive core belief and rating its strength
- Restructuring the maladaptive core belief
- Rating the impact of the maladaptive belief on emotion
- Rating the impact of new core belief on emotion
- Behavioural techniques used during therapy:

Some of the common techniques include the following:

- Rehearsal: It helps the client to anticipate challenges and to develop strategies to overcome difficulties.
- Inclusion of graded assignment on exposure.
- Training oneself to be self-reliant.
- Pleasure and mastery of skills.

- Activity scheduling to increase contact with positive activities and decrease avoidance and withdrawal.
- Diversion or distraction techniques.
- It is pertinent to allow patients to recognize how each session is structured:
  - Weekly update
  - Bridge from the previous session
  - Review previous homework assigned
  - Setting an agenda for the current session
  - Working on the agenda
  - Providing brief summaries
  - Assigning homework for the next session
  - Summarizing each session and offering feedback
- 12–16 sessions are recommended.
- In the early phase, it is pertinent for the therapist to build on the therapeutic alliance. The client needs to be educated on the model of CBT and the influence of thoughts on behaviour and emotions. Goals are set for the psychotherapy session. Negative automatic thoughts are identified. The therapist makes use of Socratic questioning to reveal the self-defeating nature of the client's thought process and identify cognitive triad.
- In the middle phase, the therapist asks the patient to keep a dysfunctional thought diary. Through the homework assignment, the therapist identifies cognitive errors and core beliefs. The therapist practices skills for reattribution by reviewing evidence and challenging cognitive errors. Behaviour therapy involves identifying safety behaviours, entering feared situations without safety manoeuvres and applying relaxation techniques, activity scheduling and assertiveness training. The therapist reviews progress and offers feedback to the client.
- The last stage of therapy involves termination. The therapist helps to identify early symptoms of relapse and predicts high-risk situations leading to a relapse. The client is taught coping strategies to overcome negative emotions, interpersonal conflicts and pressure. A plan is formulated for early intervention should relapse take place. The skills and knowledge acquired in therapy are consolidated.

STATION 95: PSYCHOTHERAPY – COGNITIVE ERRORS (PAIRED STATION A)

Information to candidates

Name of patient: Mr Patterson

You have been asked to speak to Mr Patterson. He is a 25-year-old footballer with the Manchester United team. Recently, in the last game, he failed to score a very important goal, and that resulted in the team losing the championship title. Ever since the last game, his team coach, Mark, has noticed that he is no longer able to perform on the pitch anymore and has been complaining of increased panic-like symptoms whenever he is on the pitch. Mark is very concerned about this as he used to be the star striker in the team. Mark has brought him here today for an assessment, hoping that something can be done to help him.

Task

Please speak to Mr Patterson and take a history from him. Please also try to elicit the relevant cognitive distortions that he might have. Please note that you will need to speak to the team manager in the next station to discuss with him his concerns.

Outline of station

You are Mr Patterson, and your team manager, Mark, has asked you to come for a psychiatric visitation today. You failed to score an important goal in the last game in the championship last week and that resulted in your team not getting the title. Ever since then, you have been feeling very anxious whenever you are on the pitch. You keep ruminating over thoughts that it was your fault, despite the fact that none of the team members have actually blamed you for it. In addition, despite the fact that you have been nominated as the star player for two consecutive years, you feel that it is entirely not possible for you to be the star player again in view of this mistake that you have made. You feel that you are lousy on the pitch as well as a lousy husband and father at home. You do not really think that the psychiatrist can do much to help you.

CASC construct table

The CASC construct table is formatted such that candidates will be able to cover adequately both the range and the depth of the assessment required in this station.

Starting off: 'Hello, I am Dr Melvyn, one of the psychiatrists from the mental health unit. I understand that your coach requested that you see us today. Can we have a chat?'			
History of presenting complaint	Thanks for seeing us today. Can you help me understand the difficulties that you have been facing?	Thanks for sharing with me. I understand that it must have been a very difficult time for you. About the panic symptoms: Can you tell me when they first started?	Can I clarify the bodily symptoms you experience each time you have those attacks? Are there any specific thoughts that run through your mind when you are feeling so anxious? Are you worried about the next episode happening? Is there any anticipatory anxiety?

(Continued)

Elicit cognitive distortions of minimization and magnification	You mentioned that you have been feeling this way since the time you failed to score an important goal. I'm really sorry to be hearing this. Can you tell me how you managed to play in matches prior to that miss?	It seemed that you have previous successes as well. Are those previous successes not important at all? Is it true that one miss would lead to the loss of the entire match? What was the entire season like for you?	Can you have underestimated your contribution to the team? Have you won any awards before, such as being titled the player of the year? Have you managed to score any difficult balls before? Would you not say that you were remarkable previously?
Elicit cognitive distortions of personalization and labelling	I'm sorry to learn about what happened in the last match. Who do you think is responsible for the loss?	Are you the only striker in the team? Isn't football a team sport? What about the other players? Do they not play a part in contributing to the scores? Have the other players blamed you for the recent miss in the game? It seems to me that you have attributed the failure of the team solely on yourself. Could there be any other factors that might contribute to the loss of the game?	Can you tell me what does missing a goal say about you? I hear that you're calling yourself a loser. Would you call a teammate who merely missed one ball a loser as well?
Elicit cognitive distortions of selective abstraction, overgeneralization and dichotomous thinking	Based on the information that you have provided me, it seemed to me that you have contributed a lot to the team in terms of winning games and getting the championship. How do you feel about those previous achievements?	How have things been outside of football? We all have various roles outside work, such as being a husband and a father. How do you see yourself in those different roles?	It seems to me that you feel that you would have been either a complete success if you had hit the ball, or are now a complete failure because you missed the goal. Are there any shades in between? Thanks for speaking to me. I understand that your coach is here as well. Would you mind if I were to speak to him about your condition?

Common pitfalls

a. Failure to cover the range and depth of the information required for this station

Quick recall*

- Beck proposed a cognitive model of depression from which cognitive therapy has developed. Three concepts seek to explain the psychological substrate of depression:
  - Cognitive triad: The depressed person has a negative personal view, a tendency to interpret his or her ongoing experiences in a negative way and a negative view of the future.
  - Schemas: These are stable cognitive patterns forming the basis for the interpretation of situations.
  - Cognitive errors: There are systematic errors in thinking that maintain depressed people's beliefs in negative concepts.
- Cognitive distortions include Beck's cognitive triad: self, environment and the future. Common cognitive errors in depression are catastrophic thinking, black-and-white thinking, tunnel vision, selective abstraction, labelling, overgeneralization, personalization, 'should' statements, magnification and minimization, discarding evidence or arbitrary inference and emotional reasoning.
- Cognitive bias and questions to be asked:

The questions to ask to elicit the respective cognitive bias are as follows:

Minimization	Did you play a part in any previous success?
	How do you see your role in the team?
	Do you feel that you could have underestimated your contribution?
	Have you won any awards before (such as being the star player in the team)?
	Have you hit any difficult balls before? Would you say those were remarkable?
	How many matches have you won previously?
	How many points have you scored this season? Over how many games?
	That sounds like a good average. What do you think?
Magnification	How did you play in the match before that miss?
	Aren't those successes important as well?
	Would one miss lead to the loss of an entire match?
	What about the whole season?
Overgeneralization	How have things been outside of your current job? We all have various roles outside work as a husband, as a father and as a friend. How do you see yourself in these different roles?

(Continued)

---

* Adapted from B.K. Puri, A. Hall and R. Ho (2014). *Revision Notes in Psychiatry*. London, UK: CRC Press, p. 386.

Selective abstraction	Based on what you have told me, you have contributed a lot to the team. How do you feel about the previous successes?
Personalization	I am sorry to hear that the team has lost the game. Who do you think is responsible for the loss? Are you the only striker on the team? Football is a team sport. What about the other players? Are they not responsible as well? It seems that you attribute failure of the team solely to yourself. Are there other factors contributing?
Arbitrary inference	What do your coach and teammates think about you now? How does this single miss affect the outcome of the season?
Dichotomous thinking	It seems that you're either a complete success if you had hit the ball or a complete failure if you didn't. Are there shades in between?
Catastrophic thinking	It seems like you consider your situation to be rather depressing. Is a disaster going to happen?
Labelling	What does missing the ball say about you? You're calling yourself a loser. Would you call a teammate who merely missed one ball a loser?

STATION 96: PSYCHOTHERAPY – COGNITIVE ERRORS (PAIRED STATION B)

Information to candidates

Name of patient: Mark

You had been asked to speak to Mr Patterson. Mr Patterson is a 25-year-old footballer with the Manchester United team. Recently, in the last game, he failed to score a very important goal, and that resulted in the team losing the championship title. Ever since the last game, his team coach, Mark, has noticed that he is no longer able to perform on the pitch anymore and has been complaining of increased panic-like symptoms whenever he is on the pitch. Mark is very concerned about this as he used to be the star striker in the team. Mark has brought him here today for an assessment, hoping that something could be done to help him. In the previous station, you spoke to Mr Patterson and obtained a history from him. You have managed to identify some cognitive distortions that Mr Patterson has at the moment. You understand that Mark, his team coach, is keen to speak to you more about how he can help his player.

Task

Please speak to Mark, the team coach, and explain the presence of cognitive distortions and discuss the appropriate treatment options.

Outline of station

You are Mark, the coach of the football team that Mr Patterson is in. Mr Patterson has been your star player for the last two seasons. Unfortunately, what happened this season was that he missed a very important goal during the last match of the season and that caused your team to lose the championship. You do not think that it is entirely his fault, as it was partly due to the fact that the organization of the players on the field was suboptimal too. You realize that he has been having panic-like symptoms and has not been able to go on the pitch. You want to know what forms of treatment could be offered to help him. You are concerned about starting him on antidepressant medications, as you are worried that the medications will impair performance. In addition, you do not want your player to be tested positive for drugs and run afoul of the football association rules. You are concerned when the core trainee suggests starting him on a long dose of sleeping tablets to help alleviate his anxiety and panic-like symptoms.

CASC construct table

The CASC construct table is formatted such that candidates will be able to cover adequately both the range and the depth of the assessment required in this station.

Starting off: 'Hello, I am Dr Melvyn, one of the psychiatrists from the mental health unit. I understand that you have some concerns about your player, Mr Patterson. Can we have a chat about this?'			
Explanation of current assessment	I have spoken to your player previously, and I have gathered some information about his condition. Can you help me understand what your concerns are with regard to your player? I fully understand your current concerns, and I do hope that I can help to alleviate some of his symptoms so that he can return back to the pitch as soon as possible.	Based on my assessment, it seems like Mr Patterson has some anxiety-like symptoms, as well as some cognitive distortions. Have you heard of the term 'cognitive distortions' before? Let me explain more. It seems to me that he is thinking and seeing things from negative perspectives. These cognitive distortions are errors in thinking and attributions.	I sense that he is overly concerned about the goal he recently missed scoring. However, he has previous achievements and chooses to magnify the current problem and minimize his past achievements. Also, I realize that he has taken on all the responsibilities for your team's failure to get the championship cup this season and has personalized it such that he feels entirely responsible. He feels that he has been a failure and has generalized these feelings to his other roles as a husband and also as a father.

(Continued)

Management – pharmacological	I understand that you are very concerned about how we can help him to get back to the pitch as soon as possible.	There are various options, and medications might be one option. We could start him on an antidepressant, and the one that we could use would be that of a selective serotonin reuptake inhibitor (SSRI).	These medications would help to regulate the amount of chemicals in his brain that would in turn affect his mood as well as the way he thinks about things.
Management – psychological	Apart from medications, there are other modalities of help we could offer him.	Have you heard of this form of psychotherapy, called CBT, before? CBT would be helpful for him, as it focuses on his current issues, and it would help him to understand how the way he thinks contributes to how he is feeling and his behaviour.	Our therapists can help him to identify the cognitive errors he is making in his thinking. They can help him to restructure the way he thinks about things. We usually recommend a course of therapy, and such therapy usually lasts between 12 and 16 sessions. Apart from psychological-based interventions, it is of utmost importance that your team continues to support him and provide some accommodations for him.
Address concerns	I know I have shared quite a lot of information. Do you have any questions for me?	I understand that you are quite concerned about the medications that we have recommended. Please allow me to clarify that antidepressants are not addictive in nature. Patients who are on antidepressants would not run afoul of the rules of the football association as these are not performance-enhancing drugs.	We might consider giving him some hypnotics or sleeping pills to help him to alleviate his panic-like symptoms. We do need to inform you that sleeping pills are addictive in nature, and we usually do not recommend that he take them over a protected period.

Common pitfalls

a. Failure to cover the range and depth of the information required for this station

Quick recall*

- Pharmacotherapy for panic disorders: The National Institute for Health and Care Excellence (NICE) guidelines recommend SSRI as the first-line treatment for panic disorder. Examples include citalopram, escitalopram, fluoxetine, paroxetine or sertraline. If an SSRI is unsuitable and there is no improvement, consider the usage of imipramine or clomipramine but not venlafaxine. The tricyclic antidepressants imipramine and clomipramine, monoamine oxidase inhibitors (MAOIs) and SSRIs are efficacious in the treatment of panic disorder. The downregulation of 5-hydroxytryptamine (5-HT2) receptors may be responsible for therapeutic effects, which may take up to 4 weeks to appear. Increased anxiety or panic may occur in the first week of treatment. Benzodiazepines reduce the frequency of panic attacks in the short term. There is a need to maintain treatment in the long term, with the risk of dependency.
- Psychological treatment
  - CBT should be offered to generalized anxiety disorder (GAD) and panic disorders.
  - For panic disorder, CBT should be delivered by trained and supervised therapists and closely adhere to the treatment protocols. CBT should be offered weekly with a duration of 1–2 hours and be completed within 4 months. The optimal range is 7 (brief CBT) to 14 hours in total.
- CBT involving the cognitive restructuring of catastrophic interpretations of bodily experiences is effective for panic disorder, as are exposure techniques that generate bodily sensations of fear during therapy with the aim of habituating the subject to them. Agoraphobic avoidance is treated by situational exposure and relaxation techniques.

STATION 97: AGORAPHOBIA – SYSTEMATIC DESENSITIZATION

Information to candidates

Name of patient: Mrs Brown

You have been tasked to speak to Mr Brown, the husband of Mrs Brown. Mrs Brown was seen by your consultant 2 weeks ago and has been diagnosed with an anxiety condition known as agoraphobia. Mr Brown is here today, as he wants to

---

* Adapted from B.K. Puri, A. Hall and R. Ho (2014). *Revision Notes in Psychiatry*. London, UK: CRC Press, p. 415.

know what his wife is suffering from and the causes of her current condition. He is keen to know the available treatments for her condition as well.

Task

Please speak to Mr Brown and address all his concerns and expectations.

Outline of station

You are the husband of Mrs Brown and understand that your wife was seen by the psychiatrist 2 weeks ago. You came by today as you want to know what she is suffering from. You want to have a better understanding of what the doctors are recommending for her in terms of treatment as well. If the core trainee suggests CBT, you hope that the core trainee can explain more about the therapy to you. In addition, you have concerns about how therapy might proceed in the event that your wife is not amenable to step out of her house to come to the psychologist sessions.

CASC construct table

The CASC construct table is formatted such that candidates will be able to cover adequately both the range and the depth of the assessment required in this station.

Starting off: 'Hello, I am Dr Melvyn, one of the psychiatrists from the mental health unit. I understand that you have some concerns about your wife. Can we have a chat about this?'			
Clarifying diagnosis	Can you help me to understand more about your concerns about your wife? Has any doctor told you what she is suffering from?	We saw your wife previously and assessed her condition. It seems to us that she is suffering from a condition known as agoraphobia. Have you heard of this condition before?	Basically, agoraphobia is an anxiety condition in which the patient has anxiety-like panic symptoms, usually when they are in situations which they perceive to be dangerous or uncomfortable. This is a fairly common anxiety-related disorder and can be treated.
Explaining pharmacological treatment	There are several options with regard to treatment. We could start by helping your wife understand more about anxiety and more about her condition.	We do recommend a course of antidepressants to help her with her condition.	Antidepressants would help in the regulation of brain chemicals that are involved in anxiety state and would be beneficial for your wife.

(Continued)

Explaining psychological treatment	Apart from medications, your wife might benefit from a form of talking therapy called CBT. Have you heard about this form of therapy before?	In this form of therapy, it is believed that the way we think in turn affects how we feel and behave. As the name suggests, it is important for you to realize that there are two main principles governing the therapy session.	Cognitive techniques are used during the therapy session. Apart from cognitive techniques, specific behavioural techniques are also used. Some of the common behavioural techniques that might be helpful for your wife include breathing exercises and relaxation training. One component of this therapy that is highly effective is systematic desensitization (SD).
Clarifying structure of treatment	SD usually refers to graded exposure with relaxation. It involves allowing your wife to draw up a hierarchy of her fears and then involves her performing the less anxiety-provoking behaviours first and then progressing on to those that are more anxiety provoking. The therapist would pair this together with relaxation exercises.	The total duration of therapy might take up to 12–16 sessions. We will arrange for your wife to meet up with the therapist on a weekly basis. Each session usually last for around 45 minutes to an hour. There might be some homework exercises prescribed in between the sessions.	The therapist might go through the homework exercises in the initial part of the session. He or she might also go through some of the core skills reviewed in the previous session.
Address concerns and expectations	I know that I have shared quite a lot of information. Do you have any questions for me at the moment?	I hear your concerns about how therapy could potentially progress if your wife is not able to come out of the house. We might be able to make some arrangements for the therapist to visit your wife at home to get the therapy started.	I understand that you have heard that valium might be useful for her condition. It is a hypnotic medication and could be useful for her to calm her down, but over the longer term, we are concerned about its addictive potential. With regard to antidepressants, they are not addictive in nature. I would like to offer you a brochure about CBT and SD. Please feel free to contact me if you need further clarifications.

Common pitfalls

a. Failure to cover the range and depth of the information required for this station

Quick recall*

- The concept is based on that of reciprocal inhibition.
- It holds that relaxation inhibits anxiety so that the two are mutually exclusive.
- It can be used in treating conditions associated with anticipatory anxiety.
- Patients are asked to identify increasingly greater anxiety-evoking stimuli, to form an anxiety hierarchy. During systematic desensitization, the patient is successfully exposed (in reality or in imagination) to these stimuli in the hierarchy, beginning with the least anxiety-evoking one, each exposure being paired with relaxation.
- This differs from the concept of habituation. Habituation is an important component of the behaviour treatment for OCD using exposure and response prevention. The ultimate aim of exposure techniques is to reduce the discomfort associated with eliciting stimuli through habituation.

The other components of CBT should be explained in this station

- Cognitive techniques used during therapy:

Cognitive restructuring helps the client to identify negative thoughts, dysfunctional assumptions and maladaptive core beliefs relating to their underlying problems. It also tests the validity of those thoughts, assumptions and beliefs. The goal is to produce more adaptive and positive alternatives. Features of cognitive techniques include the following:

- Identification of negative automatic thoughts
- Identification of dysfunctional or faulty assumption
- Identification of maladaptive core belief and rating its strength
- Restructuring the maladaptive core belief
- Rating the impact of the maladaptive belief on emotion
- Rating the impact of new core belief on emotion
- Behavioural techniques used during therapy include the following:
  - Rehearsal: This helps the client to anticipate challenges and to develop strategies to overcome difficulties.
  - Inclusion of graded assignment on exposure.
  - Training oneself to be self-reliant.
  - Pleasure and mastery of skills.
  - Activity scheduling to increase contact with positive activities and decrease avoidance and withdrawal.
  - Diversion or distraction techniques.

---

* Adapted from B.K. Puri, A. Hall and R. Ho (2014). *Revision Notes in Psychiatry*. London, UK: CRC Press, p. 28.

- It is pertinent to allow patients to recognize how each session is structured:
  - Weekly update
  - Bridge from the previous session
  - Review previous homework assigned
  - Setting an agenda for the current session
  - Working on the agenda
  - Providing brief summaries
  - Assigning home assignment for the next session
  - Summarizing each session and offering feedback
- Between 12 and 16 sessions are recommended.
- In the early phase, it is important for the therapist to build on the therapeutic alliance. The client needs to be educated on the model of CBT and the influence of thoughts on behaviour and emotions. Goals are set for the psychotherapy session. Negative automatic thoughts are identified. The therapist makes use of Socratic questioning to reveal the self-defeating nature of the client's thought process and identify cognitive triad.
- In the middle phase, the therapist asks the patient to keep a dysfunctional thought diary. Through the homework assignment, the therapist identifies cognitive errors and core beliefs. The therapist practices skills for reattribution by reviewing evidence and challenging cognitive errors. Behaviour therapy involves identifying safety behaviours, entering feared situations without safety manoeuvres and applying relaxation techniques, activity scheduling and assertiveness training. The therapist reviews progress and offers feedback to the client.
- The last stage of therapy involves termination. The therapist helps to identify early symptoms of relapse and predict high-risk situations leading to a relapse. The client is taught coping strategies to overcome negative emotions, interpersonal conflicts and pressure. A plan is formulated for early intervention should relapse take place. The skills and knowledge acquired in therapy are consolidated.

Further information about agoraphobia:

Based on the *International Statistical Classification of Diseases and Related Health Problems,* 10th revision (*ICD-10*) classification system, the following symptoms need to be present to make the diagnosis:

1. Symptoms are manifestations of anxiety and are not secondary to other symptoms such as delusions or obsessional thoughts.
2. Anxiety is restricted to at least two of the following: crowds, public places, travelling away from home and travelling alone.
3. At least two symptoms from automatic arousal symptoms, symptoms involving the chest and abdomen and symptoms involving the mental state need to be present.
4. Avoidance of the phobic situation is prominent.
5. There are two subtypes: agoraphobia without panic disorder or with panic disorder.

Treatment

1. Psychological approaches: Behavioural therapy is the treatment of choice. Exposure techniques are most widely used. Wolpe's systematic desensitization combines relaxation with graded exposure. Reciprocal inhibition prevents anxiety from being maintained when exposed to the phobic stimulus whilst relaxed.
2. Pharmacological approaches: SSRIs such as escitalopram, fluvoxamine, paroxetine and sertraline are the first-line treatment for phobic anxiety disorder.

STATION 98: OCD – EXPOSURE AND RESPONSE PREVENTION

Information to candidates

Name of patient: Mr Benjamin

You have been tasked to speak to Mr Benjamin, who has been referred by his GP for excessive handwashing. Your consultant has diagnosed him with OCD. He has defaulted a follow-up appointment with your consultant but is here today seeking help. He has not taken the antidepressant prescribed previously and is worried about being on medications. He hopes that you can offer an alternative to medications. He has read up online and heard that there are some psychological treatments for his condition. He wants to know more about them.

Task

Please speak to Mr Benjamin and discuss with him more about psychological treatment, in particular the specific form of behaviour therapy that might be indicated in his case. Please address all his concerns and expectations.

Outline of station

You are Mr Benjamin, and you have been referred by your GP to see the psychiatrist because of your excessive preoccupation with contamination and needing to wash as a result of your preoccupations. The psychiatrist has diagnosed you with OCD and has recommended a course of antidepressant. You are ambivalent about being on medications and have not started on the medications recommended by the consultant psychiatrist. You have searched for more information about your condition on the Internet and realize that there are alternatives to medications, such as psychological treatment. You wish to know more about the appropriate psychological treatment and hope that the doctor you're seeing today can give you a better overview of what the psychological treatment entails.

CASC construct table

The CASC construct table is formatted such that candidates will be able to cover adequately both the range and the depth of the assessment required in this station.

Starting off: 'Hello, I am Dr Melvyn, one of the psychiatrists from the mental health unit. I understand that you have some concerns about your condition. Can we have a chat about this?'			
Discuss alternatives to medication	I understand that my consultant has seen you recently and has started you on an antidepressant medication. Can I understand your concerns about your current condition?	I hear your concerns about being on medications (antidepressant) for your condition. Please let me share with you that antidepressants are not addictive in nature. We do usually prescribe antidepressants for patients who are suffering from similar condition as yours.	I hear that you wish to consider alternatives to medications. There are alternatives such as psychotherapy for your current condition. Have you heard of this therapy known as CBT before? Can you share with me more about your understanding of this form of therapy?
Explanation about cognitive aspects of CBT	In this form of therapy, it is believed that the way we think in turn affects how we feel and behave. As the name suggests, it is important for you to realize that there are two main principles governing the therapy session.	Cognitive techniques are used during the therapy session.	Cognitive restructuring helps you to identify negative thoughts, dysfunctional assumptions and maladaptive core beliefs relating to your underlying problems. It also tests the validity of those thoughts, assumptions and beliefs. The goal is to produce more adaptive and positive alternatives.
Explanation about behavioural aspects of CBT	Apart from the cognitive component of this form of therapy, there are other behavioural techniques that are used in this form of therapy.	In particular, one particular form of behavioural therapy, known as exposure and response prevention, is very helpful for your condition. Do you have any ideas about what it entails?	Exposure and response prevention involves first making a hierarchy of situations from the least anxiety provoking to the most anxiety provoking. The therapist will gradually expose you to the situation you are fearful of being in and at the same time will prevent you from performing your routine ritual.

(Continued)

Explain structure of sessions	The total duration of therapy might range from 12 to 16 sessions.	Each session usually lasts between 45 minutes to an hour. There might be some homework that is assigned in between the sessions.	You will be engaging with a therapist who has professional training in this area.
Address other concerns and expectations	I know that I have shared a whole lot of information. Do you have any questions for me?	CBT and, in particular, exposure and response prevention therapy have been known to be efficacious for patients with OCD.	I would like to offer you some brochures to take home, for you to understand more about what the psychological therapy entails. Would that be alright with you? Should you have any other questions, please feel free to fix a time with me for further discussion.

Common pitfalls

a. Failure to cover the range and depth of the information required for this station

Quick recall*

- Pharmacotherapy: Antidepressants are effective in the short-term treatment of OCD. SSRIs such as fluvoxamine, fluoxetine, paroxetine and sertraline are commonly used. Clomipramine and SSRIs have greater efficacy than antidepressants with no selective serotonergic properties. Concomitant depression is not necessary for serotonergic antidepressants to improve symptoms. There are success rates of 50%–79%. Relapse often follows discontinuation of treatment. For treatment-resistant OCD, there is some evidence that adding quetiapine or risperidone to antidepressant helps to improve efficacy, but this needs to be weighed against less tolerability and limited data.
- Psychological treatments: NICE guidelines recommend evoked response prevention (ERP) and CBT for OCD and body dysmorphic disorder.
  - For the initial treatment of OCD, ERP (up to 10 therapist hours per client), brief individual CBT using self-help materials and telephone and group CBT should be offered.
  - For adults with OCD with mild-to-moderate functional impairment, more intensive CBT (including ERP) (more than 10 therapist hours per client) is recommended.

---

* Adapted from B.K. Puri, A. Hall and R. Ho (2014). *Revision Notes in Psychiatry.* London, UK: CRC Press, p. 418.

- For children and young people with OCD with moderate-to-severe functional impairments, CBT (including ERP) is a first-line treatment option.
- With regard to the course of the illness, the favourable prognostic factors include mild symptoms, predominance of phobic ruminative ideas, absence of compulsion and short duration of symptoms. There should not be any childhood symptoms or abnormal personality traits.
- The poor prognostic factors include males with early onset, symptoms involving the need for symmetry and exactness, the presence of hopelessness, hallucinations or delusions, a family history of OCD and a continuous, episodic or deteriorating course.
- Habituation is an important component of the behaviour treatment for OCD using exposure and response prevention. The ultimate aim of exposure techniques is to reduce the discomfort associated with eliciting stimuli through habituation.

STATION 99: PANIC DISORDER AND HYPERVENTILATION

Information to candidates

Name of patient: Mr Winslow

You have been asked to review a 40-year-old male, Mr Winslow, in the emergency room. Your medical colleagues have informed you that Mr Winslow came through the emergency services after he called the ambulance when he was feeling unwell at home. He told the medics that he felt as if he was having a heart attack. The medics have done the necessary biochemical investigation and heart tracing monitoring and have ruled out an underlying cardiac issue. The medics strongly believe that Mr Winslow is feeling this way due to a possible underlying psychiatric disorder. Apart from the normal results obtained thus far, the medics are convinced that he does not have a cardiac history as he has been extensively worked up by the cardiologist in the outpatient clinic. You have been informed that Mr Winslow does have a positive family history of cardiovascular disease, and in fact, two of his relatives just passed on recently due to cardiac arrest. His daughter, Sarah, is here and wants to speak to you. She is deeply concerned about her father's issue.

Task

Please speak to Sarah, the daughter of Mr Winslow, and explain the likely diagnosis for him. Please also address all her concerns and expectations accordingly.

Outline of station

You are the daughter of Mr Winslow and are quite distressed by your father's condition. This is the fifth time this month that he has called an ambulance to take him to the hospital. You are especially worried as two of your close relatives have just passed on due to underlying cardiac issues. You understand that your father has had been extensively worked up by the cardiologist, and thus far, there have not been any abnormalities discovered. You are curious as to what is really wrong with your father now that he has been referred to see a psychiatrist. If the core trainee explains that Mr Winslow might have an underlying panic disorder or hyperventilation disorder, you expect the core trainee to explain more about the disorders. You want to know from the core trainee how best you as a carer could help support your father's current condition. You wonder whether there is any role for medications in his case. In addition, you wonder whether your father will be fit for his regular routines of golfing.

CASC construct table

The CASC construct table is formatted such that candidates will be able to cover adequately both the range and the depth of the assessment required in this station.

Starting off: 'Hello, I am Dr Melvyn, one of the psychiatrists from the mental health unit. I understand that you have some concerns about your father's condition. Can we have a chat about it?'			
Explanation of current findings and reassurance	I'm sorry to hear how difficult it has been for you. I understand that you are very worried about your father's condition. My emergency room colleagues have informed me to see your father, to see how we can jointly help him.	Based on my understanding, the medical team has done quite a comprehensive evaluation of his medical condition. Thus far, the laboratory investigations that have been done are normal, and the heart tracing is normal as well.	The medical team does not currently think that your father has an underlying heart condition or that he is having a heart attack. From my understanding, he has been seen by the cardiologist recently, who has done a very comprehensive workup as well. Thus far, everything seems fine with regard to his heart.
Clarify diagnosis of panic disorder	I hear that you're concerned as to what the underlying cause could be given that all the investigations we've done are normal. This is the reason why my medical colleagues have called upon me. At times, some patients with a psychiatric condition might experience such symptoms. Would you mind if I go on to explain more after having spoken to and assessed your father?	One of the conditions that we feel your father might have at the moment is a panic disorder. Have you heard of panic disorders before? Can I go on to explain more about panic disorder? Panic disorder usually involves recurrent unpredictable attacks of severe anxiety lasting usually for a few minutes only.	There could be a sudden onset of palpitations, chest pain, choking, dizziness, depersonalization and derealization, together with a fear of dying, losing control or going mad. It often results in a hurried exit and a subsequent avoidance of similar situations. This is in turn followed by persistent fears of another attack.

(Continued)

Clarify diagnosis of hyperventilation disorder	The other clinical diagnosis that we think applies to your father is hyperventilation syndrome. Have you heard about this condition before?	Hyperventilation syndrome results when an individual makes excessive use of accessory muscles to breathe, thus resulting in hyper-inflated lungs.	The symptoms of hyperventilation disorder can resemble panic disorder.
Management	There are various ways we can help to manage your father's symptoms.	The acute phase usually involves reassuring patients and helping them establish normal breathing patterns. Sometimes, the anxiety can be reduced through the prescription of anxiolytics.	In the longer term, the management involves teaching appropriate relaxation techniques. If the condition persists, we can consider referring your father for a form of psychotherapy or talking therapy known as CBT. Have you heard of this therapy before? Can I leave you a brochure about the therapy for you to understand it further?
Address all concerns and expectations	I understand that I have shared quite a lot of information. Do you have any specific questions you wish to ask?	With regard to medications, there are some medications available to help with his anxiety condition, apart from the hypnotics we have discussed earlier. At times, we do consider the commencement of antidepressants to help with the symptoms.	With time, I am hopeful that your father will respond well to the treatment, and he should be able to get back to activities he previously enjoyed.

Common pitfalls

a. Failure to cover the range and depth of the information required for this station

Quick recall*

ICD-10 diagnostic criteria for panic disorder

- Episodic paroxysmal anxiety not confined to a predictable situation
- Several attacks occur within 1 month

---

* Adapted from B.K. Puri, A. Hall and R. Ho (2014). *Revision Notes in Psychiatry*. London, UK: CRC Press, p. 415.

- Discrete episodes of intense fear or discomfort, abrupt onset that reaches a maximum within a few minutes and autonomic arousal symptoms with freedom from anxiety symptoms between attacks
- Symptoms involving the chest and the abdomen
- Symptoms involving mental state
- Hot flushes and chills
- The medical differential diagnosis to consider includes respiratory disorders: chronic obstructive pulmonary disease (COPD), asthma and mitral valve prolapse and endocrine disorders such as diabetes, hypoglycaemia, thyrotoxicosis and anaemia.
- Differences between panic disorder and hyperventilation syndrome:
  - Panic disorder is a recognized disorder on both the *ICD-10* and *Diagnostic and Statistical Manual of Mental Disorders,* 5th edition (*DSM-5*) diagnostic criteria. Approximately 50%–60% of patients with panic disorder or agoraphobia also have hyperventilation syndrome. Biological and psychological causes are well defined. Panic disorder has more mental symptoms compared with hyperventilation syndrome. The role of metabolic disturbances is less well established. Acute management involves reassuring the patients, establishing normal breathing pattern and reducting anxiety using anxiolytics. Long-term managements include relaxation exercises and CBT.
  - Hyperventilation syndrome is not a recognized disorder on both the *ICD-10* and *DSM-5* diagnostic criteria. Twenty-five per cent of patients with hyperventilation syndrome have symptoms of panic disorder as well. The aetiology is less well defined. Lactate, Cholecystokinin (CCK), caffeine and psychological stressors also play a role. Salient clinical features include the fact that high thoracic breathing or excessive use of accessory muscles to breathe in turn result in hyper-inflated lungs. Metabolic disturbances: acute hypocalcaemia: positive Chvostek and Trousseau signs and prolonged QTc interval/hypokalaemia with generalized weakness /respiratory alkalosis and acute hypophosphataemia leading to paraesthesia and generalized weakness. In terms of management, investigations include d-dimer and possible V/Q scan to rule out pulmonary embolism. Acute and long-term management are similar to panic disorder. De-arousal strategy is useful.

STATION 100: INTERPERSONAL THERAPY (IPT)

Information to candidates

Name of patient: Grace

You have been tasked to see Grace, a 25-year-old female, who has been referred to the specialist service by her GP. The GP noted that she has been low in her mood following the loss of her mother, as well as due to her relationship issues with her husband. The consultant psychiatrist has previously recommended a combination of medication and interpersonal psychotherapy, but Grace was not keen. She is back here for a follow-up and is keen to consider interpersonal psychotherapy. She hopes to find out more about the therapy before commencing on it.

Task

Please speak to Grace and explain more about interpersonal psychotherapy to her. Please assess to see whether she is suitable for the therapy. If she is not suitable for the therapy, please recommend other alternatives for her.

Outline of Station

You are Grace, a 25-year-old female, who has been referred to the specialist service by your GP. The consultant psychiatrist previously recommended a combination of medication and interpersonal psychotherapy for your depressive symptoms. However, you were not keen for the psychotherapy. You have returned today as you feel that you are more ready for it. Your stressors include the recent loss of your beloved mother, as well as some relationship issues with your husband. Recently, there have been some changes at the workplace as well, as your company is streamlining the business and is dismissing some staff. You would like to know more about the therapy and whether it would be suitable for you.

CASC construct table

The CASC construct table is formatted such that candidates will be able to cover adequately both the range and the depth of the assessment required in this station.

Starting off: 'Hello, I am Dr Melvyn, one of the psychiatrists from the mental health unit. I understand that you have some concerns. Can we have a chat about it?'			
History of presenting complaint	I understand that you have been seen by our consultant and have been diagnosed with depression. How long have you been feeling low? When did this first start?	Apart from your low mood, do you find yourself having less interest in things or activities which you previously enjoyed doing? How is your energy level? Do you have enough energy to get through a normal day?	How has your sleep been for you? What about your appetite? Can you manage your meals? Have things been so stressful for you that you have had unusual experiences (such as hearing voices) when you are alone? Have you felt that life is no longer worth living? Have you entertained thoughts recently with regard to ending your life?
Determination of whether her current symptoms are suitable for interpersonal psychotherapy	Did the consultant psychiatrist explain to you what mental health condition you have? Did he inform you more about the severity of your mental health condition?	Prior to this, have you seen a psychiatrist?	Interpersonal therapy is usually indicated for patients with mild-to-moderate depression and not for patients with bipolar disorder or severe depression. This is why I am checking with you regarding your history.

(Continued)

Identify recent grief	Can you share with me your recent stressors? I am sorry to learn that your mother has passed on recently.	How have you been coping with the loss? Was it a sudden event, or did you have knowledge that your mother has been ill for some time?	Did you manage to attend the funeral? How are you currently feeling with regard to your mother's death?
Identify interpersonal disputes	Besides the recent loss of your mother, have there been any other matters that have been bothering you?	Can you tell me a bit more about how your relationship with your husband has been bothering you?	How long has it been bothering you? Apart from the frequent disagreements and arguments, has your husband been physically aggressive towards you?
Identify role transitions	Have there been any other changes in your life?	You mentioned that there have been some changes at your workplace. Can you tell me more?	
Identify interpersonal role deficits	Is there someone to whom you could confide when you feel low in your mood?	How is your relationship with your family members?	What about your relationships with your friends and colleagues?
Explanation of structure of therapy	The main aim of interpersonal therapy (IPT) is to reduce your suffering and to improve interpersonal functioning. IPT focuses mainly on interpersonal relationship as a means to bring about change. The goal is to help you to improve your interpersonal relationships or change your expectations regarding interpersonal relationships.	IPT is designed to help you to recognize your interpersonal needs and to seek attachment and reassurance in the process of improving interpersonal relationships.	There are three main stages of IPT. In the first stage, the therapist tries his or her best to develop a good therapeutic relationship with you and to understand your problems. In the second stage, the therapist analyses the way you communicate with other people. The therapist gives you useful advice and helps you to develop new skills by means of role-play. In the final stage, the therapist will strengthen the skills you learned in the therapy. The therapist will help to identify resources for you to handle interpersonal problems in the future. The whole IPT takes around 16–20 sessions.

Common pitfalls

a. Failure to cover the range and depth of the information required for this
station

Quick recall*

Interpersonal therapy is based on attachment theory.

- The objectives are to create a therapeutic environment with a meaningful
  therapeutic relationship and recognition of the client's underlying attachment
  needs, to develop an understanding of the client's communication difficulties
  and attachment style both inside and outside of therapy, to identify the client's
  maladaptive patterns of communication and establishment of insight and to
  assist the client in building a better social support network and mobilizing
  resources.
- The indications are for depressive disorders (in which IPT has been
  demonstrated to be as effective as CBT) and eating disorders: bulimia
  nervosa, dysthymia and other interpersonal disputes, role transitions, grief
  and loss.
- Structure of the sessions:
  - Initial phase: Definition of depression and explaining diagnosis. There is
    a need to offer an interpersonal formation. It is pertinent to explain the
    rationales of IPT and the logistics of treatment such as treatment contract.
    It is important to identify target interpersonal problems such as grief, role
    transition, role dispute and interpersonal deficits.
  - Middle phase: It is important to identify one to two interpersonal problem
    areas. There is a need to assess the impact of interpersonal events on
    mood. Patients' expectations should be explored. An interpersonal
    inventory card needs to be filled up. Communication analysis helps to
    identify maladaptive patterns of communication. The therapist can adopt
    three stances: neutral, passive and client advocate stance on correcting
    communication patterns. Role-play and strategies need to be developed so
    that the patient is able to handle similar situations in the future. For grief,
    it is important to explore grief feelings for loss of relationship or loss of
    status, facilitate mourning of loss and develop interests and relationships
    to substitute for loss. For interpersonal disputes, it is important to
    identify the current stage of interpersonal disputes and to understand
    role expectations, modify non-reciprocal role expectations, examine
    interpersonal relationships and assumptions behind patient's behaviour
    and modify faulty assumptions. For role transitions, the therapist needs to
    help the patient to accept the loss of previous roles and develop a positive
    attitude towards the new roles and to develop a sense of mastery in new
    roles. For interpersonal role deficits, it is important to reduce social

---

* Adapted from B.K. Puri, A. Hall and R. Ho (2014). *Revision Notes in Psychiatry*. London, UK: CRC
Press, pp. 340–343.

isolation, encourage formation of new relationships and explore repetitive patterns in relationships.

- Termination phase: It is important to discuss the impact of termination. It is important to acknowledge that termination may trigger grief feelings. The patient needs to establish competency to handle interpersonal problems independently after termination. It is also important to identify social support services.

Explanation of IPT to a client

IPT is in essence a time-limited psychotherapy. The main aim of IPT is to reduce the patient's suffering and to help the patient to improve interpersonal functioning.

- IPT focuses mainly on interpersonal relationships and how this psychotherapy can help bring about change. The ultimate goal is to help patients to improve interpersonal relationships or change expectations regarding interpersonal relationships.
- The therapist helps the patient to improve their social support network so that they can be better able to manage any interpersonal distress. IPT is designed to help the patient recognize their interpersonal needs and to seek attachment and reassurance in the process of improving interpersonal relationships.
- With regard to the number of stages that IPT has, it has basically three different stages. In the first stage, the therapist tries his or her best to develop a therapeutic relationship with the patient and understand the patient's problem in greater detail. In the second stage, the therapist seeks the patient's views to work on an agreed problem area. The therapist analyses the way the patient communicates with other people. The therapist gives useful advice and helps the patient develop new skills by using role-playing. The therapist helps the patient work on issues related to loss and to develop a new role. In the final stage, the therapist strengthens the skills the patient learnt in therapy.
- The therapist, during termination, will help to identify resources for the patient to handle interpersonal problems in the future.
- The whole IPT takes around 16–20 sessions.

STATION 101: TERMINATION OF THERAPY AND TRANSFERENCE REACTION

Information to candidates

Name of patient: Mr Charlie Brown

You have been asked to see Mr Charlie Brown, who has requested to stop attending his psychotherapy sessions. He enrolled in psychodynamic psychotherapy and has since attended three sessions.

Task

Please speak to him and explore his reasons for wanting to discontinue therapy. Please advise him accordingly.

Outline of station

You are Mr Charlie Brown and were diagnosed with depression around 2 months ago. The psychiatrist recommends for you to be on an antidepressant as well as to be commenced on psychotherapy. You have attended three sessions of psychotherapy, but you are reluctant to continue on with the therapy. You do not think that you wish to continue, although you know that your depressive symptoms have not actually improved. There have not been any other changes in life causing you to want to terminate therapy. You do not have any financial concerns that would limit your attendance of psychotherapy. You wish to stop the current therapy, as you do not wish to be constantly talking about your past. You feel that the therapist is cold and unemotional and not understanding, and he seems to be critical towards you at times. This brings to mind some past relationships you have had. You are not keen to continue on with therapy no matter what the core trainee says.

CASC construct table

The CASC construct table is formatted such that candidates will be able to cover adequately both the range and the depth of the assessment required in this station.

Starting off: 'Hello, I am Dr Melvyn, one of the psychiatrists from the mental health unit. I understand that you have some concerns with regard to the therapy that you are attending. Can we have a chat about it?'			
Exploration of potential reasons leading to discontinuing of therapy – patient factors	I understand that you have some concerns about the therapy that has been recommended and organized for you. Can you help me understand more about it? How many sessions of the therapy have you attended thus far?	At times, patients do tell us that they wish to discontinue therapy for a variety of reasons. Sometimes it is because they feel that therapy has been going on well for them, and their symptoms have improved. Is this the case for you? How have you been feeling in your mood?	At times, patients wish to discontinue the therapy because they have experienced some changes in their life. Have there been any recent changes in your life? Have you moved house recently? Is there adequate time for you to attend the therapy sessions? Do you have financial concerns that might limit your attendance?

(Continued)

Exploration of potential reasons leading to discontinuing of therapy – therapist factors	Thanks for sharing with me your concerns. Sometimes, patients do tell us they wish to discontinue therapy due to therapist-related reasons.	Have you ever felt that your therapist is not competent enough to help you with your problems? Do you feel that he or she lacks the necessary competence and experience?	Is one of the reasons for you wanting to discontinue therapy that you do not have trust in the therapist? You mentioned that you have undergone three psychotherapy sessions thus far. Has there been any change of therapist in between the sessions that you have attended thus far?
Identification of core problems	You mentioned that you do not feel comfortable with the therapist. Would you mind telling me more? In what ways does the therapist makes you feel uncomfortable?	I'm sorry to hear that you feel that the therapist seemed to be critical towards you. You also mentioned that the therapist seemed to be cold and unemotional throughout the therapy sessions.	Does the attitude of the therapist remind you of any previous relationships you have had? Can you tell me more? Am I right to say that the way you are currently feeling towards the therapist is similar to the way you used to feel towards your father (who you felt was very harsh and critical towards you)?
Explanation of transference	It seems to me that the way you are feeling towards the therapist is due to a process called transference. Have you heard about this before?	Transference is the process in which a patient projects onto the therapist feelings and emotions that are derived from previous difficult relationships (in your case, it seems to me that the previous difficult relationship you have had was that with your father).	Whilst transference in itself might seem to limit the therapy, it is also crucial to work through these feelings.
Address concern and advise patient accordingly	I understand that you are not keen to continue with therapy. However, I hope that you can reconsider this. Sometimes we do advise our patients that when they are undergoing psychotherapy, they might start to feel worse before actually getting better.	It is important for you to speak to your therapist more about the feelings that you are having at the moment, as it is important to address and work through these feelings, as it might affect your future relationships with others.	Do you have any questions for me? I really hope you can reconsider and speak to your therapist. Of course, should you still feel strongly against therapy, we could arrange another session to discuss further how best we can help you with regard to the therapy.

Common pitfalls

a. Failure to cover the range and depth of the information required for this station
b. Failure to explore all possible areas for patient's wish to terminate therapy

Do not appear to be paternalistic in the approach of this station. Explore patient's concerns and expectations and respect his or her decision.

Quick recall*

Negative reactions during dynamic psychotherapy

- Resistance: The patient is ambivalent about getting help and may oppose attempts from the therapist who offers help. Resistance may manifest in the form of silence, avoidance or absences.
- Acting out: This typically refers to the poor containment of strong feelings triggered by the therapy.
- Acting in: This typically refers to the exploration of therapist's personal and private information by the client or even presenting a symbolic gift to a therapist.
- Negative therapeutic reaction: This refers to the sudden and unexpected worsening or regression in spite of apparent progression during therapy (such as premature termination of therapy by the client without any explanation despite a period of engagement).

Brief overview of dynamic psychotherapy and how to explain to patients

- Dynamic psychotherapy is helpful for a patient who wants to understand how his or her current difficulties may be related to past experiences.
- Traditional psychoanalysis involves frequent meetings (at least five times a week), whereas in brief dynamic psychotherapy, the aim is to reduce the distress reported by the client through less frequent sessions over a time-limited period (such as weekly session over a period of 6 months to 1 year).
- The therapist works with the client to identify recurrent patterns. The therapist helps the client to draw upon feelings evoked during the therapy session. The therapist promotes reflective thinking and helps the clients to make links with past experiences. The goals of therapy are to resolve conflict, to effect changes to improve quality of life and to enhance the client's capacity to handle frustration.
- In general, patients who are more articulate, psychologically inclined and able to tolerate stress are more likely to benefit from brief dynamic psychotherapy. The therapist is mostly nondirective and follows the thoughts and feelings of the client.

---

* Adapted from B.K. Puri, A. Hall and R. Ho (2014). *Revision Notes in Psychiatry*. London, UK: CRC Press, pp. 334–335, 132.

Transference and countertransference concepts

- Transference: This is an unconscious process in which the patient transfers to the therapist feelings, emotions or attitudes that were experienced and desired in the patient's childhood, usually in relation to parents and siblings.
- It is important to note that transference can be both positive and negative.
- For example, the therapist's transference represents on one hand a very powerful ally, but in consideration of the possible transference's resistance, it might be a therapeutic difficulty in itself.
- Countertransference: This is the therapist's own feelings, emotions and attitude towards his patient. In the treatment mode, the therapist needs to screen out those that are mediated only by the therapist and take note of those generated in the therapist from emotional contact with the patient.

STATION 102: DEFENCE MECHANISMS

Information to candidates

Name of patient: Robert

You have been tasked to Robert, a 40-year-old male who has been referred by his GP. His GP stated in the memo that Robert has been having much difficulty at work. He is having difficulties with meeting the deadlines at work as well as with his relationships with his work colleagues.

Task

Please speak to Robert with the aim of understanding more about his difficulties at work. Please identify the relevant psychodynamic defences that he may be using. You are expected to explain to the patient more about his condition and address all his concerns and expectations.

Outline of station

You are Robert, a 40-year-old male who has been referred by your GP for having difficulties at work. Recently, you have been having difficulties with work, especially in terms of your relationships with your colleagues. You have been married for 2 months, and things have not gone well with your current marital relationship. Your wife is keen to have a child, but you are not feeling prepared for it. You have been trying to explain to her, but it always ends up in an argument. You are not sure why this is affecting your work as well. Your colleagues have mentioned that you appear more irritable when you are working with them. You decided to see your GP as you realized that you need some help.

CASC construct table

The CASC construct table is formatted such that candidates will be able to cover adequately both the range and the depth of the assessment required in this station.

Starting off: 'Hello, I am Dr Melvyn, one of the psychiatrists from the mental health unit. I understand that you have been referred by your GP for work-related difficulties. Can we have a chat about this?'		
Presenting history	I understand from the memo that you have seen your GP for work-related difficulties. Can you tell me more about what has been troubling you at work?	I'm sorry to be hearing about this. It must be a difficult time for you. Did your colleagues comment about the change in your work attitude as well?	How long have you been having difficulties at work?
Current stressor	How has your mood been recently? Have you lost interest in things which you have previously enjoyed doing? Is there anything that is bothering you at the moment?	Have there been any problems at home with regard to finances or relationships? Can you tell me more?	I'm sorry to hear that things have been difficult for you at home. You mentioned that there have been some difficulties in terms of your relationship with your wife. Does that result in frequent arguments? How has she been treating you recently?
Identification of relevant psychodynamic defences that patient is using	It seems to me that you have been undergoing a very tough period for the last 2 months. Things have not been going well since you got married. You have been quite upset about your wife.	There is a chance that your current difficulties with your work and in terms of your relationship with your colleagues might be a resultant effect of your difficulties at home.	Sometimes, when we are undergoing stressful situations, we tend to displace and shift our emotions from one situation onto another situation. For example, a colleague who is scolded by the consultant for her performance might project her anger onto her family members or an object. This is common and is a form of defence mechanism known as displacement. Have you heard of this before?
Address concerns and expectations	I understand that your work-related issues are an additional stress for you.	I hope I can refer you to the counsellor or perhaps the psychotherapist for them to help you cope with the situation better.	Would that be fine with you? Do you have any other questions for me?

Common pitfalls

a. Failure to cover the range and depth of the information required for this station

In this station, you may want to consider using the technique of 'reflection', using examples that the patient cited to reflect the core defence mechanisms. This will help to demonstrate to the examiner that you are doing a systematic interview and that you know what the defence mechanisms are.

Quick recall*

Overview of defence mechanisms:

Repression	The pushing away of unacceptable ideas, affects, emotions, memories and drives, relegating them to unconscious. When this is successful, there remains no trace in consciousness.
Reaction formation	A psychological attitude that is directly opposed to an oppressed wish and constitutes a reaction against it.
Isolation	Certain thoughts/affects/behaviours are isolated so that links with other thoughts or memories are broken.
Undoing	An attempt to negate or atone for the forbidden thoughts, affect and memories.
Projection	Unacceptable qualities, feelings, thoughts or wishes are being projected onto another person or thing.
Projective identification	The subject sees the other as possessing aspects of the self that have been repressed but also constrains the other to take on those aspects.
Identification	Attributes of others are now taken onto oneself.
Turning against the self	An impulse meant to be expressed to another is being turned against oneself.
Rationalization	An attempt to explain, in a logically consistent or ethically acceptable way, ideas, thoughts and feelings whose true motives are not perceived. It operates in everyday life and in a delusional system.
Sublimation	A process that utilizes the force of a sexual instinct in drives, affects and memories to motivate creative activities having no apparent connection with sexuality.
Regression	Transition, at times of stress and threat, to moods of expression and functioning that are on a lower level of complexity, so that one returns to an earlier level of maturational functioning.
Denial	Denying the external reality of an unwanted or unpleasant piece of information.
Splitting	Separating good objects, affects and memories from bad ones.
Distortion	Reshaping external reality to suit inner needs.
Acting out	Expressing unconscious emotional conflicts or feelings directly in actions without being consciously aware of their meaning.
Displacement	Emotions, ideas or wishes are transferred from their original object to a more acceptable substitute.
Intellectualization	Excessive abstract thinking occurs to avoid conflicts or disturbing feelings.

---

* Adapted from B.K. Puri, A. Hall and R. Ho (2014). *Revision Notes in Psychiatry*. London, UK: CRC Press, pp. 136,137.

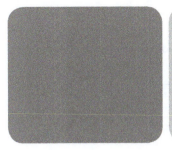

STATION 103: BORDERLINE PERSONALITY DISORDER

Information to candidates

Name of patient: Samantha

Samantha, a 25-year-old female, has been admitted to the emergency services following her attempt to overdose on medication. This is her third visitation to the emergency services within the past month. The medical team is concerned about her recurrent overdoses and have requested the on-call psychiatrist to speak to her to determine whether she has any mental health issues. You are the on-call core trainee 3, and your consultant has requested that you assess the patient first.

Task

Please speak to Samantha and obtain a complete history from her. Please get sufficient history to formulate a clinical diagnosis.

Outline of station

The purpose of providing an outline of the station is to allow candidates to be familiar with the structure of the station. This outline could also be helpful when candidates practice for the MRCPsych, joining with their colleagues to act out the station.

Please note that the outlines provided are based on the experiences of the authors. There may be variations in the actual examination.

You are Samantha and have been transferred to the accident and emergency department following an attempt to overdose again. This is your third episode of overdosing this month. You have been having stressors mainly from your relationship difficulties. You have a history of short and intense relationships. You feel abandoned and unloved in between relationships. You cut yourself or overdose at times as a way to cope with the stressors arising from these relationships. There have also been times in which you have done impulsive acts. You are willing to disclose more only if the interviewer is nice and empathetic in questioning.

CASC construct table

The CASC construct table is formatted such that candidates will be able to cover adequately both the range and the depth of the assessment required in this station.

Starting off: 'Hello, I am Dr Melvyn, one of the psychiatrists from the mental health unit. I understand that you have just been admitted to the emergency department. Can we have a chat?'			
Rapport building and history of presenting complaint and explore borderline traits – self-harm attempts	I received some information from the medical doctors. My understanding is that you have been admitted to the emergency department following an overdose. Am I right? I'm sorry to learn of that, and I understand that it must have been quite a difficult time for you.	Can you tell me more about what happened? Was there anything bothering you prior to the attempt?	Is this the first time that it has occurred? When did something similar happen? How recent was that? You mentioned that you have previously overdosed on medications. Have you done anything else? You mentioned that you have cut yourself previously. How frequently was that? What do you use to cut? What was running through your mind when you cut yourself? Were you having thoughts of ending your life, or were you cutting yourself to release the stress and tension within?
Explore borderline traits – relationships	It seems to me that the main stressor that led to you having an overdose was your relationship issues.	How do you usually cope when your relationships do not turn out well? How do you feel when your relationships end? Have you ever felt that you have been abandoned, especially in between relationships?	How many relationships have you had now? How long does each relationship last for you?
Explore borderline traits – identity disturbances and impulsiveness	Can you tell me how you feel about yourself and your future?	Some people tell me that they have this feeling of chronic emptiness. Have you had such feelings and experiences before?	How would you describe yourself? Do you think you are someone who is very impulsive?
Explore borderline traits – affective instability	How has your mood been?	Do you find that there is much fluctuation in your mood? What do others say about your mood?	

(Continued)

Explore quasi-psychotic symptoms	With all these stressors that you have been enduring, has there been a time in which you have had unusual experiences?	By that I mean hearing voices or seeing things that are not there?	Can you tell me more?

Common pitfalls

a. Failure to cover the range and depth of the information required for this station

If the patient mentions that she has been self-cutting, it would be worthwhile to offer to look at the cuts. This demonstrates empathy on your part and also allows you to assess for the severity of the cuts and possible complications (e.g. infection or abscess).

Quick recall*

The prevalence of borderline personality disorder is 1%–2%.

- The gender ratio is 1:2 (males : females).
- The age of onset is usually during adolescence or early adulthood.
- The suicide rate is 9%.

The *International Statistical Classification of Diseases and Related Health Problems*, 10th revision (*ICD-10*) classifies emotionally unstable personality disorder into impulsive and borderline type. The *Diagnostic and Statistical Manual of Mental Disorders*, 5th edition (*DSM-5*) does not propose the concept of emotionally unstable personality disorder and has only borderline personality disorder. The patient meets the general criteria for personality disorder with at least three of the following symptoms of impulsive type:

- Affect: tendency towards outbursts of anger or violence, with inability to control the resulting behavioural explosions, unstable and capricious mood
- Behaviour: marked tendency to act unexpectedly and without consideration of consequences; marked tendency of quarrelsome behaviour and conflicts with others, especially when impulsive acts are thwarted or criticized and difficulty in maintaining any course of action that offers no immediate reward

Elicit borderline personality disorder (key questions to ask):

- Do you have problems with your anger control? How often do you get into quarrels?

---

* Adapted from: B.K. Puri, A. Hall and R. Ho (2014). *Revision Notes in Psychiatry*. London, UK: CRC Press, p. 443.

- How often do you feel empty inside? What do you do when you feel empty?
- How are your relationships with other people?
- How would you feel if your friend or partner left you? Would you have a strong feeling of abandonment?
- Do you think that your friends view you as a moody person?
- How often do you hurt yourself? Why do you cut yourself? Do you want to re-experience the pain in the past?
- Commonly associated conditions include depression, post-traumatic stress disorder (PTSD), substance misuse and bulimia nervosa.

Management

Inpatient treatment and therapeutic communities	Indications for admission: 1. Life-threatening suicide attempt 2. Imminent danger to other people 3. Psychosis 4. Severe symptoms interfering with functioning that are unresponsive to outpatient treatment Risk of hospitalizations include the following: 1. Stigma 2. Disruption of social and occupational roles 3. Loss of freedom 4. Hospital-induced behavioural regression
Psychotherapy	• Long-term inpatient psychotherapy is recommended because patients can handle challenges in their daily life with the support from psychotherapists. • Dialectical behaviour therapy and mentalization-based therapy are recommended treatment for people with borderline personality disorder. • The National Institute for Health and Care Excellence (NICE) guidelines recommend that therapists should use an explicit and integrated approach and share this with their clients. • The guidelines also recommend that the therapists should set therapy at twice per week and should not offer brief interventions. • Supportive psychotherapy helps to diminish the suicidal behaviours and impulsive acts whilst awaiting a remission, since the long-term prognosis of the disorder is good. • Cognitive behavioural therapy (CBT) focuses on maladaptive cognitions about oneself and other people. Behaviour therapy improves social and emotional functioning. • Transference-focused therapy aims at correcting distorted perceptions of significant others and decreasing symptoms and self-destructive behaviour. • Family therapy is frequently offered to borderline adolescent patients and is regarded by many as the treatment of choice for these patients. • Social skills training.
Pharmacotherapy	• The psychiatrist can prescribe a selective serotonin reuptake inhibitor (SSRI, such as fluoxetine) to treat mood, rejection sensitivity and anger. If the second SSRI is not effective, the psychiatrist could consider adding on a low-dose antipsychotic for anger control and an anxiolytic for anxiety control. • Mood stabilizers such as sodium valproate medications can be added if the above-mentioned stabilizers are not effective.

Course and prognosis:

- Impulsivity improves significantly over time. Affective symptoms have the least improvement.
- Poor prognosis is associated with early childhood sexual abuse, early first psychiatric contact, chronicity of symptoms, high affective instability, aggression and substance use disorder.

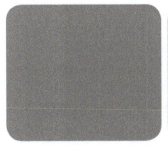

STATION 104: EATING DISORDERS (PROGNOSTIC FACTORS)

Information to candidates

Name of patient: Ms Smith

You have been tasked to see Ms Smith, a 20-year-old female who has been referred by her general practitioner (GP). During the recent routine health screening with her GP, her GP has noted that her body mass index (BMI) is on the lower limit. Ms Smith did share that she has been restricting her diet to achieve a desired body weight. The GP has referred her to your service, as the GP felt that Ms Smith would benefit from some form of help for her eating issues. She has been admitted to the inpatient unit, and her weight has stabilized after commencing gradual re-feeding. The psychologist is due to see her today but would like to know more about her background and the prognostic factors for her.

Task

Please speak to Ms Smith and elicit both the positive and negative prognostic factors.

Outline of station

The purpose of providing an outline of the station is to allow candidates to be familiar with the structure of the station. This outline could also be helpful when candidates practice for the MRCPsych, joining with their colleagues to act out the station.

Please note that the outlines provided are based on the experiences of the authors. There may be variations in the actual examination.

You are Ms Smith and have been referred initially by your GP to the mental health service. You have been admitted to the inpatient unit since. The team has commenced gradual re-feeding, and your weight has improved. You are due to see a psychologist. You understand that the core trainee is supposed to speak to you to get more information about the prognostic factors with regard to your condition. You will share the following information with the core trainee: you have had this disorder since the age of 14 years, but you have had only one hospitalization since then. There were times during which you have had bingeing behaviours, such as vomiting and purging. Your relationship with your family is not good. You do not have any other comorbid psychiatric history.

CASC construct table

The CASC construct table is formatted such that candidates will be able to cover adequately both the range and the depth of the assessment required in this station.

Starting off: 'Hello, I am Dr Melvyn, one of the psychiatrists from the mental health unit. I understand that you have been admitted to the inpatient unit recently. Can we have a chat?'			
Explore longitudinal history of symptoms	I understand that you have been diagnosed with anorexia nervosa (AN). Can you tell me more about it?	Do you remember at what age you were diagnosed with this disorder?	Were you diagnosed before the age of 15 years? Have you had any previous hospital stay for your symptoms?
Explore core symptoms for AN	Do you remember what your weight was when you were first diagnosed?	Can you tell me more about your anorexia symptoms?	Did you suffer from any physical complications as a result of AN symptoms? Did you have any difficulties with your menstrual cycle? How long have these difficulties lasted for you? How long was it before you went ahead to seek help?
Explore presence of bulimic features	Apart from the symptoms that you have mentioned, have you had any of these symptoms since the time you were diagnosed?	Do you have persistent preoccupation with eating and an irresistible craving for food, with episodes of overeating in which large amounts of food are consumed in short periods?	Have you ever made any attempts to counteract the fattening effects of food using one or more of the following: self-induced vomiting, purgative abuse, alternating periods of starvation or through the usage of drugs?
Explore social circumstances	How is your current relationship with your family?	Is your family supportive? (Or) Are there continued family problems?	Do your parents set unrealistic expectations for you?
Explore psychiatric comorbidities	Have you had any other consultations with a psychiatrist for other mental health problems?	Do you have any family history of any mental health problems?	

Common pitfalls

a. Failure to cover the range and depth of the information required for this station

Quick recall*

- AN: It is rare, with prevalence about 1–2 per 1,000 women. The epidemiological catchment area (ECA) study found only 11 cases in 20,000 persons studied.
- The peak age of onset is 15–19 years.
- The incidence is 10 times higher in females compared with males.
- There is a higher prevalence in higher socioeconomic classes and Western Caucasians and a significant association with greater parental education.

International Statistical Classification of Diseases and Related Health Problems, 10th revision (*ICD-10*) diagnostic criteria: This condition is characterized by deliberate weight loss resulting in undernutrition with secondary endocrine and metabolic disturbance. It requires the presence of all of the following:

- Body weight maintained at 15% below expected with BMI of less than 17.5.
- Weight loss self-induced by the avoidance of fattening food and one or more of the following: self-induced vomiting, self-induced purging, excessive exercise and the use of appetite suppressants or diuretics.
- Body image distortion: A specific psychopathology comprising a dread of fatness that persists as an intrusive, overvalued idea; a low weight threshold is imposed on the self.
- Amenorrhea in women, loss of sexual interest and potency in men, endocrine disorder, elevated growth hormone and cortisol levels and abnormal peripheral abnormalities of insulin secretion.
- If the onset is prepubertal, the sequence of pubertal events is delayed or arrested; puberty is often completed with recovery, but menarche is late.

Good and poor prognostic factors include

Good prognostic factors	Poor prognostic factors
• Onset less than 15 years of age	• Onset at older age
• Higher weight at onset and at presentation	• Lower weight at onset and at presentation
• Receives treatment within 3 months after the onset of the illness	• Very frequent vomiting and the presence of bulimia
• Recovery within 2 years after the initiation of treatment	• Very severe weight loss
• Outpatient treatment	• Long duration of the condition
• Supportive family	• Previous hospitalization
• Good motivation to change	• Extreme resistance to treatment
• Good childhood social adjustment	• Continued family problems
	• Neurotic personality
	• Male gender

* Adapted from B.K. Puri, A. Hall and R. Ho (2014). *Revision Notes in Psychiatry*. London, UK: CRC Press, p. 581.

STATION 105: EATING DISORDERS (HISTORY TAKING: PAIRED A)

Information to candidates

Name of patient: Amelia

You have been asked to speak to Amelia, a 25-year-old female. She has been referred by her GP to the mental health service. She has visited her GP as she has been missing her menstrual periods for the past 2 months. The GP managed to gather more information from her and realized that she has been intentionally losing weight for the past year or so.

Task

Please speak to Amelia and get a history with the aim of establishing a diagnosis. Please also assess for aetiological factors. Please note down important points, as in the next station you will be speaking to a medical student to explain more about the aetiology as well as the appropriate management of her case.

Outline of station

You are Amelia, a 25-year-old university student, and have been referred by your GP to the mental health service. You have been told by your GP that you likely have a weight problem. It is true that over the past couple of months, you have been trying to lose as much weight as possible to get to your ideal weight. You have been exercising excessively and have been skipping meals at times as well. You have a sister who has eating disorder as well. Since young, you have been a perfectionistic person. You do not have any other comorbid psychiatric disorders.

CASC construct table

The CASC construct table is formatted such that candidates will be able to cover adequately both the range and the depth of the assessment required in this station.

Starting off: 'Hello, I am Dr Melvyn, one of the psychiatrists from the mental health unit. I understand that you have been referred by your GP. Can we have a chat?'			
Explore core symptoms	I understand that your GP has referred you to see us. Can you tell me more? I'm sorry to learn of the circumstances of the referral. I'd like to understand more about your symptoms to help you with your weight issues.	Can you share with me what methods you have been adopting to lose weight? Do you tend to avoid food? Do you engage in excessive exercises?	Do you constantly think about food? Do you find yourself counting the calories of the food that you eat? How do you feel about your body? Do you constantly think that you are too fat? Has anyone questioned you about the way you have been feeling?

(Continued)

	Can you tell me what your average weight was over the past couple of months? What was your highest and lowest weight over the past couple of months? Do you have an ideal weight that you are targeting? What is your ideal weight?	Have you tried to induce vomiting before? Do you use laxatives or diuretics to help you lose weight? Have you tried any other methods to lose weight?	
Explore complications arising from AN diagnosis	I'm sorry but I do need to ask you a couple of personal questions. Can you tell me more about your periods? Have they been regular? Are they affected at all?	Have you ever had any other complications in view of your low weight? Have you ever felt faint or dizzy? Do you feel weak most of the time?	Have you required any hospitalization due to these medical issues?
Explore aetiological factors	Can you tell me more about your family? Are your family members close to you? Do you think that you have been too close to them?	How is the relationship between yourself and your siblings? Does anyone in your family have an eating disorder as well?	How do illnesses affect the dynamics in the family? Do you tend to get more attention from the rest of the family? How did your family react when they learned that you have an eating disorder? What is your family's view about food and body image? Finally, can you tell me more about your childhood? What was it like? Is there anything in particular that sticks out? Can you also briefly tell me more about your personality?
Rule out other psychiatric comorbidities	How has your mood been lately? Are you still interested in doing things that you were previously interested in doing?	How has your energy level been? How has your sleep been? Can you focus and concentrate on things you like to do?	Have you had any unusual experiences such as hearing voices when no one is there? Do you feel that life is meaningless and not worth living?

Common pitfalls

a. Failure to cover the range and depth of the information required for this station

Quick recall*

- AN: It is rare, with prevalence about 1–2 per 1,000 women. The ECA study found only 11 cases in 20,000 persons studied.
- The peak age of onset is 15–19 years.
- The incidence is 10 times higher in females compared with males.
- There is a higher prevalence in higher socioeconomic classes and Western Caucasians and a significant association with greater parental education.

ICD-10 diagnostic criteria: This condition is characterized by deliberate weight loss resulting in undernutrition with secondary endocrine and metabolic disturbance. It requires the presence of all of the following:

- Body weight maintained at 15% below expected with BMI of less than 17.5.
- Weight loss self-induced by the avoidance of fattening food and one or more of the following: self-induced vomiting, self-induced purging, excessive exercise and the use of appetite suppressants or diuretics.
- Body image distortion: A specific psychopathology comprising a dread of fatness that persists as an intrusive, overvalued idea; a low weight threshold is imposed on the self.
- Amenorrhea in women, loss of sexual interest and potency in men, endocrine disorder, elevated growth hormone and cortisol levels and abnormal peripheral abnormalities of insulin secretion.
- If the onset is prepubertal, the sequence of pubertal events is delayed or arrested; puberty is often completed with recovery, but menarche is late.

Aetiological factors:

Genetics	Family studies have found an increased incidence of eating disorders amongst first- and second-generation relatives of those suffering from AN.
Biological factors	Brain serotonin systems have been implicated in the modulation of appetite, mood, personality and neuroendocrine functions. An increase in the intra-synaptic serotonin reduces food consumption, whereas a reduction leads to increased food consumption and promotes weight gain. A lower level of dopamine in turn leads to a reduction in appetite. The levels of brain-derived neutropenic factor (BDNF) are also reduced in AN. The levels of leptin are reduced in acute AN and are associated with poor appetite. Premature birth, small for gestational age and cephalhematoma are all risk factors for AN.
Physical illness	An excess of physical illness in childhood has been found in those with AN. Physical illness may be a risk factor for the later development of AN, possibly by inducing pathology in the family dynamics.

(Continued)

* Adapted from B.K. Puri, A. Hall and R. Ho (2014). *Revision Notes in Psychiatry*. London, UK: CRC Press, pp. 575–581.

Psychological factors	Psychodynamic theories include fantasies of oral impregnation, dependent relationships with a passive father and guilt over aggression towards ambivalently regarded mother.
	Operant conditioning theories include phobic avoidance of food resulting from sexual and social tensions generated by physical changes associated with puberty.
	Anorexics have a high prevalence of defined personality disorders and an excess of obsessive, inhibited and impulsive traits. It is suggested that in an environment that emphasizes thinness as a criterion for self-worth, vulnerable individuals cope with challenges of adolescence by repetitive reward-seeking behaviour.
	Previous research has demonstrated that around 69% of eating-disordered patients did have at least one personality disorder.
	Anorexics are more likely to suffer from anxious-avoidant personality disorder, whereas dramatic-erratic personality disorders are more common in bulimics.
	Other factors include childhood obesity and teasing by classmates or teachers.
	Anorexics tend to have failure of identity formation and psychosexual development in adolescence.
Environmental factors	Relationships in families of anorexics are characterized by overprotection and enmeshment. A typical anorexic comes from an inward, often overprotected and highly controlled family. Young patients with AN may use the illness to gain control and overcome rigidity, enmeshment and overprotection in the family.
	Higher rates of childhood sexual abuse are reported by eating-disordered patients than controls. Childhood sexual abuse appears to be a vulnerability factor for psychiatric disorder in general, not for eating disorder in particular.
	Anorexics and bulimics viewing fashion images of women show 25% increase in their body size estimation afterwards. The media representation of idealized women is likely to have some effect upon eating-disordered subjects.
	Immigrants from low- to high-prevalence cultures may develop AN as thin-body ideals are assimilated. Cultural factors influence the manifestation of the disorder.

STATION 106: EATING DISORDERS (MANAGEMENT: PAIRED B)

Information to candidates

Name of patient: Amelia

You have been asked to speak to Amelia, a 25-year-old female. She has been referred by her GP to the mental health service. She has visited her GP as she has been missing her menstrual periods for the past 2 months. The GP managed to gather more information from her and realized that she has been intentionally losing weight for the past year or so. In the previous station, you spoke to Amelia and obtained a history to come to a diagnosis. You have also obtained further history regarding relevant etiological factors. You have a medical student attached to the clinic. He wants to know more about her diagnosis and your treatment plans.

Task

Please explain to the medical student her diagnosis. Please also inform the medical student more about the aetiological factors predisposing her to her current condition. Please also educate the medical student with regard to the appropriate treatment plans.

Outline of station

You are a medical student who is newly posted to psychiatry. You heard about this case from the consultant on call. You wish to know more about the diagnosis for Amelia. You wish to find out more about the aetiological factors that would predispose Amelia towards her current condition. You also wish to know more about the appropriate management for her condition. You hope that the core trainee can provide you with more information.

CASC construct table

The CASC construct table is formatted such that candidates will be able to cover adequately both the range and the depth of the assessment required in this station.

Starting off: 'Hello, I am Dr Melvyn, one of the psychiatrists from the mental health unit. I understand that you have some questions about the patient that I just saw. Can we have a chat?'			
Clarification of diagnosis	I have just seen Ms Amelia, a 25-year-old female who has been referred by her GP. She has been restricting her diet for the past couple of months to achieve an ideal body weight. Based on the history I have obtained, the main diagnosis I am suspecting at the moment is AN. Have you heard of the term 'AN' before? (Or) What is your understanding of this condition?	Please allow me to share more about the condition. AN is characterized by deliberate weight loss, thus resulting in undernutrition and with resultant endocrine as well as metabolic disturbances. The following needs to be present in order for us to make the diagnosis: a. The body weight must be maintained at 15% below that of the expected. b. There must be weight loss	Usually the peak age of onset of these symptoms is around 15–19 years. The incidence of this condition is 10 times higher in females compared with males. The condition is usually more prevalent in the higher socio-economic classes.

(Continued)

		self-induced by the avoidance of fattening food by methods such as self-induced vomiting, excessive exercise and use of appetite suppressants. c. Body image distortion. d. Changes in the menstrual cycle.	
Explain common aetiological factors	There are multiple factors that might predispose an individual towards this condition. If there is a family history of this condition, she will be at an increased risk of acquiring the disorder.	Several studies have also demonstrated the involvement of brain chemicals in this condition. An excess of physical illness in childhood may also predispose individuals towards the development of the condition.	Psychological factors might also predispose an individual towards the disorder. In addition, those who have obsessive and impulsive traits are at enhanced risk for developing the disorder. In addition, family relationships might also predispose an individual towards an eating disorder. A typical anorexic usually comes from an inward, often overprotected and highly controlled family. The culture of thinness in itself might also be a predisposing factor.
Explain treatment options	Prior to the commencement of any treatment, baseline vitals and laboratory work need to be done.	Most individuals with this condition can be treated on an outpatient basis. Inpatient care is indicated for patients who are very emaciated. There are a variety of treatment options available, which I will elaborate further. We need to get the dietician involved and aim for an average weekly gain of 0.5–1 kg. The dietician can also provide advice about re-feeding, to avoid re-feeding syndromes.	Apart from medications, psychotherapy could be of benefit: cognitive behavioural therapy (CBT), cognitive analytic therapy, interpersonal therapy and focal and even family interventions which focus explicitly on eating disorders. CBT largely targets the cognitive distortions and behaviours related to body weight, body image and eating. Based on the National Institute for Health and Care Excellence (NICE) recommendations, outpatient psychological treatment should be offered after discharge, and the duration is for at least 12 months.

(Continued)

			Usually medications are not used as the sole or primary treatment for AN.
Clarify any concerns	I understand that you have some concerns about the prognosis of the patient. Can I share more about her prognosis?	Her prognosis is considered good if she has the following prognostic factors: onset prior to the age of 15 years, higher weight at onset and at presentation, having received treatment within 3 months after the onset of illness, recovery within 2 years after initiation of treatment, supportive family and having motivation to change along with good social adjustment.	Her prognosis is considered poor if she has the following prognostic factors: onset at older age, lower weight at onset and at presentation, very frequent vomiting and presence of bulimia, very severe weight loss, long duration of AN, previous hospitalization, extreme resistance to treatment and continued family problems.

Common pitfalls

a. Failure to cover the range and depth of the information required for this station

Quick recall*

Most people with AN should be treated as an outpatient before reaching severe emaciation. If a person has very low BMI, inpatient care may become necessary, and the NICE guidelines recommend the involvement of the physician or paediatrician with expertise in the treatment of medically at-risk patients with AN. Other indications for inpatient treatment are as follows:

- Persistent decline in oral intake or rapid decline in weight in adults who are already less than 80%–85% of their healthy weight.
- Vital sign abnormalities: Heart rate less than 40 beats per minute and orthostatic hypotension (drop in blood pressure of 20 mmHg from supine to standing position).
- Low body temperature of less than 36°C.
- Severe electrolyte imbalance: presence of low potassium and sodium levels.
- Organ failure.
- Underlying psychiatric disorder (such as severe depression and suicidal ideations).

---

* Adapted from B.K. Puri, A. Hall and R. Ho (2014). *Revision Notes in Psychiatry*. London, UK: CRC Press, pp. 575–577.

- Failure of outpatient treatment.
- Pregnancy: More intensive prenatal care is required to ensure adequate prenatal nutrition and foetal development.

Recommended guidelines for weight restoration

- An average weight gain of 0.5–1 kg in inpatient settings and 0.5 kg in outpatient settings should be an aim of treatment. The weight gain should not be more than 2 kg per week. This requires about 3500–7000 kcal per week.
- As a rule of thumb, the premorbid weight or the weight at which periods stopped plus 5 kg is a guide to the healthy weight.

Recommended guidelines for feeding

- A dietician should be consulted before the initiation of feeding. There is slowed gastric emptying, and hence meals must be introduced slowly to reduce the risk of gastric dilatation or rupture.
- If the patient is very frail, liquid feeds should be started instead. Gradually build up from 1000–3500 kcal/day.
- A multivitamin supplement in the oral form is recommended for people with AN during both inpatient and outpatient weight restoration.
- Total parenteral nutrition should not be used unless there is significant gastrointestinal dysfunction.
- Feeding against the will of the patient should be the last resort.

Managing risk

- The frequency of monitoring is determined by the severity of the AN condition, and the doctor should inform the patient and their carers about the physical risk of AN.
- Rapid feeding may lead to a life-threatening condition known as re-feeding syndrome, which usually occurs in the first 4 days of re-feeding. As a result of prolonged starvation and malnourishment, there is an intracellular loss of electrolytes such as phosphates. During feeding, there will be a sudden shift from lipid to carbohydrate metabolism. The carbohydrate metabolism stimulates the cellular update of phosphate to generate ATP. When phosphate is used up for ATP production, this leads to severe low levels of phosphate and the lack of ATP for cardiac muscles. The patient will develop cardiac failure and irregular heart rhythms that lead to sudden death.

Psychotherapy

- For outpatients, cognitive analytical therapy, cognitive behavioural therapy, interpersonal therapy, focal dynamic therapy and family interventions focused explicitly on eating disorders are the treatment of choice.
- The aims of psychotherapy should reduce risk, enhance motivation, encourage healthy eating and reduce other symptoms related to AN.
- CBT targets at cognitive distortions and behaviours related to body weight, body image and eating.
- The minimum duration for outpatient psychological treatment is 6 months.

- If outpatient treatment fails, the psychiatrist can offer combined individual and family therapy and day-care or inpatient treatment.
- Psychotherapy is difficult for patients with severely low weight. Wait until the patient's weight has increased and then offer a structured symptom-focused treatment regimen focusing on eating behaviour and attitude.
- Rigid inpatient behaviour modification program should not be used.
- For inpatients, outpatient psychological treatment should be offered after discharge, and the duration is for at least 12 months.
- Family therapy is the treatment of choice, particularly for children and adolescents with AN.

Pharmacotherapy

- Medication should not be used as the sole or primary treatment for AN.
- Be aware of the cardiac side effects of the medications given.
- Olanzapine is the most extensively studied antipsychotic in AN. It is associated with greater weight gain, reduction in obsessive symptoms, reduction in anxiety and increase in compliance.
- Risperidone is associated with weight gain and reduction in anxiety when combined with an antidepressant, based on a case report.
- Quetiapine is associated with significant increase in BMI and reduction in the eating disorder examination restraint schedule scores over 8 weeks, based on an open-label study.
- Fluoxetine failed to demonstrate any benefit in the treatment of patients with AN following weight restoration, based on a randomized controlled trail.
- Oestrogen administration should not be used to treat bone density problems in children and adolescents.

Prognosis

- The course and outcome are variable.
- Some patients recover fully after a single episode.
- Some exhibit fluctuating patterns of weight gain followed by a relapse. For adolescents with AN, around 80% recover in 5 years, and 20% may develop chronic AN. For adults with AN, 50% recover, 25% have intermediate outcome and 25% have poor outcome; 50% of restrictive AN may develop bulimia after 5 years.

STATION 107: BULIMIA NERVOSA (HISTORY AND PROGNOSTIC FACTORS)

Information to candidates

Name of patient: Rebecca

You have been tasked to see Rebecca, a 20-year-old university student. She has a history of type I diabetes mellitus, and it has been recommended that she be on long-term subcutaneous insulin injection. Recently, she has been admitted to the hospital twice following episodes of hyperglycaemia. The medics have been concerned about her recurrence admissions. She did share with the medics that she has frequently been omitting insulin as she has an ideal body weight and size and is trying to achieve that. The medics have decided to get your opinion about her case.

Task

Please speak to Rebecca and elicit an eating disorder history with the aim of coming to a conclusion what subtype of eating disorder she is suffering from. Please also assess for both positive and negative prognostic factors as it will have an impact on further treatment.

Outline of station

You are Rebecca, a 20-year old university student. You have an intense morbid fear of fatness. You have persistent food craving approximately three times a week and indulge in binge eating. After your binge eating, you resort to measures to lose weight such as avoidance of foods and fluids as well as vomiting. You have a history of depression, and you have been having these symptoms for the last 5 years. Your premorbid personality is that of someone who is very introverted, with low self-esteem.

CASC construct table

The CASC construct table is formatted such that candidates will be able to cover adequately both the range and the depth of the assessment required in this station.

Starting off: 'Hello, I am Dr Melvyn, one of the psychiatrists from the mental health unit. I have received the referral letter from your GP. Can we have a chat today about your condition?'			
Eating disorder history	Can you please tell me more about what has been troubling you? I understand from your GP that you have been having some issues with your diet. Can you tell me more?	Do you find yourself being overly preoccupied with eating and having irresistible cravings for food? Have there been episodes in which you overeat large amounts of food in a short period? How frequently does this occur for you?	After your binge episodes, do you indulge in any attempt to try to counteract the fattening effects of food? Have you resorted to self-induced vomiting or misuse of purgative? I understand that you have an underlying diabetic condition. Have there been times you have missed your insulin dose? Can you tell me why you decide to miss your regular doses? Is there an ideal weight that you are trying to achieve? Do you have an ideal BMI that you are trying to achieve?

(Continued)

Eliciting psychological symptoms	What are your thoughts with regard to your body image? Are you very concerned that you are fat?	Can you tell me more about your emotions before and after your binge-eating episodes?	Do you try to restrict the amount of food you take? Do you engage in excessive exercises?
Eliciting physical signs and complications	Sometimes, patients do have bodily symptoms as a result of their eating problems.	Have you had any bodily symptoms?	
Assessing prognostic factors	Have you seen a psychiatrist before? What did the psychiatrist diagnose you with? Do you have anyone in your family who has a mental health–related disorder?	Do you remember when your symptoms first started? Have you required any hospitalizations as a result of your eating habits?	Can you tell me more about your personality? Were there any problems when you were younger? What was your childhood like? Do you use any other substances like alcohol or drugs to cope with stressors in life?

Common pitfalls

a. Failure to cover the range and depth of the information required for this station

Quick recall*

- The prevalence of bulimia nervosa (BN) amongst adolescent and young adult females is approximately 1%–3%.
- The lifetime prevalence for strictly defined BN is 1.1% in females and 0.1% in males.
- The heritability of BN is 50%.
- The social class distribution is more even compared with that of AN.
- The average age of onset is 18 years, slightly older than in AN.
- The female-to-male ratio is 10:1.
- It is reported more commonly in the Caucasians in Western Europe, North America and Australia.

ICD-10 diagnostic criteria

- BN is characterized by repeated bouts of overeating and excessive preoccupation with the control of body weight, leading to extreme measures

---

* Adapted from B.K. Puri, A. Hall and R. Ho (2014). *Revision Notes in Psychiatry.* London, UK: CRC Press, p. 580.

to mitigate against the fattening effects of food. It shares the same specific psychopathology of fear of fatness as that of AN.

- There must be persistent preoccupation with eating and irresistible craving for food as well as episodes of overeating in which large amounts of food are consumed in short periods.
- Attempts to counteract the fattening effects of food by one or more of the following: self-induced vomiting, purgative abuse (appetite suppressants, thyroid preparation, diuretics). Diabetic bulimics may neglect insulin treatment.
- Morbid dread of fatness. Patient sets weight threshold well below healthy weight. Often there is a history of AN.

The *Diagnostic and Statistical Manual of Mental Disorders* (DSM) diagnostic criteria states the following:

- Eating in a discrete period (within any 2-hour period) an amount of food that is definitely larger than most people could eat in a similar circumstances.
- A sense of lack of control over eating during the episode.
- Recurrent inappropriate compensatory behaviours (such as self-induced vomiting; misuse of laxatives, diuretics or other medications; fasting or excessive exercise) to prevent weight gain.
- Both binge-eating and inappropriate compensatory behaviour occur at least once per week for 3 months.
- Repetitive self-evaluation as a result of undue influence by distorted body shape and weight.
- The disturbances do not occur exclusively during episodes of AN.

Management of patients with BN

Most patients with BN are treated in an outpatient setting. For patients who are at risk of suicide or severe medical complications, inpatient treatment is recommended.

Psychotherapy

Behavioural, cognitive-behavioural and group therapies were all effective; 77% of patients with BN who had such therapy stopped binging. Improvements were maintained at 1 year. Behavioural therapy was the most effective, with the lowest dropout rate and earlier onset of improvement. There seemed to be no advantage in adding a cognitive element. Psychotherapy produces a wider range of changes with more stable maintenance than does drug therapy. Cognitive behavioural therapy: This includes psycho-education, self-monitoring and cognitive restructuring. Eating regular meals is very important. The course of the treatment should be aimed at 16–20 sessions over a cumulative period of 4–5 months. The aims of behavioural therapy are to stop bingeing and purging by restricting exposure cues that trigger binge/purge behaviour, developing alternative behaviours and delaying vomiting.

In the event that CBT fails, IPT could be considered. The duration is between 8 and 12 months.

Pharmacotherapy

Selective serotonin reuptake inhibitors (SSRIs), usually fluoxetine, are the drugs of first choice for the treatment of BN in terms of acceptability, tolerability and the reduction of symptoms. The effective dose of the medication is 60 mg/day. Other psychotropic medications are not recommended for the treatment of BN.

Prognosis

- The outcome of BN improves with time and is considered to be generally better compared with that for AN. The majority of patients make a full recovery or suffer only moderate abnormalities in eating attitude after 10 years.
- There is comorbidity with depression, and prominent anorectic features increase the likelihood of a poor response.
- In a 10-year follow-up of treated patients, 52% recovered fully, 39% continued to suffer some symptoms and 9% continued to suffer from the full syndrome.
- In terms of prognostic factors, there is evidence from a number of studies that the following factors may be associated with poor outcome: depression, personality disturbances, greater severity of symptoms, longer duration of symptoms, low self-esteem, substance abuse and childhood obesity. It should be noted that those with multi-impulsive personality disorder do less well than those with bulimia alone.

STATION 108: RE-FEEDING SYNDROME AND USE OF THE MENTAL HEALTH ACT

Information to candidates

Name of patient: Mr Tom Smith

You have been tasked to speak to Mr Tom Smith, the father of Rebecca. Rebecca's GP has referred her to the mental health service as she has low weight. In addition, her routine medical screen has highlighted no significant electrolyte abnormalities. Mr Smith knows that his daughter has been dieting for some time. He is very worried about his daughter's condition and hopes to speak to someone from the mental health service about her condition. He is hoping that she can be sectioned under the Mental Health Act for mandatory treatment.

Task

Please speak to the father (Mr Smith) and address all his concerns and expectations.

Outline of station

You are the Mr Tom Smith, the father of Rebecca. Rebecca is your only daughter and you have been extremely concerned about her condition. You know that she has been dieting over the past few months. You decided that she needed help and brought her to the GP 2 days ago. The GP has referred her over to the mental health services. You are hoping that a professional can help your daughter with her condition. You understand that there is a Mental Health Act and hope that the professional can apply it for treating your daughter. You are at a loss about how best to help Rebecca. You are curious whether you could force-feed her. You wish to know more about the other treatment methods. In addition, you hope to be able to clarify with the mental health professional about the criteria for admission. You are very anxious about your daughter as you have been her main caregiver since you divorced your wife 10 years ago.

CASC construct table

The CASC construct table is formatted such that candidates will be able to cover adequately both the range and the depth of the assessment required in this station.

Starting off: 'Hello, I am Dr Melvyn, one of the psychiatrists from the mental health unit. I understand that you have some concerns about your daughter. Can we have a chat?'			
Address expectations and concerns	I understand that you have been having some concerns with regard to your daughter's condition. I understand that she has been dieting over the past few months. Can you tell me more?	I understand you're deeply concerned about your daughter's condition. With regard to your concern about whether we could section your daughter for treatment, I am sorry to say that we need to still respect her personal rights. There are other circumstances in which we might consider the utilization of the Mental Health Act, such as when the individual is actively suicidal.	I hear your concerns about your daughter's current weight. We need to gradually commence re-feeding slowly. Forced feeding might be counter-therapeutic, and she might develop other complications.
Clarify criteria for admission	We will consider recommending your daughter for a course of inpatient treatment if she has one of the following features:	Persistent decline in oral intake or rapid decline in weight of more than 1 kg per week, presence of heart rate abnormalities or blood pressure abnormalities or having low body temperature.	Severe electrolyte imbalance, worsening of an underlying psychiatric disorder, or the failure of outpatient treatment.

(Continued)

Explain treatment options	There are various treatment strategies that we could adopt to help your daughter.	Weight restoration: Whilst she is an inpatient, we aim for a weight gain of 0.5–1 kg per week.	Feeding: We will work with a dietician prior to the initiation of feeding.
Explain management plans	Psychotherapy: There are various forms of psychotherapy that might be beneficial for patients. Examples of such psychotherapy include cognitive analytic therapy, cognitive-behavioural therapy, interpersonal therapy, focal dynamic therapy and family interventions.	For inpatients, we usually recommend that outpatient psychological treatment be also offered on discharge, and we recommend a total duration of therapy to be around 12 months.	Pharmacotherapy: Usually medications are not used as the sole or primary treatment for the condition. Do you have any other questions for me? Thanks for sharing your concerns with me, and I do hope that I have addressed them accordingly.

Common pitfalls

a. Failure to cover the range and depth of the information required for this station
b. Failure to adequately explain the mechanism behind re-feeding syndrome and the range of electrolyte disturbance that results from it
c. Failure to correctly advise on rate of healthy caloric increase and weight gain in management

Quick recall*

Treatment settings

- Most people with AN should be treated on an outpatient basis before reaching the state of severe emaciation. If a person is very low in body weight and BMI, inpatient care may be necessary, and the NICE guidelines recommend the involvement of a physician or a paediatrician with expertise in the treatment of medically at-risk patients with AN. Other indications for inpatient treatment include the following:
- Persistent decline in oral intake or rapid decline in weight (for example, more than 1 kg per week) in adults who are already less than 80%–85% of their healthy weights.
- Vital signs abnormalities: heart rate of less than 40 beats per minute and orthostatic hypotension (drop in BP of more than 20 mm Hg from supine to standing position).
- Low body temperature of less than 36°C.

---

* Adapted from B.K. Puri, A. Hall and R. Ho (2014). *Revision Notes in Psychiatry*. London, UK: CRC Press, pp. 575–579.

- Severe electrolyte imbalance.
- Organ failure.
- Poorly controlled diabetes.
- Underlying psychiatric disorder (severe depression and suicidal ideation).
- Failure of outpatient treatment.
- Pregnancy: More intensive prenatal care is required to ensure adequate prenatal nutrition and foetal development.

Baseline monitoring and investigations should be conducted prior to admission.

- Blood pressure and pulse rate monitoring.
- BMI.
- Weight.
- Although weight and BMI are important indicators of the severity of AN, the NICE guidelines recommended that BMI and the weight should not be considered as sole indicators of physical risk. The nature of the investigations should be adjusted to the severity of the AN.
- Full blood count: Anaemia (usually normochromic normocytic anaemia), reduced erythrocyte sedimentation rate (ESR), thrombocytopenia.
- Electrolyte disturbances.
- Metabolic alkalosis detected on arterial blood gas.
- Renal function tests: increase in urea as a result of dehydration and renal failure.
- Liver function tests: reduced albumin, raised serum amylase.
- Fasting blood: hypercholesterolaemia as a result of low oestrogen, hypoglycaemia.
- Hormones: decrease in T3, increase in corticotropin-releasing hormone (CRH), increase in cortisol, increase in growth hormone, decrease in follicle-stimulating hormone (FSH), decrease in luteinizing hormone (LH) and decrease in oestrogen.
- Imaging: Computed tomography (CT) brain – brain pseudo-atrophy.
- Bone scan: reduction in the bone mineral density.

Recommend guidelines for weight restoration

- An average weight gain of 0.5–1 kg in inpatient settings and 0.5 kg in outpatient settings should be an aim of treatment. The weight gain should not be more than 2 kg per week. This requires about 3500–7000 kcal per week.
- As a rule of thumb, the premorbid weight or the weight at which periods stopped plus 5 kg is a guide to the healthy weight.

Recommend guidelines for feeding

- A dietician should be consulted before the initiation of feeding. There is slowed gastric emptying, and hence meals must be introduced slowly to reduce the risk of gastric dilatation or rupture.
- If the patient is very frail, liquid feeds should be started instead. Gradually build up from 1000–3500 kcal/day.
- A multivitamin supplement in the oral form is recommended for people with AN during both inpatient and outpatient weight restoration.

- Total parenteral nutrition should not be used unless there is significant gastrointestinal dysfunction.
- Feeding against the will of the patient should be the last resort.

Managing risk

- The frequency of monitoring is determined by the severity of the AN condition, and the doctor should inform the patient and their carers about the physical risk of AN.
- Rapid feeding may lead to a life-threatening condition known as re-feeding syndrome, which usually occurs in the first 4 days of re-feeding. As a result of prolonged starvation and malnourishment, there is an intracellular loss of electrolytes such as phosphates. During feeding, there will be a sudden shift from lipid to carbohydrate metabolism. The carbohydrate metabolism stimulates the cellular update of phosphate to generate ATP. When phosphate is used up for ATP production, this leads to severely low levels of phosphate and the lack of ATP for cardiac muscles. The patient will develop cardiac failure and irregular heart rhythms, leading to sudden death.

Psychotherapy

- For outpatients, cognitive analytical therapy, cognitive behavioural therapy, interpersonal therapy, focal dynamic therapy and family interventions focused explicitly on eating disorders are the treatment of choice.
- The aims of psychotherapy should reduce risk, enhance motivation, encourage healthy eating and reduce other symptoms related to AN.
- CBT targets cognitive distortions and behaviours related to body weight, body image and eating.
- The minimum duration for outpatient psychological treatment is 6 months.
- If outpatient treatment fails, the psychiatrist can offer combined individual and family therapy and day-care or inpatient treatment.
- Psychotherapy is difficult for patients with severely low weight. Wait until the patient's weight has increased and then offer a structured symptom-focused treatment regimen focusing on eating behaviour and attitude.
- Rigid inpatient behaviour modification program should not be used.
- For inpatients, outpatient psychological treatment should be offered after discharge, and the duration is for at least 12 months.
- Family therapy is the treatment of choice, particularly for children and adolescents with AN.

Pharmacotherapy

- Medication should not be used as the sole or primary treatment for AN.
- Be aware of the cardiac side effects of the medications given.
- Olanzapine is the most extensively studied antipsychotic in AN. It is associated with greater weight gain, reduction in obsessive symptoms, reduction in anxiety and increase in compliance.
- Risperidone is associated with weight gain and reduction in anxiety when combined with an antidepressant, based on a case report.

- Quetiapine is associated with significant increase in BMI and reduction in the eating disorder examination restraint schedule scores over 8 weeks, based on an open-label study.
- Fluoxetine failed to demonstrate any benefit in the treatment of patients with AN following weight restoration based on a randomized controlled trail.
- Oestrogen administration should not be used to treat bone density problems in children and adolescents.

STATION 109: RE-FEEDING SYNDROME: EXPLANATION

Information to candidates

Name of patient: Sarah

You have been tasked to speak to Laura, a community practice nurse who has been following up on one of the outpatients, Sarah. During the last home visit, she noted that Sarah's mother has been forcing her child (Sarah) to binge-eat. Laura shared that Sarah has gained a total of 2 kg over the past week. During one of the routine visitations to the local GP, it was discovered that there were several abnormalities in the blood test for Sarah. Laura is at a loss as to how best to help Sarah and she hopes that you will be able to help her.

Task

Please speak to Laura, the community practice nurse who has been following up on the care of Sarah, and address all her concerns and expectations.

Outline of station

You are Laura, the community practice nurse who has been following up on an outpatient named Sarah. You have known Sarah since her last hospitalization for her eating disorder issue 1 year ago. You note that her mother has been force-feeding Sarah, because she is quite upset with sarah for constantly restricting her diet. You are aware that in the course of 1 week, Sarah has gained a total of 2 kg. During one of her routine follow-up check-ups with the local GP, it was discovered that Sarah has several blood abnormalities. You are very concerned about Sarah and wonder if she could be suffering from re-feeding syndrome. You wish to know more about this syndrome and how best to help Sarah with her condition.

CASC construct table

The CASC construct table is formatted such that candidates will be able to cover adequately both the range and the depth of the assessment required in this station.

Starting off: 'Hello, I am Dr Melvyn, one of the psychiatrists from the mental health unit. I understand that you have been following up on Sarah. Can we have a chat about her condition?'			
Explore concerns	I understand that you wanted to meet up with me as you have some concerns about Sarah's condition. Can you tell me more?	You mentioned that she has gained weight rapidly over the past week. Can you share with me more? Does Sarah have any bodily symptoms of concern?	I also understand that she has had some blood tests done with her local GP. Can you tell me more about the results of those tests? Can you share with me when Sarah was first diagnosed with eating disorder? Did she require any previous inpatient hospitalization? How long have you been following up on her condition as an outpatient?
Explain likely diagnosis of re-feeding syndrome	Thanks for sharing with me your concerns. It seems that Sarah might have developed a condition known as re-feeding syndrome. Have you heard about it before?	Can I explain more about re-feeding syndrome? This is a condition in which individuals, usually those with eating disorders, are receiving additional calories too fast.	It is usually characterized by a variety of chemical imbalances and changes in the body. Hence, this explains the abnormal blood results that Sarah has at the moment. When additional calories are introduced into the body too rapidly, the body has to switch from fat metabolism over to carbohydrate metabolism. When this happens, it is commonly associated with a shift in the electrolyte and fluid balances. Hence, electrolytes such as potassium, magnesium and phosphates are affected, and this would in turn cause a variety of clinical signs and symptoms.

(Continued)

Explain signs and symptoms of re-feeding syndrome	There are a variety of signs and symptoms that patients might have when they develop re-feeding syndrome. In Sarah's case, she has oedema of her hands and legs.	Other symptoms might include constipation, vomiting, diarrhoea, generalized lethargy as well as abnormal heart rhythm.	Some patients might also develop seizures as a result of re-feeding syndrome. In severe cases, they might also suffer from cardiac/heart failure.
Explain management plans	I need your help to arrange a consultation with Sarah. In the event that we are really certain that she has re-feeding syndrome, she cannot be managed as an outpatient.	I would need her to be admitted to the hospital for further inpatient treatment and stabilization.	We need to correct the electrolyte abnormalities and consider careful re-feeding with the help of our dietician and members of the multidisciplinary team. Do you have any other questions for me?

Common pitfalls

a. Failure to cover the range and depth of the information required for this station
b. Failure to adequately explain the mechanism behind re-feeding syndrome and the range of electrolyte disturbance that results from it
c. Failure to correctly advise on rate of healthy caloric increase and weight gain in management

Quick Recall*

Recommended guidelines for weight restoration

- An average weight gain of 0.5–1 kg in inpatient settings and 0.5 kg in outpatient settings should be an aim of treatment. The weight gain should not be more than 2 kg per week. This requires about 3500–7000 kcal per week.
- As a rule of thumb, the premorbid weight or the weight at which periods stopped plus 5 kg is a guide to the healthy weight.

Recommend guidelines for feeing

- A dietician should be consulted before the initiation of feeding. There is slowed gastric emptying, and hence meals must be introduced slowly to reduce the risk of gastric dilatation or rupture.
- If the patient is very frail, liquid feeds should be started instead. Gradually build up from 1000–3500 kcal/day.

---

* Adapted from B.K. Puri, A. Hall and R. Ho (2014). *Revision Notes in Psychiatry.* London, UK: CRC Press, pp. 575–579.

- A multivitamin supplement in the oral form is recommended for people with AN during both inpatient and outpatient weight restoration.
- Total parenteral nutrition should not be used unless there is significant gastrointestinal dysfunction.
- Feeding against the will of the patient should be the last resort.

Managing risk

- The frequency of monitoring is determined by the severity of the AN condition, and the doctor should inform the patient and their carers about the physical risk of AN.
- Rapid feeding may lead to a life-threatening condition known as re-feeding syndrome, which usually occurs in the first 4 days of re-feeding. As a result of prolonged starvation and malnourishment, there is an intracellular loss of electrolytes such as phosphates. During feeding, there will be a sudden shift from lipid to carbohydrate metabolism. The carbohydrate metabolism stimulates the cellular update of phosphate to generate ATP. When phosphate is used up for ATP production, this leads to severely low levels of phosphate and the lack of ATP for cardiac muscles. The patient will develop cardiac failure and irregular heart rhythms leading to sudden death.

Psychotherapy

- For outpatients, cognitive analytical therapy, cognitive behavioural therapy, interpersonal therapy, focal dynamic therapy and family interventions focused explicitly on eating disorders are the treatment of choice.
- The aims of psychotherapy should reduce risk, enhance motivation, encourage healthy eating and reduce other symptoms related to AN.
- CBT targets cognitive distortions and behaviours related to body weight, body image and eating.
- The minimum duration for outpatient psychological treatment is 6 months.
- If outpatient treatment fails, the psychiatrist can offer combined individual and family therapy and day-care or inpatient treatment.
- Psychotherapy is difficult for patients with severely low weight. Wait until the patient's weight has increased and then offer a structured symptom-focused treatment regimen focusing on eating behaviour and attitude.
- Rigid inpatient behaviour modification program should not be used.
- For inpatients, outpatient psychological treatment should be offered after discharge, and the duration is for at least 12 months.
- Family therapy is the treatment of choice, particularly for children and adolescents with AN.

Pharmacotherapy

- Medication should not be used as the sole or primary treatment for AN.
- Be aware of the cardiac side effects of the medications given.
- Olanzapine is the most extensively studied antipsychotic in AN. It is associated with greater weight gain, reduction in obsessive symptoms, reduction in anxiety and increase in compliance.

- Risperidone is associated with weight gain and reduction in anxiety when combined with an antidepressant, based on a case report.
- Quetiapine is associated with significant increase in BMI and reduction in the eating disorder examination restraint schedule scores over 8 weeks, based on an open-label study.
- Fluoxetine failed to demonstrate any benefit in the treatment of patients with AN following weight restoration, based on a randomized controlled trail.
- Oestrogen administration should not be used to treat bone density problems in children and adolescents.

STATION 110: POSTNATAL DEPRESSION

Information to candidates

Name of patient: Tammy

You have been tasked to speak to Tammy, a 26-year-old female. She gave birth to her baby 4 weeks ago. Her husband noted that she has been increasingly emotional and tearful lately and has not been able to care for the infant. He is very concerned about her condition and has brought her initially to the general practitioner (GP). The GP has referred her over to the mental health service.

Task

Please speak to Tammy to elicit further history with regard to her condition and perform a risk assessment.

Outline of Station

The purpose of providing an outline of the station is to allow candidates to be familiar with the structure of the station. This outline could also be helpful when candidates practice for the MRCPsych, joining with their colleagues to act out the station.

Please note that the outlines provided are based on the experiences of the authors. There may be variations in the actual examination.

You are Tammy and have given birth to your child 4 weeks ago. This is your first child after an unplanned pregnancy. There were no problems during the pregnancy, and your relationship with your spouse has been good. You find that you have become more emotional recently. You do not have much interest in caring for your child. You tend to find yourself lethargic during the day. You worry that your child is lacking good care due to your inability to take care of him. You do not have any abnormal ideas about your child. You have had passive thoughts of suicide, but you have not planned anything concrete thus far.

CASC construct table

The CASC construct table is formatted such that candidates will be able to cover adequately both the range and the depth of the assessment required in this station.

Starting off: 'Hello, I am Dr Melvyn, one of the psychiatrists from the mental health unit. I received a referral letter from your GP. Can we have a chat?'			
Presenting history	I understand that things have been difficult for you since you gave birth to your child. Can you tell me more?	I'm sorry to hear how you have been. How long have you been feeling this way?	
Elicit risk factors	Have you had similar episodes previously? Have you seen a psychiatrist before? Is there anyone in your family who has a history of any mental health issues?	Can you tell me more about your pregnancy? Is this a planned pregnancy? Is this the first time you have had a child? (If not, what is the age gap between the children?) How were things when you were having your baby? Was the antenatal check-up normal?	How was the delivery of your child? Were there any complications? Did your baby need extensive stay in the hospital after delivery? How is your relationship with your husband? Has he been supportive? Can you tell me your baby's name? Have you been able to bond with and care for your baby? Do you breastfeed your baby? Is there anyone else to help you with the care for your baby?
Assessment for depressive symptoms	You mentioned that you have been more emotional since the birth of your child. How long has this been? Does your mood vary the course of the day? Do you find yourself losing interest in things that you used to enjoy?	How have your energy levels been? Have there been any difficulties with your sleep? Can you tell me more? Do you have difficulties falling asleep or do you have difficulties staying asleep?	How has your appetite been? Have you had things that you feel guilty about?
Assessment for psychotic symptoms	I understand that this has been a very difficult time for you.	Sometimes when people are undergoing difficult situations in life they have unusual experiences, such as hearing voices or seeing things that are not there. Have you had these experiences?	Have you ever felt that someone out there was trying to do something to harm you or your baby? How certain are you about this? Do you feel that your thoughts are being interfered with? Do you feel that your emotions and actions are no longer under your control?
Risk assessment	Have you ever had thoughts that life is not worth living? Have you had any thoughts of ending your life? Have you made any plans? Have you written any last notes to your loved ones?	What do you think would keep you from thinking about harming yourself?	Have you ever felt so low in mood that you had thoughts about harming your baby? Any neglect of your baby's physical needs? Any physical abuse? Can you tell me more about your plans (if any)? Where is the baby now? Is there anyone helping with care?

It is helpful if you ask for the name of the baby early at the start of the interview. This may make the interview more personal and help the patient to open up.

Common pitfalls

a. Failure to cover the range and depth of the information required for this station

Quick recall*

- Postnatal depression is a depressive illness not much different from non-psychotic depression in other settings. It is characterized by low mood, reduced self-esteem, tearfulness and anxiety, particularly about the baby's health, and an inability to cope. Mothers may experience reduced affection for their baby and may have difficulty with breastfeeding.
- Postnatal depression occurs in 10%–15% of postpartum women usually within 3 months of childbirth.
- Those women who are emotionally unstable in the first week after childbirth are at an increased risk of developing postnatal depression.
- Postnatal depression is not associated with parity.

Clinical features

- Common symptoms seen in mother: irritability, tearfulness, poor sleep and tiredness; feeling inadequate as a mother; loss of confidence in mothering.
- Common symptoms related to the care and safety of the baby: anxieties about the baby's health; expresses concerns that the baby is malformed and does not belong to her; reluctance to feed or handle the baby; 40% of patients have had thoughts of harming the baby.

Management

- The education of health visitors and midwives is necessary to identify cases early.
- The Edinburgh Postnatal Depression Scale is a 10-item self-report questionnaire, used by health visitors to identify postnatal depression during the course of their normal contacts with new mothers.
- Nondirective counselling by health visitors individually or in groups is effective in one-third of the cases. Self-help groups and mother-and-baby groups are useful to combat isolation.
- In those with severe symptoms or those who are unresponsive to counselling, antidepressants are required.
- If the depression is severe, admission, preferably with the baby to a mother-and-baby unit, may be required.
- Suicidal mothers may have thoughts of taking their babies with them, so questions about the safety of the child should form part of the normal assessment of mothers of young children.
- Electroconvulsive therapy (ECT) may be required, particularly if worthlessness, hopelessness and despair are present.

---

* Adapted from B.K. Puri, A. Hall and R. Ho (2014). *Revision Notes in Psychiatry*. London, UK: CRC Press, pp. 563–565.

- Breastfeeding should not be routinely suspended. Tricyclic antidepressants (TCAs) are transmitted in reduced quantities in breast milk. They are, however, safe. Lithium is transmitted and should not be given to a breastfeeding mother because of the risk of toxicity to the child.

Outcomes

- If undetected, postnatal depression may last up to 2 years with serious consequences for the marital relationship and the development of the child.
- There is currently good evidence demonstrating a link between depressive disorders in mothers and emotional disturbances in their children.
- The following are more frequent in the children of mothers suffering from depression: insecure attachment, behavioural problems, difficulties in expressive language, fewer positive and more negative facial expressions, mild cognitive abnormalities, less affective sharing and less initial sociability.
- Social and marital difficulties are often associated with reduced quality of mother–child interactions.
- It has been noted that those who are suffering from a recurrence of depression are at greater risk of further non-postpartum episodes but not postpartum episodes. Those for whom the depression had arisen de novo are at raised risk for further episodes of postnatal depression but not for non-postpartum episodes.
- The relapse rate for subsequent non-psychotic depression is 1 in 6.

It is important to distinguish postnatal depression from postnatal blues. Postnatal blues is a brief psychological disturbance, characterized by tearfulness, labile emotions and confusion in mothers occurring in the first few days after childbirth. It tends to occur in around 50% of women, peaking at the third to the fifth day postpartum. Postnatal blues is associated with tearfulness, irritability and anxiety. In terms of management, the women should receive reassurance. No psychotropic medication is required, and the prognosis is good.

STATION 111: POSTNATAL PSYCHOSIS (HISTORY TAKING: PAIRED STATION A)

Information to candidates

Name of patient: Tammy

You have been tasked to speak to Tammy, who is a 26-year-old female. She has just given birth to her child 2 weeks ago. Her husband noted that she has been increasingly emotional and tearful lately and has not been able to care for her child. Apart from her low mood, she has expressed concerns that her child might be harmed by a devil. Her GP has referred Tammy to the mental health services for an assessment today.

Task

Please speak to Tammy to elicit further history with regard to her condition and perform a risk assessment.

Outline of station

You are Tammy and have given birth to your child 4 weeks ago. This is your first child after an unplanned pregnancy. There were no problems during the pregnancy, and your relationship with your spouse has been good. You find that you have become more emotional recently. You are very worried that the devil is out to harm your baby. You have been hearing voices telling you that you need to keep your baby safe from the devil.

CASC construct table

The CASC construct table is formatted such that candidates will be able to cover adequately both the range and the depth of the assessment required in this station.

Starting off: 'Hello, I am Dr Melvyn, one of the psychiatrists from the mental health unit. I received a referral letter from your GP. Can we have a chat?'			
Presenting history	I understand that things have been difficult for you since you gave birth to your child. Can you tell me more?	I'm sorry to hear how you have been. How long have you been feeling this way?	
Elicit risk factors	Have you had similar episodes previously? Have you seen a psychiatrist before? Is there anyone in your family who has a history of any mental health issues?	Can you tell me more about your pregnancy? Was this a planned pregnancy? Is this your first child? How were things during the pregnancy? Was the antenatal check-up normal?	How was the delivery of your child? Were there any complications? Did your baby need extensive stay in the hospital after delivery? How is your relationship with your husband? Has he been supportive? Can you tell me your baby's name? Have you been able to bond with and care for your baby? Do you breastfeed your baby? Is there anyone else to help you with the care of your baby?

(Continued)

Assessment for psychotic symptoms	I understand that it has been a very difficult time for you. Have you ever worried that someone wants to harm you and your baby? Can you tell me more? How certain are you that there is indeed someone who wants to do this? Is there any alternative explanation for this?	Are you worried that there is something wrong with your baby? If so, can you tell me more? Other symptoms: • Any mood swings? • Have there been times when you are confused about the time, place and person?	Have you heard voices after delivery? Can you tell me more? If so, did the voices ever give you any instructions such as telling you to harm your baby? Do you feel in control of your thoughts? Or do you feel that your thoughts are being interfered with? Do you feel as if someone else could control the way you feel and the way you think and act?
Risk assessment	Have you ever had thoughts that life is not worth living? Have you had any thoughts of ending your life? Have you made any plans? Have you written any last notes to your loved ones?	What do you think would keep you from thinking about harming yourself? Any neglect of your baby's physical needs? Any physical abuse?	Have you ever felt so low in mood that you had thoughts about harming your baby? Can you tell me more about your plans (if any)? What do you think would stop you from doing anything to your child? Where is the baby now? Is there anyone helping to take care of your baby?

Common pitfalls

a. Failure to cover the range and depth of the information required for this station

It is important to assess for orientation and signs of confusion in this patient, as they are a major sign of postpartum psychosis.

Quick recall*

- The risk of developing a psychotic illness is increased 20-fold in the first postpartum month. Certain symptoms that are distinctive include the following:
  - Sudden onset, usually within the first 2 weeks after childbirth
  - Marked perplexity but with no detectable cognitive impairment
  - Rapid changes in mental state, sometimes from hour to hour
  - Marked restlessness, fear and insomnia
  - Delusions, hallucinations and disturbed behaviour that develop rapidly

---

* Adapted from B.K. Puri, A. Hall and R. Ho (2014). *Revision Notes in Psychiatry*. London, UK: CRC Press, pp. 564–568.

- It is important to note that 80% of postpartum psychosis is affective in nature. Schizophreniform psychosis often has manic features. Those with a previous history of manic-depressive illness have a substantially higher risk than those with a history of schizophrenia or depression.
- The following factors are associated with women developing puerperal psychosis: increased rate of caesarean section, higher social class, older age at birth of first child and primiparae.
- Psychosis following childbirth is usually an affective type with a particularly high proportion of manic episodes within the first 2 weeks.
- Postpartum psychosis follows 20%–30% of births in those with pre-existing bipolar mood disorders.

Common symptoms include the following:

- Sleep disturbances in the early stages.
- Mild confusion, disorientation and perplexity.
- Affective labile mood often being present with marked agitation and mania.
- The clinical features may resemble that of affective disorders (70%), schizophreniform disorder (15%) and organic illnesses (15%).
- Common symptoms related to the care and the safety of the baby might include the delusion involving the baby and her family and suicidal and infanticidal thoughts being present.

STATION 112: POSTNATAL PSYCHOSIS (MANAGEMENT: PAIRED STATION B)

Information to candidates

Name of patient: Mr Charlie Brown

You have been previously tasked to speak to Tammy Brown, who is a 26-year-old female. She has just given birth to her child 2 weeks ago. Her husband noted that she has been increasingly emotional and tearful lately and has not been able to care for her child. Apart from her low mood, she has expressed concerns that her child might be harmed by a devil. Her GP has referred Tammy to the mental health services for an assessment today.

You have spoken to Tammy in the previous station and have obtained consent to speak to her husband. Her husband is extremely concerned about her condition and the well-being of his child.

Task

Please speak to Charlie, the husband of Tammy, and address all his concerns and expectations.

Outline of station

You are the husband of Tammy, and you are extremely concerned about your wife's condition. You understand that the psychiatrist has seen your wife and wish to know more about the assessment. You want to know what condition your wife is suffering from. You wonder whether she might be having postpartum blues or postpartum depression. You hope that the team can help your wife with her condition. If the team suggests the commencement of any medications, you will be very concerned with regard to the side effects of the medications on your child, as you know that your wife has been breastfeeding. You wonder whether there are any other alternatives to medications. You want to ensure the safety of both your wife and your child and wish to know from the team how best they can help ensure their safety.

CASC construct table

The CASC construct table is formatted such that candidates will be able to cover adequately both the range and the depth of the assessment required in this station.

Starting off: 'Hello, I am Dr Melvyn, one of the psychiatrists from the mental health unit. I understand that you have some concerns about your wife's condition. Can we have a chat?'			
Clarification about diagnosis	I understand that you are very concerned about your wife's condition. We have seen your wife and have done an assessment. Can I share with you more about our assessment?	We feel that your wife might be suffering from a condition known as postpartum psychosis. Have you heard of this condition before?	This is a condition that usually commences abruptly 2 weeks after delivery. The patient usually has some affective features, along with some unusual experiences such as delusions or hallucinations. They might feel that others are out to harm them or their child or they might hear voices as well. Do you know whether your wife has an existing mental health condition? If she does, and if she has bipolar disorder, she is more predisposed towards this particular condition.
Explain management plans	I understand that you must be finding it tough to come to terms with the condition that your wife is currently having. Please let me reassure you that this is a condition that is highly treatable. We will do our best to help your wife with her condition. Can I tell you more about how best we could offer your wife assistance with her condition?	One of the concerns that we have lies largely with the safety of her and your child. We would recommend admitting her to the mother-and-baby unit for further treatment and stabilization. The nursing staff in the unit will be able to monitor her condition, and we can also help her through the commencement of certain medications.	We would like to commence an antipsychotic medication for your wife. In the event that medications do not help your wife, one other alternative that we could consider is administration of ECT. Have you heard about this form of therapy before? Can I take some time to explain more about the therapy to you? Apart from medications, we will also provide supportive counselling to help your wife with her condition. We will work closely with a multidisciplinary team that consists of a social worker and an obstetrician to help your wife.

(Continued)

| Explain potential complications if patient is not treated | One of our concerns is that if your wife is not stabilized and treated, there might be a risk of her harming herself and her child. | Also, given her symptoms, she is not likely to be able to care for your child. | This will affect the parent–child bonding and would be detrimental for your child in the longer term. Studies have shown that it might result in emotional problems in the child. |
| Address concerns and expectations | I hope that I have managed to address all your concerns and expectations. Do you have any questions for me? | I hear that you are very concerned about the commencement of medications, given that your wife is breastfeeding. Please let me reassure you that we take this into consideration and would start her on a medication safe for use even if she is breastfeeding. Once she is better, she can have supervised meetings with the baby. We can also teach her how to better take care of the baby. | I also hear that you are very concerned about the usage of ECT for treatment of your wife's condition. ECT has been demonstrated to be a safe and effective treatment for patients who are not responding to medications. |

Common pitfalls

   a. Failure to cover the range and depth of the information required for this station

Quick recall*

Management

- The identification of high-risk patients during pregnancy is important in the planning of postnatal management.
- Admission to a psychiatric hospital is usually essential, and it is usually preferable to admit the mothers with their babies.

The following are some advantages of joint admission:

- Most psychotic mothers are capable of looking after their babies with supervision and support.
- There is evidence supporting that joint admission may reduce the duration of illness and relapse rates.

The following are some disadvantages of joint admission:

- There is a risk of non-accidental injury to the child from the mother or fellow patients. A nurse should be dedicated to the care and supervision of the child and a lockable nursery should be provided.

---

* Adapted from B.K. Puri, A. Hall and R. Ho (2014). *Revision Notes in Psychiatry*. London, UK: CRC Press, pp. 565–568.

- Joint admission requires higher staffing levels.
- The long-term effects of admission upon the development of the child are not known.
- The women's partner needs support and education.

Treatment

- Phenzothiazines and lithium are effective in the treatment of manic episode. Control of lithium in the immediate postpartum period can be difficult because of fluid and electrolyte changes.
- ECT is particularly effective in the treatment of psychosis and accelerates recovery in all the diagnostic categories. It is used generally if the drug treatment has failed.
- In breastfeeding mothers, lithium is contraindicated because it is excreted into breast milk and is toxic to the baby.
- Neuroleptics can be administered to breastfeeding mothers, but high doses should be avoided, and the baby should be observed for signs of drowsiness, such as failure to feed adequately.
- Neuroleptics should be maintained for at least 3 months following recovery. If there are further manic or depressive episodes, lithium should be considered.
- Following discharge from the hospital, the mother will require close support and follow-up. An assessment of the mother–baby interaction should be made prior to discharge. The initial prognosis is quite good. Cases often settle within 6 weeks, and most are fully recovered by 6 months. A few, however, have a protracted course.
- After one episode of postpartum psychosis, the risk of a further episode in each subsequent pregnancy is between one in three and one in five. For those with a previous psychiatric history or a family history, the risk is higher; for those whose episode was associated with life events or C-section, the subsequent risk is lower.

Summary of the Maudsley's guideline recommendation of psychotropic medications for breastfeeding:

1. Bipolar disorder: Valproate can be used, but advise the mother to ensure adequate contraception to prevent pregnancy.
2. Depressive disorder: Paroxetine and sertraline can be used. For TCA, they are present in breast milk at relatively low levels.
3. Schizophrenia: sulpiride and olanzapine could be used.
4. Anxiety and insomnia: lorazepam for anxiety and zolpidem for insomnia. Advise mother not to sleep with her baby to avoid a suffocation accident of the newborn.
5. Substance abuse: Methadone is compatible with breast-feeding, but the dose should be kept to a minimum.

Suggested Reference: D. Taylor, C. Paton and S. Kapur (Eds) (2012). *The Maudsley Prescribing Guidelines in Psychiatry* 11th Edition. Chichester, UK: Wiley-Blackwell.

TOPIC 11
CONSULTATION
LIAISON
PSYCHIATRY

STATION 113: CONVERSION DISORDER (HISTORY TAKING AND DISCUSSION)

Information to candidates

Name of patient: Anna

Anna is a 28-year-old female who has been admitted to the emergency services for acute onset of left-sided lower-limb weakness. Both the medical doctors and the neurologist have seen her, and they do not think that she has any active medical illness. They understand from her mother that she has been through tremendous stress recently, and they feel that a psychiatric assessment is warranted.

Task

Please speak to Anna and obtain a relevant history to arrive at a diagnosis. Please perform an appropriate neurological examination. You will need to discuss your findings and your management plans with her mother in the next station. Please take down pertinent information that will be of help for you.

Outline of station

The purpose of providing an outline of the station is to allow candidates to be familiar with the structure of the station. This outline could also be helpful when candidates practice for the MRCPsych, joining with their colleagues to act out the station.

Please note that the outlines provided are based on the experiences of the authors. There may be variations in the actual examination.

You are Anna, and you have been brought into the emergency department following an acute onset of lower limb weakness. You were at your father's funeral when this happened. The significant stressor was that you were involved in a road traffic accident 3 days ago, in which you were the driver and your father was killed. No one in the family has since blamed you for the accident, but you have been feeling very guilty for it, as you feel that you could have been more cautious that day.

CASC construct table

The CASC construct table is formatted such that candidates will be able to cover adequately both the range and the depth of the assessment required in this station.

Starting off: 'Hello, I am Dr Melvyn, one of the psychiatrists from the mental health unit. I received some information as to why you have been admitted. Can we have a chat?'			
History of current presenting complaint	I understand from the medical doctors that you have been admitted today. Can you tell me more about what happened this morning? You mentioned that you have been feeling weak in one of your legs. Which leg is this?	Do you remember what you were doing when you had this sudden onset of numbness? Were there any other disturbing symptoms? Say, for example, did you have numbness or any tingling sensation? Any physical symptoms, e.g., pain or deficits elsewhere?	Have you experienced something similar to what you experienced in the past?
Stressors precipitating onset of symptoms	Have there been any changes in life recently? (Or) Have you been under any stress recently? Can you tell me more?	I'm sorry to hear that. You mentioned that you were at your father's wake when this happened.	Was your father's passage expected or was it sudden? How do you feel about it?
Eliciting la belle indifference and checking for secondary gains	Since the time that you were admitted, the medical doctors and the neurologists have checked up on you, and they have run some tests on you. Thus far, from my understanding, the test results are negative.	How do you feel about this sudden onset of weakness? Are you concerned about this? Are you relieved by the investigation findings? Do you believe what the doctors said?	How have your family members responded when they learned of the fact that you are having a weakness of your legs? Are they concerned? Have they made any alternative arrangements or accommodations for you?
Assess for comorbid psychiatric condition	Recently, how have you been feeling in your mood? Do you feel depressed or anxious? Are you still able to enjoy things that you used to enjoy?	How has your energy level been? What about your sleep and appetite?	Have you had any unusual experiences recently? Are things so troubling for you that you have entertained thoughts that life is not worth living?
Relevant personal and medical history	Have you been seen by a psychiatrist before? Does anyone in the family have any mental health conditions that I need to know of?	Do you have any other chronic medical conditions that we need to know of?	Do you take any drugs or substances to help you cope with the stress you are experiencing?
Neurological examination	*Perform a neurological examination of the lower limbs*		

Common pitfalls

a. Failure to cover the range and depth of the information required for this station

It is important to rule out other differential diagnoses, such as hypochondriasis, somatoform disorders and malingering.

Ask in a tactful manner how things have changed for the patient since developing of the physical symptoms.

Quick recall*

- Conversion disorders are presumed to be psychogenic in origin. They are associated with traumatic events, insoluble problems or disturbed relationships.
- The unpleasant affect associated with these conflicts is transferred and converted into symptoms.
- Diagnostic guidelines are as follows: (1) no evidence of physical disorder that may explain symptoms and (2) evidence for psychological causation – a clear association in time with stressful events.

Examples of specific dissociative conditions include the following:

- Dissociative amnesia: Loss of memory of an important event is not due to organic disorder, fatigue or ordinary forgetfulness. Partial and selective amnesia is usually centred on traumatic events. The extent varies from day to day. A persistent core cannot be recalled when awake. Perplexity, distress or calm acceptance may accompany the amnesia. It begins and ends suddenly, following stress. It rarely lasts more than a couple of days, and recurrence is unusual. It is more common in young adults but rare in the elderly. Recovery is complete.
- Dissociative fugue: There are all the features of dissociative amnesia, plus an apparently purposeful journey away from home. A new identity may be assumed. It is precipitated by severe stress. There is amnesia for the duration of the fugue, but self-care and social interaction are maintained. It lasts for hours to days, but recovery is abrupt and complete.
- Dissociative stupor: The sufferer is noted to be stuporose with no evidence of a physical or other psychiatric cause. Onset is sudden and stress related. The person sits motionless for long periods, with speech and movement being absent. Muscle tone, posture, breathing and eye movements indicate that the individual is neither asleep nor unconscious.
- Dissociative disorders of movement and sensation: There is loss of movement or sensations, usually cutaneous, with no physical cause. Symptoms often reflect the person's concept of disorder, which may be at variance with physiological or anatomical principles. The resulting disability helps the person

---

* Adapted from B.K. Puri, A. Hall and R. Ho (2014). *Revision Notes in Psychiatry*. London, UK: CRC Press, pp. 433–435.

to escape conflict or express dependency or resentment indirectly. There is calm acceptance (la belle indifference) not common and not diagnostic. This is also seen in normal people facing serious illness. Premorbid personality and relationships are often abnormal.

- Dissociative convulsions: pseudo-seizures that mimic epileptic seizures, but tongue biting, serious bruising and incontinence of urine are uncommon. Loss of consciousness is absent or replaced by stupor or trance.

Aetiology

- Freud introduced the term 'conversion' to describe the unconscious rendering of threatening ideas by conversion into physical symptoms, which have symbolic significance. This results in the relief of emotional conflict (primary gain) and the direct advantages of assuming a sick role (secondary gain). Levels of psychological distress are highly correlated with dissociative experiences.

STATION 114: CONVERSION DISORDER (DISCUSSION OF MANAGEMENT PLANS)

Information to candidates

Name of patient: Anna Smith

Anna Smith is a 28-year-old female who has been admitted to the emergency services for acute onset of left-sided lower-limb weakness. Both the medical doctors and the neurologist have seen her, and they do not think that she has any active medical illness. They understand from her mother, Mrs Smith, that she has been through tremendous stress recently, and they feel that a psychiatric assessment would be warranted. You have previously spoken to Anna and have obtained a history to arrive at a diagnosis. You have also performed a neurological examination. Her mother is waiting to speak to you outside the consultation room.

Task

Please speak to Anna's mother, Mrs Smith, and explain to her more about her daughter's current condition. Please address all her concerns and expectations.

Outline of station

You are the mother of Anna. You are very concerned about your daughter's condition. You wish to know more about her diagnosis, as you understand from the medical doctors as well as the neurologists that there is nothing wrong with her with regard to the biochemical and the radiological investigations. You would also like to know what is the potential cause of her condition, and how you can manage her condition. You also wish to know how best you can help her with her current condition, and you tell the core trainee that you wish to know more about her condition.

CASC construct table

The CASC construct table is formatted such that candidates will be able to cover adequately both the range and the depth of the assessment required in this station.

Starting off: 'Hello, I am Dr Melvyn, one of the psychiatrists from the mental health unit. I understand that you have some concerns about your daughter's condition. Can we have a chat about this?'			
Summarize findings	I understand that you have some concerns about your daughter's condition. I have assessed your daughter previously. Can I share my assessment with you? (Or) Can I tell you more about her condition?	The medical team and the neurologists have done some blood work as well as imaging to find a cause for her sudden onset of lower-limb weakness. I'm glad to inform you that thus far, those findings are negative.	I understand from Anna that she has been under tremendous stress recently. I'm sorry to learn of the family situation recently. We have also done a complete neurological examination during our interview.
Explain diagnosis and causes	I understand that you are concerned about the diagnosis of your daughter. We feel that your daughter has a condition known as conversion disorder. Have you heard about this before?	In essence, there is a close inter-relationship between our body and our mind. Hence if one is affected, so is the other. For example, if you have experienced a lot of stress at work, it is not uncommon for you to have a physical symptom such as headache. In Anna's case, it seems like the tremendous stress she has experienced has been converted into a physical symptom, which in her case is the weakness of her lower limb.	Do you have any questions for me at the moment? The stress that she is experiencing is very real. However, this condition is usually temporary and will gradually improve with time. The stressors that cause this disorder are usually tremendous traumatic events, insolvable problems and problematic relationships.

(Continued)

Explain management – pharmacological	There is a range of ways in which we can offer to help Anna with her current condition. As all the relevant investigations have been done and are negative, there is no further need to conduct any other investigations.	We would advise that she come back regularly, and we could monitor her mood. If her mood is low or she develops other psychiatric illnesses, we could treat them accordingly with medications.	Some patients do experience changes in their mood and might become depressed. In those circumstances, medications such as antidepressants are indicated.
Explain management – psychological	Apart from medications, there are other modalities of therapy that have been shown to be helpful.	Such therapies might include talking therapies such as cognitive behavioural therapy (CBT). Have you heard of this?	The family is advised to avoid reinforcing Anna's weakness/inability to do things.
Address concerns and expectations	I understand that I have shared quite a lot of information. Do you have any questions for me?	I totally understand how concerned you are with regard to her condition. As her mother, I think the most important thing for you to do is to acknowledge that she has a real problem – she is dealing with a tremendous stressor. Your support is important for her.	With regard to the prognosis, over time, people do recover well from the condition. I would like to offer you some leaflets from the Royal College of Psychiatrists for you to have a better understanding of her condition.

Common pitfalls

a. Failure to cover the range and depth of the information required for this station

Quick recall*

Management

- It is important not to confront the individual. Complete physical investigations should be conducted to emphasize that a serious illness is excluded. It is important to minimize the advantages of a sick role and praise healthy behaviour.

---

* Adapted from B.K. Puri, A. Hall and R. Ho (2014). *Revision Notes in Psychiatry*. London, UK: CRC Press, pp. 433–435.

Course

- Dissociative states tend to remit after a few weeks or months. Chronic states of more than 1 or 2 years are often resistant to therapy. Those with acute, recent onset, a good premorbid personality and resolvable conflict have a better prognosis.

STATION 115: HEALTH ANXIETY DISORDER (HISTORY TAKING)

Information to candidates

Name of patient: Mr Charlie Smith

You have been tasked to speak to Mr Charlie Brown, a 35-year-old man, who has been referred by the neurologist. He previously has been referred to multiple neurologists for his headaches. He has done multiple investigations, which to date all have been normal.

Task

Please speak to Mr Smith to obtain more history with regard to his symptoms. Please assess adequately to formulate a diagnosis.

Outline of station

You are Mr Charlie Smith. You have been having persistent headaches for the past couple of months. Several neurologists have seen you, and they have done basic blood work for you as well as radiological imaging scans. You have been told that there is nothing abnormal, but that only brings you temporary reassurance. You recently sought a consultation with another neurologist, who has decided to refer you to a psychiatrist. You have been told that your headaches might be stress induced, and hence the referral.

CASC construct table

The CASC construct table is formatted such that candidates will be able to cover adequately both the range and the depth of the assessment required in this station.

Starting off: 'Hello, I am Dr Melvyn, one of the psychiatrists from the mental health unit. I understand that your neurologist has referred you. Can we have a chat to understand your condition better?'

History of presenting complaint	I understand from the memo from your neurologist that you have been troubled by headaches recently. Can you tell me more about your headaches? When did these headaches first start for you? How have the headaches progressed since then?	Can you tell me whether there is anything that would make it better? Are there things that might make it worse than usual? Over this entire period, do you have other symptoms, such as weakness or nausea or vomiting?	I understand that you have previously consulted multiple neurologists. What have they told you? Have they done any blood tests or investigations? Did they share with you more about the results? Are you convinced by the results of the tests that you have undergone? How long did you feel reassured by the test results, before you needed to seek the advice of another doctor? Are you concerned that you might have an underlying brain issue? What brain condition do you think you have? What makes you feel that you are at risk with regard to this condition?
Impact on current life	Do you find yourself preoccupied with thoughts that you might have an underlying brain condition? Have you been spending a lot of time reading up more about the various conditions? From whereabouts have you been getting your information? Do you find yourself needing to get constant reassurance from your family members? (Or) What have your family members said to you regarding your condition?	How has this affected your life in general? Has this condition affected you in terms of your functioning? Are you able to do things like how you used to be able to? How is your relationship with your family members, loved ones and your friends?	Has this condition affected you in terms of your work at all? Are you able to perform like how you used to be able to at work?

(Continued)

Previous medical history, social and personal history	Can I check whether you have any past medical conditions that I need to know of? Do you have any long-term illnesses? Are you on any long-term medications?	How was your childhood? Were you frequently sick? How did your family respond whenever you fell ill? Did they take you to the doctors every time for every single symptom?	Do you have any family members who have long-term conditions? Do you have family members who have been diagnosed with the condition that you have spoken about? Can you tell me more? When did you learn that they have been suffering from such a condition? Was it just recently, over the past couple of months or so?
Other comorbidities	With all this going on and its impact on your life, how has your mood been? Are you able to maintain interest in things that you used to enjoy doing?	How have your energy levels been? Are you able to sleep? How has your appetite been?	Sometimes when people are undergoing stressful experiences, they do report of unusual experiences. Have you ever had these experiences before? Do you find that with your current condition life is no longer worth living and that you might be better off dead?

Common pitfalls

a. Failure to cover the range and depth of the information required for this station
b. Failure to ascertain adequately the degree of conviction of the thoughts – whether they are overvalued ideas or delusional in intensity

Quick recall*

- The prevalence of health anxiety disorder in the general population is 1% and in medical patients is 5%.
- The onset is between 20 and 30 years of age. It occurs in both men and women, with no familial characteristics.
- It is usually associated with lower economic status and history of medical illness.
- The aetiology of the disorder includes social learning theory, and patients may adopt a sick role to avoid obligations. From the psychodynamic perspective, aggression is being transformed into these health anxiety ideations.

---

* Adapted from B.K. Puri, A. Hall and R. Ho (2014). *Revision Notes in Psychiatry*. London, UK: CRC Press, pp. 470–472.

- *International Statistical Classification of Diseases and Related Health Problems,* 10th revision (*ICD-10*) diagnostic criteria: There is persistent belief in the presence of at least one serious physical illness, despite repeated investigations revealing no physical explanation of presenting symptoms, or persistent preoccupations with presumed deformity. There is a persistent refusal to accept the advice of several different doctors that there is no physical illness underlying the symptoms. Attention is usually focused on one- or two-organ systems only. Anxiety disorder and depressive disorder are common comorbid.
  Diagnostic and Statistical Manual of Mental Disorders, 5th edition (*DSM-5*): The name of the condition has been changed to illness anxiety disorder. To fulfil the diagnostic criteria, the patient is preoccupied with having a serious illness that is clearly excessive or disproportionate. Somatic symptoms are usually not present and if present, only mild in intensity. The person also exhibits high levels of anxiety and is easily alarmed about health and performs excessive health-related behaviours. The duration of the illness is at least 6 months. There are two types of illness-anxiety disorder, the care-seeking subtype and the care-avoidant subtype.

STATION 116: HEALTH ANXIETY DISORDER (MANAGEMENT)

Information to candidates

Name of patient: Mrs Smith

You have been tasked to speak to Mr Charlie Smith, a 35-year-old man, who has been referred by the neurologist. He previously has been referred to multiple neurologists for his headache. He has done multiple investigations, which to date all have been normal. You have previously spoken to Mr Smith to obtain a history of his presenting complaint as well as more information about his previous medical and personal histories. You managed to arrive at a diagnosis at the end of the interview. Mrs Smith, his wife, is currently waiting outside the consultation room. She is very keen to speak to you to understand more about her husband's condition.

Task

Please speak to Mrs Smith with regard to her husband's condition. You are expected to discuss more about his diagnosis as well as the management options for her husband. Please address all her concerns as well as her expectations.

Outline of station

You are Mrs Smith, the wife of Mr Smith. You understand that his neurologist has referred him over to a psychiatrist. You are curious about the reason for the referral. You hope that the core trainee can tell you more about your husband's diagnosis. In addition, you want to know what has caused him to be feeling this way. You are keen to learn more about management options for your husband, as you are keen for him to get better as soon as possible. You know that your husband needs you to be there to render him support emotionally most of the time. You wonder what else you could do to help your husband to get well sooner.

CASC construct table

The CASC construct table is formatted such that candidates will be able to cover adequately both the range and the depth of the assessment required in this station.

Starting off: 'Hello, I am Dr Melvyn, one of the psychiatrists from the mental health unit. I understand that you have some concerns about your husband's condition. I have seen him. Can we have a chat about his condition?'			
Establishing rapport and discussing diagnosis	I'm sorry to hear that you have been through quite a difficult time. It must have been very tough for you in the past few months. I received information from the neurologists that he has been seeing that his blood tests and brain scans have been normal. They do not feel that your husband has any neurological or medical condition at the moment, given the findings of the results.	I have previously spoken to your husband and have assessed him accordingly. It seems to me that your husband has a condition known as health anxiety disorder or hypochondriasis. Have you heard of this condition before?	The condition that your husband has is actually a very common condition. For some people, they tend to believe or fear that they have a medical condition, despite the fact that their results are normal. Hence, it is not uncommon for them to repeatedly see various doctors and request for more tests as they are doubtful about the results. In addition, they are constantly preoccupied with their condition and very often constantly seek out more information. They also tend to need constant reassurances.
Explaining causes	There has not been an established cause identified for this particular disorder.	Sometimes, it might be a resultant effect of someone who is living in a family who is very health conscious.	At times, stress could also be a trigger for someone to have such a condition. Chemical imbalances, particularly with regard to a brain chemical called serotonin, might contribute to the condition as well.
Explain management – pharmacological	There are various ways in which we could help your husband. Medications might be one option which we could consider.	The medications that we feel might benefit your husband are antidepressants.	Antidepressants help to regulate the amount of serotonin in the brain and would help with his symptoms.

(Continued)

Explain management – psychological	Apart from medications, another option which we could consider is engaging your husband in psychotherapy or talking therapy such as cognitive behavioural therapy, or CBT. Have you heard of this before?	As the name implies, there are two components in CBT. There is the cognitive component as well as the behavioural component. The goals of cognitive therapy are aimed towards reattribution and developing alternative explanations of symptoms and concerns of serious illness. Cognitive restructuring can modify dysfunctional assumptions.	The goals of behavioural therapy are aimed towards self-monitoring of worries, negative thoughts and illness-related behaviours. It also involves exposure and response prevention and reducing repeated reassurance-seeking behaviours. The therapist would also help your husband to cope with his worries by teaching him relaxation techniques.
Address concerns and expectations	I understand that it is very stressful for you when your husband requests further evaluation. Given that he has been through multiple tests and investigations, further investigations would not be warranted currently.	I understand that it is very distressing for you given that he is constantly seeking reassurances from you. The reason he needs reassurance is that it helps to provide temporary relief from his anxiety. This acts as a reward for him, and he is more likely to seek further reassurances from you.	Hence, it might be important for you to recognize his concerns and continue to support him in the best way you can. We would advise him to continue back routinely for his follow-up with the psychologist. In addition, he should be maintained on the medications at the moment.

Common pitfalls

a. Failure to cover the range and depth of the information required for this station

For hypochondriasis, it is important in the management to mention that containment of patient to only one or two specialists to ensure consistency in the care and to prevent doctor hopping to get more investigations done.

Quick recall*

- Management: Psychiatrists should advice medical colleagues or general practitioners (GPs) to gradually reduce the frequency of visits and unnecessary investigations by increasing the duration between appointments.

---

* Adapted from B.K. Puri, A. Hall & R. Ho (2014). *Revision Notes in Psychiatry*. London, UK: CRC Press, pp. 470–472.

Antidepressants such as selective serotonin reuptake inhibitor (SSRI) are useful. Psychotherapy is useful to treat the disorder:

- Cognitive therapy: reattribution and developing alternative explanations of symptoms and concerns of serious illness. Cognitive restructuring can modify dysfunctional assumptions.
- Behavioural therapy: self-monitoring of worries, negative thoughts and illness-related behaviours. It also involves exposure and response prevention and reducing repeated reassurance-seeking behaviours.
- Relaxation techniques.

Course and prognosis: The course of the disorder is usually episodic, and patients may present with a different idea each time. Around 30%–60% of patients have good prognosis. Good prognostic factors include good past health, high socioeconomic status and sudden onset of these ideations.

STATION 117: SOMATOFORM PAIN DISORDER

Information to candidates

Name of patient: Mr Huston

You have been tasked to speak to Mr Huston, a 30-year-old man. He has a chronic history of back pain and has been previously seen by multiple pain specialists for his chronic pain. He has done all the necessary blood investigations as well as imaging investigations, all of which have been normal thus far. His pain specialist has referred him over to your service for further assessment.

Task

Please speak to Mr Huston and obtain more history of his pain symptoms to come to a diagnosis.

Outline of station

You are Mr Huston, and you have a chronic history of back pain. You have visited multiple pain specialists and have undergone multiple investigations, all of which have been normal thus far. You are not sure why one of your pain specialists has decided to refer you to a psychiatrist and do not feel that you have any mental health condition, and you are reluctant to engage initially. You will share more about your pain symptoms only if the psychiatrist is empathetic in questioning. The main stressor currently is that your wife is very eager to have children, but you are not keen to have children at the moment.

CASC construct table

The CASC construct table is formatted such that candidates will be able to cover adequately both the range and the depth of the assessment required in this station.

Starting off: 'Hello, I am Dr Melvyn, one of the psychiatrists from the mental health unit. I understand that your pain specialist has referred you to us. Can we have a chat?'			
History of presenting complaint	I understand that you must be feeling frustrated for your pain specialist to refer you to our service, given that you believe that you do not have any mental health condition. However, I understand that you have been having this pain for quite some time and clearly you have been quite distressed by it. I might be able to help you to cope with this stressor if only I could find out more about your symptoms. Would you be willing to share more about your symptoms with me?	I understand that this pain was been troubling you for quite some time. Can you tell me when it first started? How would you describe the pain that you first experienced? Was the pain localized to any areas of your body? How has the pain been since then? Has it been progressively worsening in nature? Can you tell me more about the pain currently?	Can you share with me whether there are any factors that could make the pain better? Can you share with me whether there are any factors that could make the pain worst? I understand that several specialists have seen you for your pain symptoms. Can you tell me whether they have done any specific investigations to look for the causes of your kind? Do you happen to know the outcomes of those tests? Given the findings of the tests, what do you think is the possible cause for your pain symptoms?
Aetiological factors precipitating pain symptoms	Sometimes, stressors in life might contribute to pain symptoms as well. Have there been any changes in life recently prior to the onset of the pain symptoms?	Have there been any problems with relationships at home (with your loved ones and also with your family members)?	Have there been any major stressors from work? (Or) How have you been coping up with work? Do you have any financial concerns recently? Do you have other medical conditions that I need to know of? Were you told of your medical condition just recently?
Impact of current symptoms on life	I'm sorry to hear that this pain has been bothering you for so many months. I'm sorry to learn of the circumstances prior to the onset of your pain symptoms.	Has your current condition affected your lifestyle? (Or) Did your lifestyle change as a result of your current pain condition?	

(Continued)

| Ruling out other psychiatric disorders | With all these going on, how has your mood been in the past month or so? Are you still able to enjoy things that you previously used to enjoy? | What about your energy levels? Do you feel lethargic easily? How has your sleep been? How has your appetite been? Do you have difficulties with concentration or attention? | Sometimes, when people are undergoing stressful circumstances, they do report of having some unusual experiences, such as hearing voices or seeing things that are not there. Does this sound like what you have experienced before? Have things been so stressful for you that you feel that life has no meaning? Have you contemplated ending your life in view of your current problems? How have you coped with the problems so far? Do you use any substance such as alcohol or street drugs to help you cope with the symptoms? |

Common pitfalls

a. Failure to cover the range and depth of the information required for this station

It is important to differentiate somatoform disorder (preoccupied with bodily symptoms) from health anxiety disorder (preoccupied with having a serious illness). Ask broadly for various physical symptoms from across different body systems, e.g., neurological, gastrointestinal and genitourinary.

Quick recall*

- Somatization disorder: There are multiple, frequently changing physical symptoms. Most patients have multiple contacts with primary and specialist medical services. There are many negative investigations. Gastrointestinal and skin symptoms are the most common. Sexual and menstrual complaints are also common. Onset after the age of 40 years may indicate the onset of affective disorder.
- There is 0.2%–0.5% prevalence in the United Kingdom.
- It is a far more common condition in women than men (F:M = 5:1).
- It is more common in people with lower education and from lower socioeconomic classes.

---

* Adapted from B.K. Puri, A. Hall and R. Ho (2014). *Revision Notes in Psychiatry*. London. UK: CRC Press, pp. 469–472.

- It usually starts in early adult life, except somatoform pain disorder that starts later in life.
- *ICD-10* requires the presence of all of the following:
  - Two years of multiple and variable physical symptoms with no physical explanation found.
  - Persistent refusal to accept the advice of several doctors.
  - Impairment of functioning attributable to symptoms and resulting behaviour.
- The possibility of developing an independent physical disorder should be considered.
- The emphasis on symptoms and their effects distinguishes this from hypochondriacal disorder where the emphasis of concern is on possible underlying disease.
- Briquet's syndrome is also known as multiple somatization disorder.
- Somatization disorder has been renamed as somatic symptom disorder in the *DSM-5*. Patients suffer from somatic symptoms that cause distress and result in significant disruption in life. Patients also have disproportionate and persistent thoughts about the seriousness of somatic symptoms. The symptoms lead to a high level of anxiety. As a result, excessive time and energy are devoted to the symptoms concerned. The duration of the symptoms must be at least 6 months. Specific features includes predominant pain.
- Comorbidities include depressive disorder, anxiety disorder, adjustment disorder, psychotic disorder, histrionic personality disorder, dissocial personality disorder, substance misuse and other somatoform disorders.
- Persistent somatoform pain disorder: This presents with persistent, severe, distressing pain, not explained by physical disorder. Pain occurs in association with emotional conflict and results in increased support and attention. The prevalence of persistent pain is 3%. The onset of somatoform pain disorder is usually between 40 and 50 years. The female-to-male ratio is 2:1. Acute pain (less than 6 months) is associated with anxiety disorder. Chronic pain (more than 6 months) is associated with depressive disorder. The onset of somatoform pain is usually abrupt. Treatment involves antidepressants, gradual withdrawal of analgesics, CBT and relaxation techniques. In general, acute pain carries a better prognosis than chronic pain.

STATION 118: TRAUMATIC BRAIN INJURY (PART A)

Information to candidates

Name of patient: Mr Jordan

You have been tasked to speak to Mr Jordan. He was involved in a traumatic car accident about 2 years ago, in which he sustained a head injury that required surgery. Post-operatively, he recovered well and managed to gradually get back to his premorbid functioning. However, recently, his wife has noted that Mr Jordan has been different in terms of his behaviour and personality. She is very concerned about the recent changes. She has brought him to the GP, who has in turn referred her to your service. She is here with him.

Task

Please speak to Mr Jordan's wife and elicit a history of personality change. Please take sufficient history to come to a formulation.

Outline of station

You are the wife of Mr Jordan. You have been married to Mr Jordan for 5 years. Two years ago, he was involved in a major car accident and sustained an injury to his head for which he needed surgery. You were thankful that post-operatively he managed to recover well. Your only concern currently is that he seems different in terms of his behaviour and personality over the past few months. At times, he seems to be quite disinhibited and would be overfamiliar and make inappropriate remarks. Due to this, you have not attended church for a while as he did made inappropriate remarks whilst in church. You have noticed at times he appears to be more aggressive and irritable. His memory is not as good as it used to be. He has not vocalized any other symptoms to you. You are concerned about his changes in personality and hope that someone can advise you of the reasons for the changes in his behaviour.

CASC construct table

The CASC construct table is formatted such that candidates will be able to cover adequately both the range and the depth of the assessment required in this station.

Starting off: 'Hello, I am Dr Melvyn, one of the psychiatrists from the mental health unit. I understand that your GP has referred your husband to us. Can we have a chat about his problems?'			
History of presenting complaint	I understand that your GP has referred your husband, Mr Jordan, for an assessment. I understand you have some concerns. Would you mind telling me more?	I'm sorry to learn how difficult things have been for you recently. Can you tell me when you first observed these changes? Was it immediately after the accident or just recently? How have things progressed since the time from which you first noticed until now? Have things been worsening?	Can you tell me more about the accident in which Mr Jordan was involved? What injuries did he sustain? Did he lose consciousness at all? You mentioned that he needed to undergo a surgery. Can you tell me more about what surgery has been done? Did the neurologist or the surgeon follow up on his care? What have they said about his current condition?

(Continued)

Explore personality changes	Can you tell me more about your husband's personality prior to the recent accident? Could you tell me more with regard to how his personality has changed?	Does he seem to be more disinhibited? Has he done anything that is sexually inappropriate?	Does he seem to be more overfamiliar at times with strangers? Does he seem to be more impulsive in nature? Could you give me some examples?
Explore behavioural changes	Can you tell me more with regard to how his behaviour has changed?	Does he seem to be easily annoyed? Does he get frustrated easily?	Has he been verbally aggressive at home? Has he been physically aggressive at home?
Explore judgement	How has his attention and concentration been?	Does he have any difficulties with making decisions?	What about his judgement?
Explore memory difficulties	How has his memory been? You mentioned that he has been having some difficulties in his memories.	Does he have any difficulties with his short-term memory? What about his long-term memory? Any problems with planning of activities? Does he have any problems with task shifting?	Is he able to recognize people whom he has not seen for some time? Does he seem to muddle up the dates and days in a week? Does he have any difficulties with expenses and finances? Does he have any difficulties with finding the right words? Does he tend to repeat the words that he has already said? Is he still able to handle and manage himself? Does he need any form of assistance currently?
Exclude other psychiatric disorders	How has his mood been? Any mood swings? Is he still able to have interest in things that he used to enjoy?	How is his energy level? How has his sleep been? What about his appetite?	Have there been any other abnormal behaviours that you have noticed?
Risk assessment	Has he expressed any ideations of ending his life?	Has he expressed any ideations to hurt or harm anyone in particular?	

Common pitfalls

a. Failure to cover the range and depth of the information required for this station

Quick recall*

- Ten per cent of all visits to the emergency department are due to underlying head injury.
- Incidence of head injury: 1,500 per 10,000.
- The male-to-female gender ratio is 2:1.

Classification of head injury

- Primary head injury: Primary head injury is a result of either rotational or horizontal acceleration or deceleration. Rotational acceleration or deceleration results in diffuse shearing of long central fibres and micro-haemorrhages in the corpus callosum and rostral brainstem. This will result in diffuse axonal injury. The rotational acceleration or deceleration also causes centrifugal pressure waves to spread out so that the brain undergoes repeated buffeting against the skull and tentorium where there are sharp bony edges or corners. The frontal poles, orbitofrontal regions, temporal poles and medial temporal structures are particularly vulnerable.
- Secondary head injury: It is caused by haemorrhage, reactive brain swelling, acute fluid collections, raised intracranial pressure and coning of the brainstem.

Neuropsychiatric sequelae of head injury

- Post-concussion syndrome occurs in 50% of the patients after 2 months and 12% after 1 year.
- Depression and anxiety are common.
- Secondary mania occurs in 9% of the patients.
- Schizophreniform disorder occurs in 2.5% of the patients.
- Paranoid psychosis occurs in 2% of the patients.
- Psychotic depression occurs in 1% of the patients.
- Impulsive personality as a result of a decreased level of 5-Hydroxyindoleacetic acid (5-HIAA) after head injury.
- Dementia is usually non-progressive.
- Memory deficit is the most frequent chronic cognitive disturbance.
- Head injury in children is associated with restlessness, overactivity, disobedience and temper tantrums.
- Seizure occurs in 5% of head injury victims. If dura mater is penetrated, the risk of epilepsy is 30%.

Aetiological factors and severity of head injury

- Biological factors include the age at the time of the injury, the extent and the location of the brain injury, post-traumatic epilepsy.
- Psychological factors include premorbid personality, premorbid intelligence and psychological reactions to the injury.
- Social factors include premorbid social functioning, social support and mild head injury.

---

* Adapted from B.K. Puri, A. Hall and R. Ho (2014). *Revision Notes in Psychiatry*. London, UK: CRC Press, pp. 469–472.

- In mild head injury, the Glasgow Coma scale (GCS) is between 14 and 15. Pay attention if the patient shows neurological signs: has haematoma, a history of coagulopathy, drug or alcohol consumption, epilepsy and past neurosurgery and is more than 60 years old.
- In moderate head injury, the GCS is 9–13. The mortality is less than 20%, although the morbidity is more than 50%. Positive neuroimaging finding in 40% of patients; 8% require neurosurgery.
- In severe head injury, the GCS is less than 9. Outcomes: It accounts for 10% of all head injuries, with a mortality of 40%.
- Post-concussion syndrome occurs after minor head injury. Post-concussion syndrome is associated with premorbid physical and social problems. It usually lasts from several weeks to 3 months and is more likely to be persistent in women. Common physical symptoms include headache, nausea and sensitivity to light and noise. Common psychological symptoms include cognitive impairment, poor concentration and irritability.
- Neuropsychiatric sequelae of frontal lobe injury: Frontal polar damage leads to poor judgement and insight, apathy and impaired problem solving. There is often no understanding of the impact of the disability on others. Orbitofrontal damage is associated with personality changes, impaired social judgement, impulsivity, hyperactivity, disinhibition, lability of mood, excitability and childishness or moria (childlike interest). Dorsolateral damage is associated with executive dysfunction, apathy, psychomotor retardation, preservation, poor initiation of tasks and memory impairment. Dorsolateral damage is associated with akinetic mutism. Left frontal lesion is associated with impairment in verbal recall.

STATION 119: TRAUMATIC BRAIN INJURY (PART B)

Information to candidates

Name of patient: Mr Jordan

You have been tasked to speak to Mr Jordan. He was involved in a traumatic car accident about 2 years ago, in which he sustained a head injury and needed an operation for. Post-operatively, he recovered well and managed to gradually get back to his premorbid functioning. However, recently his wife has noted that Mr Jordan has been different in terms of his behaviour and personality. She is very concerned about the recent changes. She has brought him to the GP, who has in turn referred her to your service. She is here with him. In the previous station, you spoke to his wife and clarified the history.

Task

Please speak to Mr Jordan and get his consent to assess his memory. Please perform a comprehensive cognitive examination based on the history elicited.

CASC construct table

The CASC construct table is formatted such that candidates will be able to cover adequately both the range and the depth of the assessment required in this station.

Starting off: 'Hello, I am Dr Melvyn, one of the psychiatrists from the mental health unit. I understand that your GP has referred you to us. I have spoken to your wife just now. Can I get you to help me with some memory tests?'			
Assess for orientation	Before we begin, could I check whether you have any visual or hearing impairment? Can you see and hear me clearly?	Do you know where we are at the moment? What level are we on? Which part of the county is this? What is the greater country that we are in?	Do you know what time it is at the moment? Do you know what year this is? Can you tell me what season, month and the day and date today?
Assess for registration	I would like you to remember three objects, which I will ask you to repeat immediately and 5 minutes later.	The three objects I would like you to remember are 'apple, table and penny'.	Can you repeat the three objects that I have told you?
Assess for attention and calculation	Can I trouble you to spell the word 'world' for me?	Can you please spell the word 'world' backwards for me?	*(If the patient is unable to spell, assessment can be done using calculation/ numbers instead.)*
Assess for recall, naming, repetition, comprehension	Can you tell me the three objects that I asked you to remember earlier?	Can you name these objects for me? *(Show the patient a pen and a watch.)*	Can you please repeat this phrase: 'No ifs, ands or buts'. Please listen to my instructions and follow them. I would like you to take this piece of paper with your right hand, fold it in half and place it on the floor.
Assess for reading, writing and copying	*(Write 'Close your eyes' on a piece of paper.)* Can you please read this sentence and do what it says?	Can you help me to write a complete sentence that has a subject and a verb?	*(Draw two intersecting pentagons.)* Can you please help me to copy this figure?
Assess for word fluency	Can you please name as many English words as possible starting with the letter 'F', 'A' and 'S'?	(Or) Can you name as many animals as possible in 1 minute?	
Assess for abstract thinking	Can you tell me the meaning of this proverb: 'A rolling stone gathers no moss'?		

(Continued)

Assess for cognitive estimates	Can you tell me on average how tall an average Englishman is?	Can you tell me how many elephants are there in London?	
Assess for judgement	Can you tell me what you will do for the following case?	If you find a letter on the floor and there is a stamp attached to it, what will you do?	
Luria's hand test and alternative sequence test	*(The doctor will demonstrate the Luria hand test to the subject.)*	*(After the subject has mastered the technique, he or she is expected to do it with one hand for at least five times.)*	*(Then the subject has to repeat with the other hand.)* *(For the alternating sequence test, the candidate draws alternative shapes and asks the person being examined to continue without telling them that there is a pattern.)*

Common pitfalls

a. Failure to cover the range and depth of the information required for this station

For verbal fluency, you will need to really take 1 minute to assess. Thus, do wear a watch for the examination! Remind the patient not to repeat words, as those with frontal lobe abnormalities tend to repeat.

Quick recall*

Category	Findings in patients without frontal lobe impairment	Findings in patients with frontal lobe impairment
Word fluency	Expected response is that they should be able to say 12–15 words in 1 minute. Some people may develop strategies to help them to find words. A person may think of a category of items starting with 'F' and then move on to other categories.	The person can only mention a few words. Very often, they repeat those words that they have already mentioned. Finally, the person stops and cannot provide more words or items.
Abstract thinking	They are able to interpret the deeper meaning and not just focus on the words superficially.	The patient cannot appreciate the deeper meanings and just focuses on the words superficially.
Cognitive estimates	Even though the patient may not know the exact number, he or she is able to give a reasonable estimate.	The patient is unable to give a reasonable estimate and usually gives an answer beyond the normal estimates.

(Continued)

* Adapted from B.K. Puri, A. Hall and R. Ho (2014). *Revision Notes in Psychiatry*. London, UK: CRC Press, p. 113.

Judgement	The patient will give logical actions.	The patient may give various responses but not conform with the logical actions proposed by people without frontal lobe impairment.
Luria's hand test	A subject without frontal lobe impairment can appreciate the three different hand positions and demonstrate them accordingly.	Patients with frontal lobe impairments will not be able to appreciate the different hand positions and cannot alternate from one to another, as a result of motor perseveration.
Alternative sequence test	Patients without frontal lobe impairment will recognize and continue with three alternative shapes.	Patients with frontal lobe impairment will continue with the last shape. The failure to appreciate the alternative pattern is a result of perseveration.
Elicit primitive reflexes	The expected normal response is that there are no primitive reflexes.	Patients with frontal lobe impairment show emergence of primitive reflexes.

STATION 120: POST-MYOCARDIAL INFARCTION DEPRESSION (PART A)

Information to candidates

Name of patient: Mr Brown

You have been tasked to speak to Mr Brown, a 55-year-old man, who has been recently admitted to the cardiac inpatient unit following a myocardial infarction. Since his discharge from the hospital, the cardiologist has linked him up with the cardiac rehabilitation program. He has managed to participate in two sessions thus far but has been missing the scheduled sessions recently. He has mentioned to his GP that he has been feeling low in his mood recently. His GP hence initiated a referral to the mental health service.

Task

Please speak to Mr Brown and take a history with the aim of establishing a clinical diagnosis. Please also assess his current social circumstances and assess his current understanding with regard to his condition. Please note that in the next station you will need to speak to your consultant to discuss the appropriate management plans, so please take down notes if needed.

Outline of station

You are Mr Brown and have just been admitted inpatient for a myocardial infarction. You have been treated, and your cardiologist has recommended that you participate in the cardiac rehabilitation program after your discharge. You have managed to make it for two sessions thus far but have been missing the remaining sessions. You find that your mood has been low, and you do not have much interest in doing things you used to enjoy. You do know the importance of participating in the program and adhering to the recommendations of the cardiologist with regard to diet. Ever since your heart issue, you have not been able to get back to your normal work. You previously worked as a physical education teacher. Your wife is supportive, but recently she also needs to work overtime, so there is no one at home. You have been feeling useless and helpless at home.

CASC construct table

The CASC construct table is formatted such that candidates will be able to cover adequately both the range and the depth of the assessment required in this station.

Starting off: 'Hello, I am Dr Melvyn, one of the psychiatrists from the mental health unit. I understand that your GP has referred you to us. Can we have a chat?'			
Elicit information about recent hospitalization and plans on discharge	I understand from the referral memo that you have recently been admitted inpatient following a heart attack. I'm sorry to learn of that. Can I understand more about your recent admission?	Can you tell me more about what happened prior to your admission to the cardiac unit? What were the symptoms you had that caused you to suspect that you had had a heart attack?	Can you tell me what treatment the cardiologist has given you so far? How has your recovery been? How long did you need to stay inpatient? Did the doctors prescribe any medications for you to take on a long-term basis on discharge? Did the doctors recommend that you take part in any specific programs on discharge? Can you tell me more? Have you been going for the programs on discharge?
Elicit core symptoms of depression	You mentioned that you have attended some of the sessions, but recently have missed the scheduled sessions because you have been feeling low. How long have you been feeling low in your mood? Does your mood vary across the course of a day?	Are you still able to enjoy things that you used to enjoy? How has your energy levels been? How has your sleep been? What about your appetite? How have your attention and concentration been?	Sometimes, patients do mention that they do experience unusual experiences when their mood is low. Have you ever had such experiences before? I'm sorry to learn that you have been through a very tough time. Do you ever feel that life is not worth living?
Elicit current stressors	Is there anything in particular that is a stressor for you ever since you were discharged?	How have things been at home? Have there been any relationship difficulties? Do your family members and loved ones understand your condition?	Did you use to work before this? Have you been able to get back to work since the heart attack? Did they make any special accommodations for you at work? Do you have any other concerns such as finances?

(Continued)

| Elicit patient's understanding with regard to his condition | You mentioned that the cardiologist recommended that you take part in the cardiac rehabilitation program. Did he tell you more about the program? | Has the cardiologist given you any other advice about how best to manage your current condition? Did the cardiologist tell you the reasons as to why there is a need to modify some area of your current lifestyle? | It seems to me that your mood is low at the moment. We can help you with this. Do you think you will still be keen to continue on with the recommended program if your mood is slightly better? |

Common pitfalls

a. Failure to cover the range and depth of the information required for this station

Quick recall*

Cardiology and psychiatry

- Stressful life events lead to appraisal of the current situation. Primary appraisal assesses the threatening nature of a life event. Secondary appraisal assesses the adequacy of coping strategies.
- There will be three phases of responses. Phase 1 is an alarm reaction, phase 2 is the resistance stage and phase 3 is the exhaustion stage.
- The sympathetic system is activated by stressful life events. The patient will experience dilation of pupils, dry mouth, palpitations and sweating.
- Chronic mental stress–associated ordinary life events are the most common precipitant of myocardial ischaemia in patients with coronary artery disease. Type A behaviour (aggression, impatience and hostility) is associated with the incidence of recurrent myocardial infarction and cardiac death in patients with previous myocardial infarction; 20% of people with acute myocardial infarction suffer from depressive disorder.
- Psychosocial stress increases the levels of adrenaline and noradrenaline, which causes an increase in peripheral vascular resistance, resulting in hypertension and hypertrophy of the heart.
- An acute emotional trigger such as provoking anger is the immediate precipitant of irregular heart rhythms in patients who are in a chronic state of helplessness. Helplessness is an underlying sense of entrapment without possible escape.

Relationship between depression and ischaemic heart disease

- Twenty per cent of patients with ischemic heart disease (IHD) have comorbid depression.
- Major depression is an independent risk factor for IHD.
- After an acute myocardial infarction, major depression predicts mortality in the first 6 months. The impact of a depressive episode is equivalent to the impact of a previous infarct.

---

* Adapted from B.K. Puri, A. Hall and R. Ho (2014). *Revision Notes in Psychiatry*. London, UK: CRC Press, pp. 472–473.

The impact of depression on heart disease

- Poor compliance to cardiac treatment.
- Autonomic disturbances in depression may lead to heart rate changes and irregular heart rhythm.
- Serotonin dysfunction in depression: platelet activation and thrombosis.

Antidepressant trials in patients suffering from IHD

- Sertraline Antidepressant Heart Attack Randomized Trial (SADHART): This study found sertraline to be a safe treatment for depression after myocardial infarction, but there was little difference in depression status between groups receiving sertraline and placebo after 24 weeks of treatment. However, the effect of sertraline was greater in the patients with severe and recurrent depression. This study was not designed to assess the effects of treatment on cardiovascular prognosis, but severe cardiovascular events during the 6-month treatment tended to be less frequent in the sertraline group. The effect of sertraline on chronic depression was not evaluated.
- Enhancing Recovery in Coronary Heart Disease (ENRCHD): In this trial, the effects of CBT on depression and cardiac outcomes were evaluated. No significant differences in the cardiac outcomes were evaluated. No significant difference in cardiac outcomes was found between the intervention and the care-as-usual arms. Although substantial improvement in the severity of depression was observed 6 months after initiation of CBT, the difference between both arms diminished over time and was no longer present after 30 months.
- Myocardial Infarction and Depression-Intervention Trial (MIND-IT): Antidepressant treatment did not alter the course of chronic depression after myocardial infarction status or improve the cardiac outcomes.

STATION 121: POST–MYOCARDIAL INFARCTION DEPRESSION (PART B: MANAGEMENT)

Information to candidates

Name of patient: Mr Brown

You have been tasked to speak to Mr Brown, a 55-year-old man, who has been recently admitted to the cardiac inpatient unit following a myocardial infarction. Since his discharge from the hospital, the cardiologist has linked him up with the cardiac rehabilitation program. He has managed to participate in two sessions thus far but has been missing the scheduled sessions recently. He has mentioned to his GP that he has been feeling low in his mood recently. His GP hence initiated a referral to the mental health service. You have in the previous station spoken to the patient and elicited a history to come to a diagnosis. You have also explored his recent stressors and his motivation to engage in the cardio rehabilitation program.

Task

Please speak to the consultant psychiatrist and discuss with the consultant the most appropriate management plan for this patient.

Outline of station

You are the consultant psychiatrist and want to know more details with regard to the patient that the core trainee has just assessed. You wish to know the patient's understanding of his current condition, as well as his attitude towards his medical condition. You wish to discuss with the trainee the prevalence of depression amongst individuals with IHD as well as the mortality rates. You hope that the trainee has formulated a management plan in accordance with the guidelines and in consideration of the IHD history.

CASC construct table

The CASC construct table is formatted such that candidates will be able to cover adequately both the range and the depth of the assessment required in this station.

Starting off: 'Hello, I am Melvyn. I have just spoken to and assessed Mr Brown. Can I discuss the case with you?'			
Summary of case	Mr Charlie Brown is a 55-year-old gentleman who has been recently admitted for a myocardial infarction. He currently has low mood with reduced interest and poor engagement with his cardiac rehabilitation program.	His ongoing stressor includes him not being able to go back to work and function like what he used to be able to.	Clinically, he is depressed, and he fulfils the ICD-10 diagnostic criteria for depressive disorder. He does have an understanding as to why he needs to continue on with the cardiac rehabilitation program, and he is still motivated to engage if his mood symptoms are better sorted out. My current diagnosis for him is a post-myocardial infarction depressive disorder.
Prevalence and associated mortality rates	Based on my understanding, the prevalence of depressive disorder in post–myocardial infarction patients is around 20%.	Compared with normal individuals, the mortality rate is enhanced, at a rate of 2–6 times higher.	

(Continued)

Management – pharmacological	With these in mind, I would like to propose both pharmacological and non-pharmacological approaches to help him with his depressive disorder and to get him back into his cardiac rehabilitation program.	With regard to medications, we need to take into consideration the recommendations of the SADHART. The trial proposed that sertraline is more suitable for patients post–myocardial infarction.	I would be cognizant not to start him with antidepressants such as the tricyclic antidepressants or venlafaxine, as tricyclics could cause irregular heart rhythms, and venlafaxine could cause an elevated blood pressure.
Management – non-pharmacological	In addition to medications, I would like to refer the patient for psychological treatments, such as CBT.	In addition to psychological treatment, counselling services might also be beneficial for him, as they could educate him about life-style changes he needs to make.	
Management – others	I would liaise closely with the cardiologist and update the cardiologist about the treatment we have started for the patient.	Eventually, we hope that we could get the patient back on board the cardiac rehabilitation program, so that he could get back to his normal functioning in due course.	We will together with the multidisciplinary team. Also involve the dietician in educating the patient about a healthy balanced diet. Ensure that he has adequate physical exercise.

Common pitfalls

a. Failure to cover the range and depth of the information required for this station

Quick recall*

Antidepressant trials in patients suffering from IHD

- SADHART: This study found sertraline to be a safe treatment for depression after myocardial infarction, but there was little difference in depression status between groups receiving sertraline and placebo after 24 weeks of treatment. However, the effect of sertraline was greater in the patients with severe and recurrent depression. This study was not designed to assess the effects of treatment on cardiovascular prognosis, but severe cardiovascular events during the 6-month treatment tended to be less frequent in the sertraline group. The effect of sertraline on chronic depression was not evaluated.

---

* Adapted from B.K. Puri, A. Hall and R. Ho (2014). *Revision Notes in Psychiatry*. London, UK: CRC Press, pp. 472–473.

- ENRCHD: In this trial, the effects of CBT on depression and cardiac outcomes were evaluated. No significant differences in the cardiac outcomes were evaluated. No significant difference in cardiac outcomes was found between the intervention and the care-as-usual arms. Although substantial improvement in the severity of depression was observed 6 months after initiation of CBT, the difference between both arms diminished over time and was no longer present after 30 months.
- MIND-IT: Antidepressant treatment did not alter the course of chronic depression after myocardial infarction status or improve the cardiac outcomes.

STATION 122: ANTIDEPRESSANT-INDUCED SEXUAL DYSFUNCTION (PAIRED STATION A)

Information to candidates

Name of patient: Mr Brown

You have been tasked to speak to a 40-year-old male, Mr Brown. He has been recently diagnosed with depression and has been started on fluoxetine 20 mg by the mood disorder team. He has requested an early review today, as he claimed that he has been experiencing some problems since the commencement of the antidepressant. He has been on the medications for the past 6 months.

Task

Please speak to him and explore more about his concerns with regard to the antidepressant. Please try to obtain further history from him regarding his current concerns. Please be informed that you will have to address his wife's concerns in the next station.

Outline of station

You are Mr Brown, and you were diagnosed with depression approximately 6 months ago. The team has recommended that you be commenced on an antidepressant called fluoxetine. You have been compliant with the medication thus far. However, you have been concerned, as the sexual side of your relationship appears to be affected as well. You thought that this might be due to your depression, but you personally feel that your mood symptoms have improved since the commencement of the medications. Prior to this, you did not have any difficulties with the sexual side of your relationship. You do not have any underlying medical conditions that might account for the current difficulties. You appear to be initially reluctant to discuss this with the doctor. You will be willing to discuss more only if the doctor is empathetic.

CASC construct table

The CASC construct table is formatted such that candidates will be able to cover adequately both the range and the depth of the assessment required in this station.

Starting off: 'Hello, I am Dr Melvyn. I hear that you wish to come off the antidepressant that we have recently started you on. Can we have a chat about it?'			
Explore rationale for commencement of antidepressant	I understand that we have started you on fluoxetine just recently. Can you tell me more about when it first started for you? Can I understand more about what happened back then that caused you to feel down? *Onset of symptoms:* Which came first – low mood or sexual dysfunction?	It has been some time since you have been on the antidepressant. Were there any initial difficulties with the medications? How has your mood been?	Do you feel that the medication has helped you? I understand that you wish to stop the medications currently. Can you please let me know why you wish to do so?
Explore current mood symptoms	I'm sorry to hear that you have been having some difficulties with your relationship since you have been on the medications. How has your mood been? What score would you give your mood currently?	Are you able to enjoy things which you used to enjoy? Can you give me some examples? How have your energy levels been? How has your sleep been for you? Have there been any difficulties with your appetite?	Have you had thoughts that life is not worth living and that the future is hopeless? Have you ever had thoughts of ending your life? What are your plans forward? It's good to hear from you that your mood has been more stable since the commencement of the antidepressant.
Explore relationship difficulties	It is not uncommon for some individuals to experience some side effects from the medications. I'm sorry to hear that the medication has been causing you some issues with your relationship. In addition, this is something that we deal with on a regular basis, so please be assured that you can find a solution to help you with it.	I might need to speak to you and your partner about this. Would this be alright for you? I'm sorry that I might need to ask you some very personal questions. I understand that you have been having some relationship difficulties, in particular, with the sexual side of your relationship. Can you please tell me more about your current difficulties?	Are there any problems with your interest in sex? Are there problems with you having an arousal or an erection? Are you able to perform and ejaculate during intimacy? Can you share with me more about how things were prior to the commencement of the antidepressant? In addition, have there been any other difficulties with your relationship with your partner?

(Continued)

Exclude other causative factors	Can I check whether you do have any other medical problems that I need to know of? Are you on regular medications?	Can you tell me more about the control of your chronic conditions? How has your diabetes control been?	Since the onset of your depression, has it affected your relationship with your wife?
Explore and address patient's concerns	Thanks for sharing with me your concerns. Given the recent onset of your depression, I would recommend that you be kept on treatment for the next couple of months. I hear that you have some concerns about how the antidepressant might have an effect on the sexual side of your relationship.	Given that you have responded well to this medication, I strongly feel that you should be kept on the medications. What we could do is to consider perhaps a drug holiday over the weekends and see if your symptoms get better.	Alternatively, we could consider switching you to an alternative antidepressant with lesser impact on the sexual side of your relationship. Do you have any other questions for me? Would you mind if I discuss further with your wife?

Common pitfalls

a. Failure to cover the range and depth of the information required for this station

Quick recall*

- With sexual dysfunction, the individual is unable to participate in a sexual relationship he or she wishes to have. Both psychological and somatic processes are usually involved in the causation of sexual dysfunction. Women present more commonly with complaints about the subjective quality of sexual experience; men present with a failure of specific sexual response.

ICD-10 classification

- Lack or loss of sexual desire: This is not secondary to other sexual difficulties. It does not preclude sexual enjoyment or arousal but makes the initiation of sexual activity less likely.
- Sexual aversion: Sexual interaction is associated with strong negative feelings of sufficient intensity that sexual activity is avoided.
- Lack of sexual enjoyment: Sexual responses and orgasm occur normally, but there is lack of pleasure. This is much more common in women.
- Failure of genital response: In men, this is primarily erectile dysfunction. In women, it is primarily due to vaginal dryness.
- Orgasmic dysfunction: Orgasm does not occur or is delayed. It is more common in women than men.
- Premature ejaculation: This is the inability to control ejaculation sufficiently for both partners to enjoy the sexual act.

---

* Adapted from B.K. Puri, A. Hall and R. Ho (2014). *Revision Notes in Psychiatry*. London, UK: CRC Press, p. 589.

- Non-organic vaginismus: This is the occlusion of the vaginal opening caused by spasm of the surrounding muscles. Penile entry is either impossible or painful.
- Non-organic dyspareunia: Pain during intercourse may occur in both sexes. The term is used only if an organic cause is not present and if there is no other primary sexual dysfunction.
- Excessive sexual drive: This usually occurs in men or women during late teenage or early adult years. If it is secondary to mental illness (such as mania), the underlying disorder is coded.

The effects of depression and sexual dysfunction

- It has been proposed that both depressed mood and the medications used to treat it could cause disorders of desire, arousal an orgasm.
- The onset and chronology of the onset of the sexual problems need to be clarified.
- Antidepressants could cause sedation, hormonal changes, disturbances of cholinergic, adrenergic balance and inhibition of nitric oxide and increased serotonin neurotransmission.
- The above factors have been speculated to be involved in sexual dysfunction.
- Sexual dysfunction has indeed been reported as one of the side effects of all classes of antidepressants, although the incidence rate varies.
- Previous research has highlighted a dose-dependent relationship between the dose of the antidepressant and the severity of its impact on sexual dysfunction.
- It should be noted that the sexual dysfunction that arises due to antidepressant usage could be reversed.

The following lists the antidepressant and its approximate prevalence in inducing sexual-related problems:

- Venlafaxine: 70%
- SSRI: approximately 60%–70%
- Duloxetine: 46%
- Monoamine oxidase inhibitors (MAOIs): 40%
- Tricyclic: 30%
- Mirtazapine: 25%
- Reboxetine: 5%–10%

STATION 123: ANTIDEPRESSANT-INDUCED SEXUAL DYSFUNCTION (PAIRED STATION B)

Information to candidates

Name of patient: Mr Charlie Brown

You have been tasked to speak to Mr Brown in the previous station and explore his concerns pertaining to him wanting to discontinue his antidepressant. His wife is also here and hopes to know more about your assessment and how you can manage his condition.

Task

Please speak to Mrs Brown and explain your assessment and diagnosis for Mr Brown. Please address all her concerns and expectations.

Outline of station

You are the wife of Mr Brown and are very concerned about his current condition. You know that he has been seen by the psychiatrist some months ago and has been commenced on an antidepressant. You do find that his mood has since improved after the commencement of the antidepressant. You are puzzled as to why he has been requesting to stop the antidepressant. You wish to hear from the psychiatrist his assessment, recommendations and further management plans.

CASC construct table

The CASC construct table is formatted such that candidates will be able to cover adequately both the range and the depth of the assessment required in this station.

Starting off: 'Hello, I am Dr Melvyn. I understand that you have some concerns about your husband's condition. Can we have a chat?'			
Explain current assessment	I have just seen your husband and understand that you have some concerns about his condition. He has given me permission to speak to you about it. He shared with me that he is keen to be off his antidepressants, as he has been experiencing side effects from it. He claimed that the sexual side of your relationship is affected. Can you share with me more?	Can I ask you more about your perception of his mood symptoms? Would you be able to tell me more about how his mood has been prior to him starting the antidepressant therapy? How would you say his mood has been currently? Does he complain that he feels lethargic and easily fatigued throughout the day? How do you find his appetite and sleep to be? Has he vocalized any thoughts that life is not worth living?	From my previous assessment, it does seem to me that the antidepressant therapy has been efficacious for him, and his mood has improved after the commencement of the antidepressant. I'm sorry to hear about the difficulties that you have been experiencing with your husband in terms of the sexual side of your relationship. Can I check with you whether your husband has any other medical conditions that I need to know of?

(Continued)

Address concerns and expectations	Are there any concerns that you want me to address? I hear your concerns about the medication. The common side effects of antidepressant like fluoxetine include nausea, headaches, and, in the longer term, sexual-related side effects. You are right that the medication might have contributed to his current sexual difficulties.	However, his current difficulties might also be due to the fact that his depressive symptoms have not been fully treated, and hence he should be maintained on an antidepressant.	I hear your concerns about the medications. I am concerned that if your husband is taken off the medications, he might suffer a relapse of his condition.
Explain management plans	Given that we recommend that your husband will best benefit from a continuation of his antidepressant, we could try an alternative antidepressant that would have a lesser side effect on his sexual and intimate relationship. Alternatively, we could also try strategies such as a drug holiday and see whether there is an improvement with regard to his problems.	There are other alternatives that we could also consider. Given that your husband does not have any underlying medical condition, such as any underlying cardiovascular disease, we could also consider a trial of Viagra to see if it works out well for him.	I would like to offer other forms of psychological therapies, such as couple-based therapy, which I think would be helpful in addressing this issue. Do you have any other questions for me?

Common pitfalls

a. Failure to cover the range and depth of the information required for this station

Quick recall*

Management of antidepressant-induced sexual dysfunction

- A thorough history should be taken with regard to the sexual dysfunction, to exclude potential physical health condition as a contributing factor.
- Some of the common physical health factors that could lead to sexual dysfunction include diabetes and cardiovascular disease.

---

* Adapted from B.K. Puri, A. Hall and R. Ho (2014). *Revision Notes in Psychiatry*. London, UK: CRC Press, p. 589.

- At times, psychological and relationship factors are linked to sexual-related dysfunction as well.
- It should be noted that, at times, there might be spontaneous remission, whereas in a small proportion of the cases, there might be partial remission.

Consideration of alternative management would be indicated if the problem persists. This would include the following:

- Reduction of the antidepressant dose
- Discontinuing the antidepressant
- Having drug holidays (however, clinicians need to take into account that some patients may suffer from a relapse or experience some of the antidepressant discontinuation symptoms)
- Considering a switch to another drug that has a relatively lower potential to cause sexual-related problems
- Consideration of other medications, such as sildenafil, to help with the sexual dysfunction

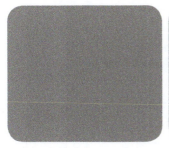

STATION 124: ASSAULT IN WARD (PAIRED STATION A)

Information to candidates

Name of patient: Stephen

You have been tasked to assess Stephen, a 40-year-old male. Stephen was admitted 2 days ago for a relapse of his underlying psychiatric condition. This morning, he assaulted one of the other patients. The nursing team is very concerned about his aggression and have requested an immediate assessment.

Task

Please speak to Stephen and find out more information with regard to the assault this morning. Please also perform a mental state examination as well as a risk assessment.

Outline of station

The purpose of providing an outline of the station is to allow candidates to be familiar with the structure of the station. This outline could also be helpful when candidates practice for the MRCPsych, joining with their colleagues to act out the station.

Please note that the outlines provided are based on the experiences of the authors. There may be variations in the actual examination.

You are Stephen and have a history of schizophrenia. You were admitted to the inpatient unit 2 days ago and brought into the hospital by the assertive outreach team. You have not been concordant with your medications recently. You have been bothered by the increasing frequency of auditory hallucinations. You suspect that others on the ward might have plotted against you. This morning, another patient stared at you, and you were convinced that he is the mastermind behind this plot. You felt you needed to do something to stop others from troubling you. You do not think you are responsible for what happened this morning. You just did what was right to protect yourself.

CASC construct table

The CASC construct table is formatted such that candidates will be able to cover adequately both the range and the depth of the assessment required in this station.

Starting off: 'Hello, I am Dr Melvyn, one of the psychiatrists from the mental health unit. I received news about what happened this morning. Can we have a chat?'			
Obtain further information about assault	I received some news about what happened this morning. Would you be able to tell me more? Did anything happen before the incident? Was there any trigger before the incident?	Can you tell me more about what you did this morning? Did you make plans for this? (Or) Was this an impulsive act?	Do you know what happened to the other patient? Do you know whether he is injured? Was any weapon used? How do you feel about what happened this morning? Do you feel remorseful with regard to your acts?
Mental state examination	Can you share with me why you have been admitted to the hospital? Have you been compliant with your medications before you came into the hospital?	How has your mood been? How has your sleep been? How has your appetite been? Do you still have interest in things that you used to enjoy? Have you been troubled by any abnormal experiences such as hearing voices when no one is around or seeing things that no one else can see?	Do you feel that others around you are trying to harm you or play tricks on you? How certain are you about this? Is there any alternative explanation for this? Do you feel safe in the ward? Do you feel that others can interfere with your thoughts? Can you give me an example of this? Do you feel in control of your emotions? Do you feel in control of your actions? Any commanding voices?
Risk assessment	I'm sorry to hear how troubled you have been. Do you feel that life is no longer worth living? Have you made plans about ending your life?	Do you still feel threatened by others around you? Do you have any thoughts of harming others around you? Have you made any plans?	Has something similar to what happened in the morning happened before? Have you been involved with the police previously? Can you tell me more? Do you drink? Do you have access to any drugs or substances? Do you feel that you are responsible for what happened this morning?

Common pitfalls

a. Failure to cover the range and depth of the information required for this station

Quick recall*

- Dangerous individuals are people who have caused or who might cause serious harm to others. The features of dangerousness include repetition, incorrigibility, unpredictability, untreatability and infectiousness.
- The best predictor of future dangerous behaviour is the individual's past behaviour. Shorter-term prediction is better than long-term prediction.
- Dangerousness is associated with the availability of weapons, morbid jealousy and sadistic murder syndrome.
- Schizophrenic patients usually assault a known person, but if they assault a stranger, the arresting police officer is the most common target. The delusional ideas often motivate the violent behaviours, and the patients usually admit experiencing command hallucinations after the violent offenses.
- Schizophrenic patients with negative symptoms commit violent offenses inadvertently and neglectfully.
- In clinical practice, psychiatrists should be aware that schizophrenic patients may display persistence of their normal selves, especially patients without history of violence.

Important factors for forensic psychiatric assessment

- Full history and mental state of the patient, including fantasies and impulses to offend.
- Objective account of the offense, such as from the arresting police officer or from statements (depositions) in Crown Court cases.
- Objective accounts of past offenses, if any, such as a list of previous convictions.
- Additional information gathering, such as interview with informants and reading a social inquiry report from a probation officer (if prepared).
- Review of previous psychiatric records, to ascertain relationship of mental disorder to previous behaviour and to psychiatric treatment and need for security.

Clinical risk assessment and risk management planning

- The aim is to get an understanding of the risk from a detailed historical longitudinal overview, obtaining information not only from the patient, who may minimize his or her history, but also from informants. Ideally, it should not be a one-off single-interview assessment.
- Reconstruct in detail what happened at the time of offense or behaviour causing concern.

---

* Adapted from B.K. Puri, A. Hall and R. Ho (2014). *Revision Notes in Psychiatry*. London, UK: CRC Press, pp. 723–724.

- Independent information form statements of victims or witnesses or police records should be obtained when available. Do not rely on what the offender tells you or the legal offense category – for example, arson may be of a wastepaper bin in a busy ward or with the intent to kill. Possession of an offensive weapon may have been prelude to homicide.
- Offense = offender × victim × circumstance/environment.
- Also consider protective factors. Practical risk assessment (history, mental state and environment) can be supplemented by standardized instruments of risk, including actuarial risk instruments based on static risk factors, such as the Violence Risk Appraisal Guide (VRAG), and dynamic risk instruments, such as the Historical, Clinical, Risk Management-20 (HCR-20), based on factors that can be changed or be managed, for example, symptoms of mental illness and noncompliance.

Ultimately, in conclusion, the aim is to answer how serious the risk is (the nature and magnitude): Is it specific or general, conditional or unconditional, immediate, long term or volatile? Have the individuals or situational risk factors changed? Who might be at risk?

From a risk assessment, a risk management plan should be developed to modify the risk factors and specify the response triggers. This should ideally be agreed upon by the individual. Is there a need for more frequent follow-up appointments, an urgent care program approach meeting or admission to the hospital, detention under the Mental Health Act, physical security, observation or medication? If the optimum plan cannot be undertaken, reasons for this should be documented and a backup plan specified.

Risk assessments and risk management plans should be communicated to others on a 'need to know' basis. On occasions, patient confidentiality will need to be breached if there is immediate grave danger to others. The police can often do little unless there is a specific threat to an individual, whereupon they may warn or charge the subject. Very careful consideration needs to be given before informing potential victims to avoid their unnecessary anxiety. Their safety is often best ensured by the management of those at risk.

STATION 125: ASSAULT IN WARD (PAIRED STATION B)

Information to candidates

Name of patient: David

You have been tasked previously to assess Stephen, a 40-year-old male. Stephen was admitted 2 days ago for a relapse of his underlying psychiatric condition. This morning, he assaulted one of the other patients. The nursing team is very concerned about his aggression and have requested an immediate assessment.

In the previous station, you assessed the mental state of the patient and did a risk assessment.

The ward manager, David, has requested to speak to you regarding Stephen.

Task

Please speak to David and explain to him your assessments. Please formulate a joint management plan with the ward manager. Please address all his concerns and expectations.

Outline of station

You are David, the ward manager of the psychiatric ward. You are aware that Stephen, one of your patients, assaulted another patient this morning. You are very worried that the victim's family will file a complaint. You hope to discuss the management plans with the core trainee. You wish to know about the patient's current mental state and risk assessment. You expect the core trainee to suggest some management plans to help contain Mr Stephen's aggression.

CASC construct table

The CASC construct table is formatted such that candidates will be able to cover adequately both the range and the depth of the assessment required in this station.

Starting off: 'Hello, I am Dr Melvyn. I understand that you have some concerns about what happened this morning in the ward. Can we have a discussion about how best to manage Stephen?'			
Explain mental state and risk assessment	I have seen the patient, and I hope to be able to answer the concerns that you have. I do understand that this is indeed a very difficult time for you and your colleagues in the ward.	When I interviewed the patient earlier, he shared with me that he assaulted another patient as he felt that the other patient was attempting to harm him. He is convinced of this just by the way the other patient looked at him.	I understand that he was just admitted to the ward around 2 days ago. It seems to me that he is not very settled with his current medication regiment and is still quite paranoid and psychotic. Currently, he tells me that he no longer harbours any thoughts or plans to deal with any other patients or your staff. I understand from his records that he has no previous forensic history and has not abused any substances such as alcohol or drugs.

(Continued)

Discuss pharmacological management plans	Given that he is still quite unwell, we might need to consider increasing the dose of the antipsychotic medication that he is currently on.	In addition, we might want to consider using antipsychotics per the rapid tranquilization protocol of the hospital. We could use sedating oral antipsychotics such as olanzapine or consider other intramuscular options such as intramuscular haloperidol or even intramuscular Ativan should he act out again.	We do, however, need to watch his vitals carefully following the administration of these medications. We should only use these medications in the event that he is extremely agitated and cannot be managed by de-escalation or seclusion techniques.
Discuss alternatives to pharmacological management	There are other viable alternatives to medications. He might benefit from being more closely monitored and, ideally, if he could be constantly monitored by a staff that he is familiar with.	We could also house him in the seclusion room to allow him to settle in the event that he is irritable or agitated.	The other alternative is to provide him with activities such as games to keep him engaged.
Discuss forensic issues pertaining to fitness to plead	I understand the concerns that you have with regard to the incident this morning; in particular, with regard to whether the victim's family might file a complaint.	We might need to get our forensic colleagues to assess the patient if there are complaints made against the patient.	However, even though he has an existing mental health disorder, it does not negate the fact that he still needs to take responsibility for his actions and is still fit to be interviewed by the police should there be a complaint and there be further investigations. Do you have any other questions for me?

Common pitfalls

a. Failure to cover the range and depth of the information required for this station

Quick recall*

Ultimately, the aim is to answer how serious the risk is (the nature and magnitude): Is it specific or general, conditional or unconditional, immediate, long term or

---

* Adapted from B.K. Puri, A. Hall and R. Ho (2014). *Revision Notes in Psychiatry*. London, UK: CRC Press, pp. 723–724.

volatile? Have the individuals or situational risk factors changed? Who might be at risk?

From a risk assessment, a risk management plan should be developed to modify the risk factors and specify the response triggers. This should ideally be agreed upon by the individual. Is there a need for more frequent follow-up appointments, an urgent care program approach meeting or admission to the hospital, detention under the Mental Health Act, physical security, observation or medication? If the optimum plan cannot be undertaken, reasons for this should be documented and a backup plan specified.

Risk assessments and risk management plans should be communicated to others on a 'need to know' basis. On occasions, patient confidentiality will need to be breached if there is immediate grave danger to others. The police can often do little unless there is specific threat to an individual, whereupon they may warn or charge the subject. Very careful consideration needs to be given before informing potential victims to avoid their unnecessary anxiety. Their safety is often best ensured by the management of those at risk.

STATION 126: FIRE-SETTING BEHAVIOUR – ASSESSMENT

Information to Candidates

Name of Patient: Catherine

You have been tasked to speak to a 17-year-old female, Catherine. She has been arrested by the police for arson and has been brought in to the emergency department for an assessment. The police might consider charging her, but they hope that a psychiatric evaluation can be conducted first, as she seemed to be quite hysterical when she was remanded to the police.

Task

Please speak to Catherine and elicit a history with regard to the arson that she has been involved in. Please obtain as much history as you can in order for you to formulate a diagnosis.

Outline of station

You are Catherine, a 17-year-old female, and you have been arrested by the police for setting fire to the apartment that you are currently living in. This is not the first time you have set fire to your apartment. What happened today was that you chanced upon a television program on BBC which showed how young children have been physically bullied by their caregivers. This reminded you of your past childhood experiences. You felt frustrated after watching the show and needed a channel to vent your frustration. You found a lighter in your room and made use of it to light up some papers in the wastepaper basket. You did not expect the fire to spread so quickly and neither did you expect your neighbours to call upon the police. You realize that it was wrong for you to do this. You have no previous mental health problems, and you did not use alcohol or any substances when you set your apartment on fire.

CASC construct table

The CASC construct table is formatted such that candidates will be able to cover adequately both the range and the depth of the assessment required in this station.

Starting off: 'Hello, I am Dr Melvyn. I understand that the police have brought you in to our emergency services. I have only a limited understanding of what happened this morning. Would you mind sharing with me more?'			
Establish rapport and explore antecedents prior to the incident	I understand that it has been a difficult time for you.	Can you tell me what happened that caused you to be arrested by the police?	Are you able to tell me more? What actually happened before you started the fire?
Explore the fire-setting behaviour	Can you share with me more about how you started the fire?	Did you make any plans prior? (Or) Was it just out of impulse?	
Explore consequences of actions	Do you remember what happened after you started the fire?	Do you know who called upon the police? Did you think about the consequences – risk to self, others and property?	Are you regretful now of your actions?
Exclude comorbid psychiatric conditions	Thanks for sharing with me. Can I clarify: Is this the first time you have been involved in fire setting?	How did you feel before you set the fire? Were you feeling tensed up? How did you feel after that? Did you feel that there was a sudden release of tension? Were there times when you felt sexually aroused whilst setting the fire? Did you have intention to end your life when you set the fire?	How has your mood been recently? Do you find that you still have interest in things that you used to enjoy? Has there been a time in which you had abnormal experiences? By that, I mean hearing things that are not there or seeing things that are not there?
Explore underlying triggers/past childhood issues	It seemed that what happened today reminded you of your past.	I understand that it might be difficult for you to share, but I'm hoping you could tell me if there were incidents in the past that were particularly significant, even up to today.	Were you bullied when you were much younger?
Rule out substance history	Did you use any alcohol prior to the recent incident?	What about other substances?	

Common pitfalls

a. Failure to cover the range and depth of the information required for this station

The patient in this station may be difficult to engage. Thus, it is important for you to be empathetic and gently probe about the circumstances of the fire. Sometimes, if she refuses to talk, it may be helpful to go around the topic and ask about more neutral topics (e.g., personality) before going back to the pertinent issues. Her tone of voice may also be soft. Therefore, you may get her permission to sit slightly closer to talk to her.

Quick recall*

- There are about 30,000 episodes of arson in England and Wales per year.
- The most common motives are revenge and fraud insurance claims.
- The other causes include anger and the need to relieve tension by fire setting.
- There is a higher representation of men with learning disability (intelligence quotient [IQ] of 70–79) because they display passive aggression and a sense of power or excitement during arson.
- Twenty to thirty per cent of individuals involved have psychiatric disorders such as alcohol misuse and schizophrenia.
- Pyromania is a rare condition in which the arsonist derives sexual satisfaction through fire setting.
- Most cases of arson (80%) do not lead to criminal conviction and only a tiny proportion lead to psychiatric disposition (more common in women).
- The recidivism rates for arson are around 10%.
- If it is a gang crime, the recidivism rate is low for the gang members but high for the gang leader.

STATION 127: MORBID JEALOUSY – (PAIRED STATION A: ASSESSMENT)

Information to candidates

Name of patient: Mr Charlie Brown

You have been tasked to speak to Mr Charlie Brown. Mr Brown was arrested this morning, as his wife called upon the police after he used a knife to threaten her. He has been suspicious about his wife's coming home late and has attributed it to her having an extramarital affair.

---

* Adapted from B.K. Puri, A. Hall and R. Ho (2014). *Revision Notes in Psychiatry*. London, UK: CRC Press, pp. 722–734.

Task

Please speak to Mr Brown and try to elicit as much history as possible to come to a diagnosis. In addition, please perform an appropriate and comprehensive risk assessment.

Outline of station

You are Mr Charlie Brown and are very upset that the police have detained you and sent you over to a mental health service for an assessment. You should vocalize your unhappiness at how the police have managed the situation and go on to mention more about your wife's problem. You have noticed that she has been coming home late these days. You went through her personal belongings a couple of days ago, and, to your surprise, you found the name card of a male business partner. You firmly believe that she must be having an affair, which would explain why she has been coming home late and also explain why she has not been interested in intimacy of late. You planned to make use of the knife today to threaten her into admitting her mistake. You do not have any plans to make use of the knife to hurt her. You use alcohol on a daily basis, but you do not use any other drugs. You do not have any previous forensic records of note.

CASC construct table

The CASC construct table is formatted such that candidates will be able to cover adequately both the range and the depth of the assessment required in this station.

Starting off: 'Hello, I am Dr Melvyn. I understand that the police have brought you in to our emergency services. I have only a limited understanding of what happened this morning. Would you mind sharing with me more?'			
Assessment of morbid jealousy symptoms	I can imagine that you have gone through a very difficult period. Can you share with me when you started to suspect your wife of having an affair?	Can you describe your recent relationship with your wife? Is there any event that triggered your suspicion? How did you arrive at the conclusion that your wife is unfaithful? Can you share with me your evidence? Do you know the identity of the third party? Do you follow your wife? If yes, how often? How often do you call your wife? Do you search her belongings (such as hand phone, text messages, underwear, handbag and credit card bill)?	Can there be other possible explanations for her infidelity? If I give you a scale from 1 to 10, 1 means that you do not believe that your wife is unfaithful, and 10 means you are completely convinced: How do you rate your belief? I can imagine that you have gone through a tough time. What is your plan for your marriage? Are you going to divorce your wife? Are you going to confront her? How do you cope with the current situation?

(Continued)

Risk assessment	Have you thought of harming yourself? If yes, how would you do it? What would you do to your wife if she denies the affair? Will you be more aggressive?	Are you going to take any action against the third party? If yes, how would you do it? Do you have any children? How old are they? What are their views on the current situation? Have you ever thought of harming them?	Do you have access to weapons? If yes, what kind of weapons do you have? Do you carry weapons with you? When will you use them?
Psychiatric comorbidity	Can you take me through how much you drink in a day? Has there been an increase in alcohol intake recently? Have you developed further problems as a result of drinking? When people are stressed, they often turn to recreational drugs. Have you tried those drugs?	Have you encountered any sexual problem (such as inability to maintain erection during sex)? If yes, how long did you have this problem? Was it related to diabetes? Can you tell me more about your past relationships? Did you suspect your partners or girlfriends in the past? Have you been unfaithful to your partners in the past?	How is your mood at the moment? Do you feel sad? Can you tell me more about your sleep, appetite and energy? How do you see your future? Do you feel guilty? How is your confidence level? Do you experience anxiety? Can you tell me more about your fear (such as losing your wife)? Do you have unusual experience such as hearing voices when no one is around? Do the voices give instructions? Do you feel that someone wants to harm you at this moment? Do you think that there is a plot behind your wife's infidelity? How do other people describe you as a person? Do they say that you are more suspicious? Do you have problems with your friends or neighbours? Do you trust them?
Past history	Did you have any encounter with the police? If yes, for what reason? What was the consequence? Have you ever appeared in court? If yes, were you sentenced to the correctional service?	Is this your first marriage? If not, how did it end last time? How about your previous romantic relationships? Can you tell me more about your family? Is there any family history of violence?	

Common pitfalls

a. Failure to cover the range and depth of the information required for this station

Important to assess risk of harm to self, wife, the third party and children. Ascertain if the patient has any concrete plans and when he plans to do it.

Quick recall*

- Pathological jealousy: This is also called the Othello syndrome, morbid jealousy, erotic jealousy, sexual jealousy, psychotic jealousy or conjugal paranoia. The person holds the delusional belief that his or her sexual partner is being unfaithful and will go to great lengths to find evidence of infidelity. Underclothing may be examined for semen stains, belongings may be searched and the partner may be interrogated and followed. It is more common in men.

  Pathological jealousy may be associated with the following conditions:

- Organic disorders and psychoactive substance use disorders (such as alcohol dependence, cerebral tumour, endocrinopathy, dementia, cerebral infection, use of amphetamines or cocaine)
- Paranoid schizophrenia
- Depression
- Neurosis or personality disorder
- Treatment should be directed at the underlying disorder.
- If no primary cause is identified, pharmacotherapy with a neuroleptic and/or psychotherapy may be helpful.
- There may be a risk of violence to the partner, and it may be best to recommend that the couple separate.

STATION 128: MORBID JEALOUSY (PAIRED STATION B: MANAGEMENT)

Information to candidates

Name of patient: Mrs Brown

You have assessed Mr Brown in the previous station. Mrs Brown is here in the hospital, and she is hoping to speak to you as she wants to know what is wrong with her husband.

Task

Please speak to Mrs Brown and explain to her about her husband's diagnosis as well as the appropriate management plan for him.

* Adapted from B.K. Puri, A. Hall and R. Ho (2014). *Revision Notes in Psychiatry*. London, UK: CRC Press, pp. 720–721.

Outline of station

You are the wife of Mr Charlie Brown and are very concerned about his sudden outrage and aggression today. You're worried as you feel that he is not his normal self. You understand that the psychiatrist has seen him and would like to hear more about the diagnosis that the psychiatrist has given him. In addition, you also wish to find out more about the management should he have a psychiatric condition.

CASC construct table

The CASC construct table is formatted such that candidates will be able to cover adequately both the range and the depth of the assessment required in this station.

Starting off: 'Hello, I am Dr Melvyn. I have just seen and assessed your husband. I understand that you have some concerns that you would like to discuss with me today. Can we have a chat?'			
Clarification of the diagnosis	I understand that this has been much of a surprise for you, and I also understand how difficult you must have felt in that situation. I understand your concerns about your husband's condition. I have seen him and have done the necessary assessment.	From what he has shared, he has a strong belief and conviction that you are having an extramarital affair. Are you alright with me going on? I have tried to challenge the beliefs your husband has, but he remains strongly convinced.	He has a condition known as morbid jealousy, a subtype of a delusional disorder. Have you heard about this condition before? In such a condition, an individual usually has a firm and unshakable belief that is out of keeping with the cultural norms.
Clarification of risk issues	I am quite concerned about the risk issues that your husband possesses. Throughout the conversation, he remains quite convicted about his beliefs. I am also concerned about your safety.	In addition, I also gathered that your husband has been using alcohol on a daily basis, which might predispose him to further violence. I understand that he does not have any previous convictions or forensic involvement. Is that true?	Given what has happened today, I will recommend that your husband be detained under the Mental Health Act for a period of treatment in view of him being unwell currently and the further risk he might pose.
Provide an overview of management plans	I hear your concerns about the treatment options that he will be put through if he is detained. With regard to treatment, there are medications available to help him with his condition.	When he is more stable, psychological treatment might be suitable to help him with his condition. The medications that we are considering for your husband are antipsychotics. These medications would help with the fixed convictions that he currently harbours against you.	As discussed, when he is more stable, we could try to engage him with psychological therapies or talking therapies. A common psychological therapy we routinely recommend to our patients is cognitive behavioural therapy (CBT). Do you have any questions about the management of your husband's condition on the ward?

(Continued)

| Provide an overview of longer-term management plans if he is discharged to the community | In the longer term, we need to consider gradual reintroduction of your husband back into the community. We would consider granting him Section 17 home leave when he is better and have a community nurse accompany him home. | You could tell us how his condition is, and we will discuss how best we can help your husband's condition with the rest of our multidisciplinary team members. | When he is eventually discharged home, we hope to be able to continue engaging him with our community mental health team. I know that I have provided you with quite a lot of information. Please let me know if you have any questions for me. |

Common pitfalls

a. Failure to cover the range and depth of the information required for this station

In this station, the wife may be very insistent for the patient to be discharged. Therefore, it is important to highlight to her the high risk that he poses.

Use patient's symptoms to highlight the characteristics of morbid jealousy. Explain to the wife in layman terms what 'delusion' means.

Quick recall*

Pathological jealousy may be associated with the following conditions:

● Organic disorders and psychoactive substance use disorders (such as alcohol dependence, cerebral tumour, endocrinopathy, dementia, cerebral infection, use of amphetamines or cocaine).
● Paranoid schizophrenia.
● Depression.
● Neurosis or personality disorder.
● Treatment should be directed at the underlying disorder.
● If no primary cause is identified, pharmacotherapy with a neuroleptic and/or psychotherapy may be helpful.
● There may be a risk of violence to the partner, and it may be best to recommend that the couple separate.

STATION 129: EROTOMANIA AND STALKING BEHAVIOUR

Information to candidates

Name of patient: Benjamin

You have been tasked to speak to Benjamin, who has turned up at the emergency department of one of the hospitals today looking for a nurse who treated him 3

---

* Adapted from B.K. Puri, A. Hall and R. Ho (2014). *Revision Notes in Psychiatry*. London, UK: CRC Press, pp. 722–734.

weeks prior. He was arrested by the police as he wielded a knife against the security staff that prevented him from looking for the nurse.

Task

Please speak to the patient and elicit his abnormal beliefs. Please also conduct a detailed risk assessment.

Outline of station

You are Benjamin and have just been arrested by the police. You merely turned up at the emergency department to look for the nurse, Sarah, who treated you weeks ago. From your brief encounter with her, you strongly believe that she has given you cues that she is in love with you. You know some details with regard to where she lives and her contact number. There was also an occasion on which you stalked her. However, you decided to look for her in the hospital's emergency department today as you knew that she would be on her shift. You have made plans for tonight, including how you would want to engage her in intimacy. You were arrested when you wielded a knife at the security staff who tried to stop you from seeing her. This is not the first time you have gotten involved with the police. When you were with your previous girlfriend, something similar happened. You are not very willing to engage with the psychiatrist as you believe that the police have got the wrong person, and that you have every right to see her. You are convinced that the nurse is in love with you.

CASC construct table

The CASC construct table is formatted such that candidates will be able to cover adequately both the range and the depth of the assessment required in this station.

Starting off: 'Hello, I am Dr Melvyn. I understand that you have been to the hospital today to look for one of the nurses and the police have since arrested you. Can we have a chat?'			
Assess current behaviour	Can you tell me why you are under police custody at this moment? What is your relationship with the nurse? What have you done to her thus far? Do you know her name? How do you feel towards her?	How much do you know about her? Do you know her number? If you do, how often do you call upon her? Would you resort to leaving a voice message if she does not respond to your call? Do you mind telling me the contents of your voice message? Do you happen to know where she lives? How did you find this out?	Why do you need to take the above actions? Do you want to be close to her? From your view, how does your behaviour affect her daily life?

(Continued)

Risk assessment	Are you planning to do anything to the nurse? If so, would you mind telling me the details? Do you plan to harm her? If yes, what would you do? Is this part of your fantasy?	Have you ever applied force on her? What was her reaction? Did she defend herself? Will you do it again in the future?	Have you thought of harming yourself? (Or) Are you so stressed up with the current situation that you have had thoughts of ending your life? Has anyone tried to stop you from following her? If yes, what did you do? Do you carry a weapon? Will you use it to harm others who try to stop you?
Differentiation between types of stalker	Incompetent stalker: Did you encounter any difficulty having a relationship in the past? Does the nurse remind you of the unpleasant past? Rejected stalker: When you are ignored or rejected by the nurse, how do you feel? Do you feel that both of you were in a relationship? Do you hope to reconcile by following her?	Intimacy seekers and erotomania Are you in love with her? Do you think she is in love with you? Do you think she will love you? How certain are you that she is in love with you? Could it be a misunderstanding? Do you have sexual feeling towards her? Resentful stalkers: Have you tried to frighten her? Are you taking revenge on her?	You have followed her a lot. Do you feel stressed? Do you want to continue this behaviour? Have you thought of changing yourself? Do you think you need treatment?
Forensic and psychiatric history	Did you have trouble with the police in the past? If yes, what was the reason? Were you charged subsequently? Did you break any court order in the past? Have you seen a psychiatrist in the past?	How often do you drink? What kind of alcohol do you drink? What would you do if you were drunk? Do you also use any recreational drugs?	

Common pitfalls

a. Failure to cover the range and depth of the information required for this station

Quick recall*

- In this condition, the person holds the delusional belief that someone, usually of a higher social or professional status or a famous personality or in some other way 'unattainable', is in love with him or her. The patient may make repeated attempts to contact that other person.
- Eventually, rejections may lead to animosity and bitterness on the part of the patient towards the object of attention.
- In hospital and outpatient clinical psychiatry, patients are more likely to be female than male, whereas in forensic psychiatry, male patients are commoner.
- Overall, females outnumber males.

Overview of delusional disorder

- According to *International Statistical Classification of Diseases and Related Health Problems,*10th revision (*ICD-10*), a delusional disorder is an ill-defined condition, manifesting as a single delusion or a set of related delusions, being persistent, sometimes lifelong and not having an identifiable organic basis.
- There are occasional or transitory auditory hallucinations, particularly in the elderly.
- Delusions are the most conspicuous or only symptoms and are present for at least 3 months. For the diagnosis, there must be no evidence of schizophrenic symptoms or brain disease.
- *ICD-10* includes the previously used term 'late paraphrenia', although there is some evidence that there are differences between persistent delusional disorder and late paraphrenia.
- Magnetic resonance imaging (MRI) scans in a group of late-onset schizophrenics and late-onset delusional disorders showed that the lateral ventricle volumes in the delusional disorder patients were much greater than those of schizophrenics and almost twice those of controls.
- Mono-delusional disorders feature a stable, encapsulated delusional system, which takes over much of a person's life. The personality is preserved.
- There is a point prevalence of 0.03% and a lifetime risk of 0.05%–0.1%.
- The mean age of onset is 35 years for males and 45 years for females.
- Onset is usually gradual and unremitting in 62%.
- Equal sex ratio of sufferers.
- Sufferers are often unmarried, with high marital breakdown and low reproductive rates.
- Introverted, long-standing interpersonal difficulties might predispose individuals towards delusional disorder.
- Family history of psychiatric disorder but not that of delusional disorder or schizophrenia is a predisposing factor.
- There is evidence of minimal brain disorder in 16% of the patients.

---

* Adapted from B.K. Puri, A. Hall and R. Ho (2014). *Revision Notes in Psychiatry.* London, UK: CRC Press, p. 370.

STATION 130: EROTOMANIA AND STALKING (DISCUSSION)

Information to candidates

Name of patient: Sarah

You have been tasked to speak to the nurse, Sarah. She understands that you have since assessed the patient (who is the one who turned up to look for her). She wants to find out more information. She wants to know the risks involved and what she ought to do.

Task

Please speak to Sarah and explain to her the current situation. In addition, please inform her about the relevant risks involved and address all her concerns and expectations.

Outline of station

You are a senior nurse working in the emergency department of a local hospital. You were told by the management that there was a man who turned up at the emergency department today, and requested to speak to you. He claimed that you knew him. You have treated many patients over the course of the past few weeks and have no recollection of who this patient is. You were told by the management that the patient has informed them that he strongly wishes to see you as he believes that you're in love with him. You were told that when he was prevented from seeing you, he wielded a knife at the security staff. The police were called in, and he was subsequently arrested. You understand that the psychiatrist has since seen him. However, you also learned from the management and the police that he was subsequently released by mistake and is currently in the community. You're very worried about the associated risks. You wish to know what precautions you ought to be taking.

CASC construct table

The CASC construct table is formatted such that candidates will be able to cover adequately both the range and the depth of the assessment required in this station.

Starting off: 'Hello, I am Dr Melvyn. I understand that you have heard about what happened this morning. I understand that you do have some concerns. Can we have a chat?'

Explain assessment	I understand that it must have been very distressing for you. I assessed the patient before he was released. I hope I can share my assessment. I hear your concerns about you not knowing him. I have spoken to him at length, and based on the information that he has shared, I have to break confidentiality and share some of my assessment with you.	He did share with me that he received treatment from you a few weeks ago, when he was in the observation ward for panic symptoms. From that particular meeting with you, he strongly believes that you're in love with him. I do understand that you would have treated him just like any other patient.	During my assessment, I have attempted to challenge those beliefs that he has. These beliefs that he has are quite fixed and cannot be challenged. My assessment is that he might be suffering from a condition known as delusion of love or 'erotomania'. Have you heard of this before? This is a condition in which an individual has a firm belief that others are in love with them. The belief is typically firmly held and not challengeable.
Explain associated risks involved	I hear your concerns with regard to the fact that he is currently out in the community. I'm sorry to hear about this. I believe the police are doing their best to try to locate him based on the information they have about him.	When I spoke to him, he did share with me some other information, which I think you do need to be aware of. I'm actually quite concerned about the risk he might pose to you. During the assessment, he did share that he actually knows where you stay and that he has your contact number. In addition, he claimed that there was an occasion in which he talked to you and followed you home.	Moreover, during the assessment, he also shared that he does have sexual fantasies about you, and he desires for intimacy with you. Is it alright for me to go on?
Address concerns – immediate plans for the nurse	I know you're deeply concerned about the risk he poses. We are also deeply concerned about your safety.	Given that he does know where you live and has your contact number, I do not advise that you head home for the time being. Do you have friends or family with whom you could potentially stay?	I will also inform the management about my assessment briefly and advise them that they allow you to go on a short period of leave, as it would be dangerous for you to return back to work currently.

(Continued)

		Thanks for sharing with me your alternative accommodation plans. I understand you are quite concerned about leaving the hospital and getting to your accommodation. We will speak to the management as well as the police, who could potentially provide you with some assistance in the meantime.	Do these plans sound reasonable for you? Are there other concerns that you have at the moment?
Address concerns – management plans for the patient	We will advise the police to continue their search for him. If the police manage to find him, he is likely to be detained for further assessment.	Should there be a need, we might need to apply the Mental Health Act on him, to detain him for further assessment and treatment.	Please be assured that it is not likely that he will be detained in the hospital that you work in, in view of the current risks posed.
Provide reassurance	Thanks for speaking to me, and I hope that I have addressed all your concerns and expectations.	I know that you are deeply troubled by the current situation, but we will work jointly with you, the management and the police to ensure your safety.	Do you have any other concerns that you would like to raise?

Common pitfalls

a. Failure to cover the range and depth of the information required for this station

Quick recall

Please refer to the first part of this paired station for further information.

STATION 131: VIOLENCE RISK ASSESSMENT (PAIRED STATION A: MSE EVALUATION)

Information to candidates

Name of patient: Christopher

You have been tasked to speak to a 32-year-old male, Christopher. He was arrested by the police and transferred to the emergency department for further evaluation.

He was arrested because he broke into the house of his ex-girlfriend. He has a known history of schizophrenia and was released from the prison 8 months ago.

Task

Please speak to him and perform a mental state examination. Please also attempt to perform a comprehensive risk assessment.

Outline of station

You are Christopher and have just been arrested by the police. You were caught for breaking into the house of your ex-girlfriend. You were released from prison around 8 months ago. You were previously arrested and convicted for housebreaking as well. Since your release, you have not been taking the medications that were prescribed for you whilst you were in prison. Recently, you started to experience auditory hallucinations as well as paranoia. You decided to break into your ex-girlfriend's house as you believe that she is part of this plot in which others are against you.

CASC construct table

The CASC construct table is formatted such that candidates will be able to cover adequately both the range and the depth of the assessment required in this station.

Starting off: 'Hello, I am Dr Melvyn. I understand that you have just been arrested by the police. Can we have a chat so that I can understand how best I can help you?'			
Explore circumstances of current offence	I received some limited information from the police with regard to what has happened today. Would you be able to tell me more?	Thanks for sharing. Did you make any plans prior to your current attempt? What plans did you make? Can you tell me how you managed to break into the house? What intentions did you have?	Did you drink any alcohol before your attempt? Did you use any substance before your current act?
Explore MSE – delusions	Can you tell me more about why you feel this way? Can there be any other alternative explanations for this?	Do you feel that other people are trying to harm you in any way? Do you feel that other people are talking about you?	Do you feel that you have some special powers or abilities? Do you feel that certain things have special meaning for you?

(Continued)

Explore MSE – hallucinations	Auditory hallucinations: Do you hear sounds or voices that others do not hear?	Second person auditory hallucinations: Do they speak directly to you? Can you give me some examples of what they have been saying to you?	How do you feel when you hear them?
	How many voices can you hear? Are they as clear as our current conversation? What do they say?	Third person auditory hallucinations: Do they refer to you as 'he' or 'she', in the third person? Do they comment on your actions? Do they give you orders or commands as to what to do? Are you able to resist them?	Can there be any alternative explanation for these experiences that you have been having?
Explore MSE – thought disorders	Thought interference: Do you feel that your thoughts are being interfered with? Who do you think is doing this?	Thought insertion: Do you have thoughts in your head that you feel are not your own? Where do you think these thoughts come from?	Thought broadcasting: Do you feel that your thoughts are being broadcasted, such that others would know what you are thinking? Thought withdrawal: Do you feel that your thoughts are being taken away from your head by some external force?
Explore MSE – passivity experiences	Do you feel in control of your own actions and emotions?	Do you feel that someone or something is trying to control you?	Who or what do you think this would be?
Risk assessment and insight	With all these troubling experiences, have you thought of ending your life?	Have you thought of taking revenge on the people you think are troubling you?	Can you share with me your plans (should you have any)? Do you have access to any weapons?
Personal history	I understand that you have previously seen a psychiatrist. Do you know what diagnosis the psychiatrist has given you? Do you know the rationale for you to be on medications? Do you have family members who have mental health–related issues as well?	Do you drink? If you do drink, how often do you drink and how much? Do you use any illicit substances?	Have you been involved with the police before? Can you tell me more? Have you ever stalked anyone before? Thanks for speaking to me today.

Common pitfalls

a. Failure to cover the range and depth of the information required for this station

Quick recall*

Violence in patients with schizophrenia

- Violence in people with schizophrenia is uncommon, but they do have a higher risk than the general population.
- Prevalence of recent aggressive behaviour amongst outpatients with schizophrenia is 5%.
- The types of violence and aggression are classified as follows: verbal aggression (45%), physical violence towards objects (30%), violence towards others (20%) and self-directed violence (10%). Family members are involved in 50% of the assaults, with strangers being attacked in about 20%.
- Psychiatrists need to be competent in identifying patients at risk and protecting both patients and others.

Dangerousness

- The best predictor of future dangerous behaviour is the individual's past behaviour.
- Shorter-term prediction is better than long-term prediction.
- Dangerousness is associated with the availability of weapons, morbid jealousy and the sadistic murder syndrome.
- Schizophrenic patients usually assault a known person, but if they assault a stranger, the arresting police officer is the most common target.
- The delusional ideas often motivate the violent behaviours, and the patients usually admit experiencing command hallucinations after the violent offenses.
- Schizophrenic patients with negative symptoms commit violent offenses inadvertently and neglectfully.
- In clinical practice, psychiatrists should be aware that schizophrenic patients may display persistence of their normal selves, especially patients without history of violence.

The following are crucial in a forensic psychiatric assessment:

- Obtaining a full history and mental state of the patient, including fantasies and impulses to offend
- Objective account of the offense, from arresting police officer or from statement in Crown Court cases.
- Objective accounts of past offenses, if any, such as to obtain a list of previous convictions

---

* Adapted from B.K. Puri, A. Hall and R. Ho (2014). *Revision Notes in Psychiatry*. London, UK: CRC Press, p. 368.

- Additional information gathering, such as interviews with informants (relatives), or reading a social inquiry report from a probation officer
- Review of previous psychiatric records, such as to ascertain relationship of mental disorder to previous behaviour and to psychiatric treatment and the need for security

STATION 132: VIOLENCE RISK ASSESSMENT (PAIRED STATION B: DISCUSSION AND MANAGEMENT)

Information to candidates

Name of Patient: Dr Richard

You have been tasked to speak to the consultant, Dr Richard, about the case that you have just assessed.

Task

Please speak to the consultant and discuss the management plans for this case.

Outline of station

You are the consultant psychiatrist in charge of the inpatient unit. The nurse manager has informed you about this case, and you are aware that the core trainee has done the necessary assessment. You wish to find out more information from the core trainee and determine whether the patient requires further inpatient management.

CASC construct table

The CASC construct table is formatted such that candidates will be able to cover adequately both the range and the depth of the assessment required in this station.

Starting off: 'Hello, I am Dr Melvyn. I would like to discuss with you the case which I have just assessed in the emergency department'.			
Explain events leading to admission	Based on the history shared by the patient, he claimed that he planned for the housebreaking today. He claimed that his thoughts were no longer within his control, and he suspects his ex-girlfriend is involved in a plot to harm him.	He wanted to break into the house to get back his belongings, as well as to leave a message to threaten the victim. He denied harbouring any homicidal ideations of harming others.	He was arrested today for housebreaking as he was spotted by passers-by.

(Continued)

Summarize mental state observation	I have briefly also assessed his mental state.	In addition, for the past month, he reports that he has been increasingly bothered by auditory hallucinations.	He has quite limited insight into his existing mental health condition. He recalls that he has been diagnosed with schizophrenia and has been on medications whilst he was previously convicted.
	He has overt paranoid ideations towards others, as he has been thinking that others around him are intending to harm him.	He also reports that he does not feel in control of his actions.	He claimed that he has since recovered from his previous episode of schizophrenia. He mentions that he is no longer keen to be on medications.
Discuss risk assessment	I have done a risk assessment as well, in view of the current circumstances leading up to admission.	The patient denies harbouring ideations to harm others. In addition, he denies harbouring any ideations to harm himself. Also, he was not intoxicated nor was he using any drugs when he attempted the housebreaking.	However, he was recently released from prison for a similar offence. He has no other history of any violent behaviours.
Explain management approach	Given his poor insight and his current risk assessment, I would like to recommend that he be admitted for further stabilization in the inpatient unit.	There is a high risk of him not being compliant with the recommended treatment if we were to engage him as an outpatient. We could potentially reconsider the introduction of antipsychotics for him and consider other strategies to ensure his compliance.	When he is more settled inpatient and due for discharge, we could consider engaging him with the community psychiatric nurse to reinforce his compliance to medications as well as monitor his mental state.

Common pitfalls

a. Failure to cover the range and depth of the information required for this station

In this station, you will need to stratify the patient's risk of violence and highlight the risk factors. It would be impressive if you could also mention what are some of the questionnaire tools you can use to assess violence risk, e.g., HCR-20 and Psychopathy Checklist-Revised (PCL-R).

Quick recall*

Clinical risk assessment and risk management planning:

- The aim is to get an understanding of the risk from a detailed historical longitudinal overview, obtaining information not only from the patient, who may minimize his or her history, but also from informants. Ideally, it should not be a one-off single-interview assessment.
- Reconstruct in detail what happened at the time of offense or behaviour causing concern.
- Independent information from statements of victims or witnesses or police records should be obtained when available. Do not rely on what the offender tells you or the legal offense category – for example, arson may be of a wastepaper bin in a busy ward or with the intent to kill. Possession of an offensive weapon may have been prelude to homicide.
- Offense = offender × victim × circumstance/environment.
- Also consider protective factors. Practical risk assessment (history, mental state and environment) can be supplemented by standardized instruments of risk, including actuarial risk instruments based on static risk factors, such as the VRAG, and dynamic risk instruments, such as the HCR-20, based on factors that can be changed or be managed, for example, symptoms of mental illness and noncompliance.

Ultimately, in conclusion, the aim is to answer how serious the risk is (the nature and magnitude): Is it specific or general, conditional or unconditional, immediate, long term or volatile? Have the individuals or situational risk factors changed? Who might be at risk?

For a risk assessment, a risk management plan should be developed to modify the risk factors and specify the response triggers. This should ideally be agreed upon with the individual. Is there a need for more frequent follow-up appointments, an urgent care program approach meeting or admission to the hospital, detention under the Mental Health Act, physical security, observation or medication? If the optimum plan cannot be undertaken, reasons for this should be documented and a backup plan specified.

Risk assessments and risk management plans should be communicated to others on a 'need to know' basis. On occasions, patient confidentiality will need to be breached if there is immediate grave danger to others. The police can often do little unless there is specific threat to an individual, whereupon they may warn or charge the subject. Very careful consideration needs to be given before informing potential victims to avoid their unnecessary anxiety. Their safety is often best ensured by the management of those at risk.

---

* Adapted from B.K. Puri, A. Hall and R. Ho (2014). *Revision Notes in Psychiatry.* London, UK: CRC Press, p. 724.

STATION 133: SEXUAL OFFENCE ASSESSMENT

Information to candidates

Name of patient: Mr Brown

You have been tasked to assess Mr Brown. He was brought in by the police for an assessment, as there is an allegation that he has been sexually inappropriate with a child. The police are awaiting your assessment before they proceed with the necessary charges against him.

Task

Please speak to Mr Brown and explore more about the circumstances of the alleged offence. Please take an appropriate history to come to a diagnosis.

Outline of station

You are Mr Brown and have just been arrested for an alleged sexual offence. You know that you are due to see the psychiatrist for an assessment. You are aware that your neighbour has called upon the police with regard to the alleged offence. You do know the victim and have been taking care of the victim on several occasions. When questioned about the alleged offence, all you will share is that you were playing a game with the victim, and he accidentally brushed himself against your groin area. You will be cooperative otherwise and will share more about your psychosexual history. You are married, but you are not in a good relationship with your wife. Otherwise, you will deny any interest in pornography and other sex materials. You have received a previous warning for a similar offence.

CASC construct table

The CASC construct table is formatted such that candidates will be able to cover adequately both the range and the depth of the assessment required in this station.

Starting off: 'Hello, I am Dr Melvyn. I'm sorry to hear that the police have arrested you today. Can we have a chat about it?'			
Elicit circumstances leading to current arrest	I'm sorry to hear that you have been arrested by the police. Are you aware of the reasons for the current arrest? Given the nature of the current allegations, I do need to ask you some personal questions. Would that be alright with you?	Can you describe to me what actually happened today? Can you tell me more about your relationship with the victim? How long have you known him or her for? Can you share with me more about how frequent you have cared for the child?	Would you mind telling me more about where you were when the incident happened? Was there anyone else present at that moment? I received news that the allegation involved you being intimate with the child. Can you tell me more?

(Continued)

Explore patient's view about alleged offence	Thanks for sharing with me the account of what has happened. You mentioned that the child brushed against you. What happened after that?	Did you get sexually aroused when that happened? I'm sorry but I do need to ask you some personal questions. Did you feel sexually aroused when that happened today? If you did, what did you do thereafter? Did you have an erection? Did you masturbate thereafter?	Given the current allegation made against you, how do you feel currently about all that has happened today? Very often, we do come across news about sexual offenders. What is your view on that?
Explore psychosexual history	Are you currently in any relationship? Can I know how long you have been married? Can you tell me more about how your relationship with your wife has been? I'm sorry to hear that you have been having some difficulties with your relationship currently.	Before being married, were you in any other relationships? Can you tell me more about those past relationships? Do you remember at what age you achieved puberty? Do you remember at what age you had your first masturbation? Would you mind sharing with me more about your intimacy? At what age did you first have an intimate experience with a partner?	Sometimes, when people are having difficulties with the sexual side of their relationship, they turn to other materials to fulfil their needs. Do you watch any pornography to satisfy your desires? Can you tell me more? Have you ever engaged in any other behaviour to achieve sexual arousal? Do you find yourself particularly attracted to children?
Explore psychiatric and forensic history	Have you seen a psychiatrist before? Is there any history of any mental health disorders in your family?	Have you been involved with the police or the legal system before? Can you please tell me more?	For the previous offence, what was the charge? Can you share with me what happened thereafter? Currently are you in contact with any children?
Explore substance usage	Have you used any drugs before?	What about alcohol? How often do you use alcohol?	Thanks for sharing with me.

Common pitfalls

a. Failure to cover the range and depth of the information required for this station

**It is important to remain empathic towards the patient and not appear judgemental.

**It is important to assess any other risk that the patient may have (e.g., current contact with children, as there may be other victims).

Quick recall*

- Definition: It is defined as the sexual preference for children, usually prepubertal or pubertal. Some are attracted to either one or both sexes.
- The overall prevalence is less than 3%. More than 90% of those diagnosed are men, and it is rare in women; 95% of them are heterosexual; 50% of them consumed alcohol at the time of the offence.
- Clinical features: Included in this diagnosis are men who retain a preference for adult sex partners, but when frustrated in their efforts turn to children as substitutes. They may have previously committed exhibitionism and other sexual offences. They tend to have low self-esteem and feel more accepted by young children.
- The *ICD-10* specifies that the individual is at least 16 years old and at least 5 years older than the child victim.
- The proposed *Diagnostic and Statistical Manual of Mental Disorders,*5th edition (*DSM-5*) criteria specify minimum 6-month duration, and the individual is at least 18 years old and at least 5 years older than the child victim. There are three subtypes:
  - Classic type: sexually attracted to prepubescent children
  - Hebephilic type: sexually attracted to early pubescent children
  - Paedohebephilic type: sexually attracted to both groups of young people
- In particular, adolescent offenders have been noted to have better prognosis compared with older offenders.
- The mentally immature offender with poor social skills may prefer child sexual partners because they are the only people with whom the person can relate at a general level.
- The persistent middle-aged offender often has evidence of personality problems with poor relationships and unstable work patterns. These offenders usually have low rather than high sex drives. There is often an emotional bond between them and their child victims.
- Some offenders are more dangerous compared with those described earlier. These offenders usually have evidence of a serious personality disturbance affecting more aspects of his or her life than the choice of a sexual outlet.
- Killing a child as part of a sexual offence is rare. It usually results from a state of panic and a desire to dispose of the evidence.

Treatment options for antisocial sexual behaviour:

- In a critical review of the existing literature, it has been concluded that treatment programs have been effective with paedophiles.
- In examining the value of the various treatment approaches, they concluded that comprehensive CBTs were most likely to be effective. There was also a

---

* Adapted from B.K. Puri, A. Hall and R. Ho (2014). *Revision Notes in Psychiatry.* London, UK: CRC Press, p. 724.

clear value in the use of anti-androgens in those offenders who engage in excessively high rates of sexual activity.

- More information about the 'Sex offender treatment program (SOTP)': It aims at increasing the responsibility and motivation of the sexual offender to change. SOTP involves anger management, CBT, relationship skill training, relapse prevention, sex education, social skill training, stress management and thinking skill program. Sex offenders are encouraged to develop victim empathy by understanding the consequences of their actions and minimize denials. Behaviour treatments include aversion, sensitization and biofeedback with penile plethysmography that measures the penile blood flow with thoughts of illegal sexual practices.

Pharmacological treatment

- The aim of pharmacological treatment is to reduce sexual drives and prevent future sexual offences especially in sex offenders who fail to respond to SOTP.
- Baseline investigations include FBC, LFT, RFT and glucose.
- Hormonal investigations include LH, FSH and serum testosterone.
- Baseline weight and blood pressure.
- Subsequent monitoring after initiation of treatment includes weight and blood pressure during each visit, monthly testosterone for the first 4 months and every 6 months afterward, LFT, RFT and prolactin every 6 months and bone scan for patients being prescribed with leuprolide.
- Selective serotonin reuptake inhibitor (SSRI): commonly prescribed with fewer side effects; no consent is required, but consent is required for the drugs described below.
- Cyproterone is a testosterone antagonist. The range dose is between 100 and 500 mg/day (oral) or 100 and 600 mg/week (intramuscular injection). Cyproterone is contraindicated in patients with chronic liver diseases and thromboembolic diseases. Side effects include depression, fatigue, gynaecomastia and weight gain.
- Medroxyprogesterone provides negative feedback to the production of FSH and LH and reduces testosterone production. The range of dose is between 100 and 600 mg/day (oral) or 100 and 700 mg/week (intramuscular). It is contraindicated in patients suffering from chronic liver diseases and thromboembolic disorders. Side effects include anxiety, depression, excessive sweating, fatigue, hypertension, insomnia, oedema and weight gain.
- Leuprolide is a GnRH analogue that controls the release of LH and FSH and subsequently reduces the testosterone production. The intramuscular dose is between 3.75 and 7.5 mg/month IM or 11.5 and 22.5 mg every 3 months. Leuprolide is contraindicated in patients suffering from osteopenia. Side effects include excessive sweating, hot flushes, myalgia, oedema and osteopenia.
- Finasteride is a 5 alpha reductase inhibitor and reduces sexual drive by inhibiting the peripheral conversion of testosterone to dihydrotestosterone.

STATION 134: FITNESS TO PLEAD ASSESSMENT

Information to candidates

Name of patient: Mr Thomas

You have been tasked to speak to Mr Thomas. He was just arrested by the police following a shop theft at the local store. Whilst he was in the remand cell, he vocalized to the police officers that he has been on regular follow-up with the local mental health service and has been on psychotropic medications.

Task

Please speak to Mr Thomas and explore more about the circumstances leading to the current offence. Please perform a brief mental state examination and assess whether he is currently fit to plead.

Outline of station

You are Mr Thomas. You have been arrested for your involvement in a shop theft. You told the police that you have been on regular psychotropic medications and have been on regular follow-up with the local mental health service. They have since referred you for further assessment. You do have residual auditory hallucinations, but otherwise, you do not have any first-rank symptoms. You carefully planned for the current offence by making sure that you stored items in an area that was not covered by the CCTV. You do understand the current charges pressed against you and do understand the differences between pleading guilty and not guilty. You have a basic understanding of the court proceedings, as you have been to the court just 6 months ago for the same offence.

CASC construct table

The CASC construct table is formatted such that candidates will be able to cover adequately both the range and the depth of the assessment required in this station.

Starting off: 'Hello, I am Dr Melvyn. I'm sorry to hear that the police have arrested you today. Can we have a chat about it?'			
Explore circumstances leading to current arrest			
Explore MSE – delusions	Can you tell me more as to why you feel this way? Could there be any other alternative explanations for this?	Do you feel that other people are trying to harm you in any way? Do you feel that other people are talking about you?	Do you feel that you have some special powers or abilities? Do you feel that certain things have special meaning for you?

(Continued)

Explore MSE – hallucinations	Auditory hallucinations: Do you hear sounds or voices that others do not hear? How many voices can you hear? Are they as clear as our current conversation? What do they say?	Second person auditory hallucinations: Do they speak directly to you? Can you give me some examples of what they have been saying to you? Third person auditory hallucinations: Do they refer to you as 'he' or 'she', in the third person? Do they comment on your actions? Do they give you orders or commands as to what to do?	How do you feel when you hear them? Could there be any alternative explanation for these experiences that you have been having?
Explore MSE – thought disorders	Thought interference: Do you feel that your thoughts are being interfered with? Who do you think is doing this?	Thought insertion: Do you have thoughts in your head that you feel are not your own? Where do you think these thoughts come from?	Thought broadcasting: Do you feel that your thoughts are being broadcasted, such that others would know what you are thinking? Thought withdrawal: Do you feel that your thoughts are being taken away from your head by some external force?
Explore MSE – passivity experiences	Do you feel in control of your own actions and emotions?	Do you feel that someone or something is trying to control you?	Who or what do you think this would be?
Explore fitness to plead	Can you tell me more about what the police are intending to charge you for? What do you think are the possible consequences for such an offence?	Can you tell me your understanding with regard to 'pleading guilty'? Can you tell me your understanding with regard to 'pleading not guilty'?	Have you been in court before? Do you know who the people are who will be there? Can you tell me more? Do you know the process of the court hearing? Do you have a legal counsel who is representing you? Do you know how to instruct the lawyer to represent you? Thanks for sharing with me.

Common pitfalls

a. Failure to cover the range and depth of the information required for this station

Quick recall*

Assessment of fitness to plead

- Understanding of the charge and its implications (Do you understand what the police say you have done wrong?)
- Understanding and appreciating the importance of entering a plea (Do you know the difference between saying guilty and not guilty?)
- Ability to instruct counsel (Can you tell your solicitor your side of the story?)
- Ability to challenge the juror (Do you know what it means if they say you can object to some of the members of the jury in your case?)
- Ability to challenge a witness (If you disagree with what a witness is saying in court, what can you do about it?)
- Ability to follow the course of the trial and understand the evidence (Will you be able to follow the procedures in the court?)
- There are instruments to assess fitness to stand trial, such as the following:
  - Fitness interview test – revised: a reliable and sensitive semi-structured instrument to screen for fitness to stand trial
  - The Nussbaum Fitness Questionnaire: a 19-item self-report measure focusing on legal issues typically addressed during fitness interviews
- Mental state at the time of the offense is irrelevant to the fitness to plead.
- Although the prevalence of mental illness is high amongst the defendants, the number of cases found unfit to plead and given a restriction order is less than 50% in the United Kingdom.
- Rates of mental illness are higher in remanded prisoners compared with sentenced prisoners as ill offenders are often diverted. Amongst those on remand, female prisoners show more behavioural disorder than male prisoners.

Some important concepts in forensic psychiatry

- McNaughton rules: In this defence, the offender is arguing that he or she is not guilty by reason of his or her insanity. The offender meets the rules if he or she fulfils the following criteria:
  - That by reason of such defect from disease of the mind, the person did not know the nature of the quality of his or her act.
  - The person did not know what he or she was doing was wrong.
  - If the person was suffering from a delusion, his or her actions would be judged by the relationship to the delusion; that is, if he or she believed his

---

* Adapted from B.K. Puri, A. Hall and R. Ho (2014). *Revision Notes in Psychiatry*. London, UK: CRC Press, p. 728.

or her life to be immediately threatened, then he or she would be justified in striking out, but not otherwise.

In the legal concepts, the term 'disease of the mind' is divided into two parts. 'Mind' refers to the mind for reasoning, memory and understanding and 'disease' refers to the organic/functional, permanent/temporary, treatable/not treatable and is internal.

- Diminished responsibility: In the case of a charge of murder, a defence of diminished responsibility may be brought in, whereupon it has to be shown that, at the time of the offense, the offender suffered from such abnormality of mind, whether caused from a condition of arrested or retarded development of mind or any inherent causes or induced by disease or injury, as substantially impaired mental responsibility for his or her act.

  Diminished responsibility is determined by the court (usually by the jury or by the judge if both the prosecution and defence agree on plea). Examples of diminished responsibility include killing a spouse in a state of depression. The abnormality of mind substantially impairs criminal responsibility of the person's acts. If a person is found to have diminished responsibility, it may imply that the court will return such a person to society earlier than a responsible offender.

- Automatism: Under the British law, automatism is a legal concept. Automatism is different from automatic behaviour, which is a clinical concept, and there is no relationship between these two terms. The defendant pleads that his or her behaviour was automatic at the time of the offense (that is, no guilty mind or no decision making). Automatism refers to the unconscious, involuntary, non-purposeful acts where the mind is not conscious of what the body is doing. There is a separation between the mind and the act. Sane automatism is a once-only event, resulting from external causes, for example, hypoglycaemia caused by insulin. Insane automatism is caused by diseases of the mind, such as mental illness or brain disease (intrinsic factors), for example, epilepsy, dissociative fugue states and sleepwalking and night terrors in slow-wave sleep. Insane automatism tends to recur. Voluntary intoxication by itself does not constitute a defence.

STATION 135: EXHIBITIONISM – PAIRED STATION A

Information to candidates

Name of patient: Jonathan

You have been tasked to assess Jonathan. He has been brought into the emergency room after he was arrested by the police for exposing himself in public.

Task

Please speak to Jonathan and obtain a history to establish a clinical diagnosis. His wife is here as well and has indicated her desire to speak to you in the next station.

Outline of station

You are Jonathan and have just been arrested by the police. The police have arrested you as your neighbour has lodged a police report after she witnessed you exposing yourself in the garden. You are angry at your neighbour for making the police report. You deny feeling any sexual arousal during the incident. You are willing to cooperate much later into the interview and will answer the questions posed by the psychiatrist accordingly.

CASC construct table

The CASC construct table is formatted such that candidates will be able to cover adequately both the range and the depth of the assessment required in this station.

Starting off: 'Hello, I am Dr Melvyn. I have received some information about what has happened. Can we have a chat about it?'			
Explore history of current presentation	Thanks for agreeing to speak to me. I have received some information about what has happened that led to your current situation. In order for me to help you, I would need to ask you some other questions. Would that be alright with you?	Can you tell me more details with regard to what has happened today? Can you tell me what you were doing when the incident took place?	Were you aware that your neighbour might be there? Has something similar to this happened before?
Explore patient's attitude towards current presentation	I'm sorry but I do have to ask you some personal questions. I hope you can answer them accordingly. How do you feel about this entire incident?	Due to the ongoing police investigations with regard to you having exposed yourself, I need to ask if you felt any pleasure/arousal when you exposed yourself?	In addition, did you have an erection during the incident?

(Continued)

Explore psychosexual and forensic history	Can you tell me more about your relationships? Are you currently married? How long have you been married for? Do you have children?	How is your relationship with your wife? Have there been any difficulties with your relationship with your wife? Have there been any difficulties with the sexual side of your relationship with your wife? Did you have any other relationships before you got married? Can you tell me more about those relationships? Do you remember the first time you were sexually active? Do you remember when you first maturbated?	Pardon me for asking, but I would like to understand whether you have been previously involved with the police? Can you tell me more about what happened previously? Did the police charge you for the offence? What happened after that?
Explore psychiatry history and current mental state	Can I check whether you have seen a psychiatrist before? Is there anyone in the family who has a history of mental health–related disorder? Do you use alcohol or any other substances? Can you tell me more?	Over the past month, how has your mood been for you? Do you find yourself losing interest in things that you previously used to enjoy? Are there any difficulties with your sleep or appetite? Have you had have any unusual experiences? By that I mean do you hear voices or see anything unusual when you are alone?	Do you feel that there are others out there who are trying to harm you? Do you feel in control of your thought processes? Do you feel in control of your emotions and actions?
Explore other possible diagnosis – cognitive decline and dementia	How has your memory been recently? Do you find yourself having difficulties remembering appointments or important tasks? Any accompanying physical symptoms (e.g., urinary incontinence, gait instability)? Any head injury/trauma?	Have others around you commented about your memory? How about others commenting about any change in your personality?	Do you find yourself having difficulties with your daily activities? Do you find yourself having difficulties with your finances? Is there anything else you wish to share with me? I understand that your wife is here and wishes to speak to me about your current condition. Would it be alright for me to speak to her?

Common pitfalls

a. Failure to cover the range and depth of the information required for this station

**In the case of an elderly patient, you need to assess whether there is any cognitive impairment that may affect his judgement and impulse control. In a younger person, you would want to rule out any organic brain syndrome.

**Differential diagnoses in this case include paraphilia, psychosis, dementia, organic brain syndrome and influence under substances.

Quick recall*

- Indecent exposure is an offence under the 1824 Vagrancy Act.
- Exhibitionism, the exposing of the genitals to the opposite sex, is characterized into the following two main groups:
  - Type I: inhibited young men of relatively normal personality and good character who struggle against the impulse but find it irresistible. They expose with a flaccid penis and do not masturbate. They expose to individuals, not seeking a particular response. The frequency of exposure is often related to other sexual stresses and anxieties, such as marital conflict or pregnancy in the spouse.
  - Type II: less inhibited, more sociopathic men. Individuals expose with erect penis in a state of excitement and may masturbate. Pleasure is obtained, and little guilt is shown. The person is more likely to expose to a group of women or girls and may return repeatedly to the same place. The person seeks a response from the victim, either shock or disgust. There are fewer attempts to resist the urge to expose. The behaviour is associated with other psychosexual disorders and other types of offences. Thus may lead to more serious mental illness.
- Eighty per cent do not reoffend if they are charged with a first offence. The chances of reconviction rises dramatically with the second offence. There is a small group of recidivists who persist, but these tend to reduce in their 40s. It is generally a harmless nonviolent offence, except in a minority who may progress to more violent offences.
- There is a good prognosis associated with being married, good social relationships and good work record.

* Adapted from B.K. Puri, A. Hall and R. Ho (2014). *Revision Notes in Psychiatry*. London, UK: CRC Press, p. 607.

STATION 136: EXHIBITIONISM – PAIRED STATION B

Information to candidates

Name of patient: Sarah

You have previously assessed Jonathan following his arrest by the police after he exposed himself in his garden. His wife is here, and she is keen to find out more from you with regard to your assessment. She has some concerns that she would like to clarify with you. In the previous station, her husband (Mr Jonathan) has consented for you to speak to her.

Task

Please speak to Sarah and address all her concerns and expectations.

Outline of station

You are Sarah and are very concerned about your husband's condition. You are concerned as this is not the first time this has happened. In the past year or so, this has happened at least thrice. There was another occasion last month when your husband nearly exposed himself in front of your grandchildren. You are very concerned about the safety of your grandchildren as they do come over regularly over the weekend. You are extremely worried about the confidentiality of the information shared and want the core trainee to reassure you that all the information shared will be confidential. You do not want your grandchildren to be taken away or your access to your children be restricted. If the core trainee explains that there are times in which confidentiality needs to be broken, you will appear to be extremely upset and low in your mood. You would like to understand from the core trainee what form of help might be available for your husband. You then share with the core trainee that you have been feeling low in your mood in view of your husband's condition. You do have most of the clinical symptoms of depression, and the core trainee needs to ask you about these symptoms in the consult.

CASC construct table

The CASC construct table is formatted such that candidates will be able to cover adequately both the range and the depth of the assessment required in this station.

Starting off: 'Hello, I am Dr Melvyn. I have just spoken to your husband. I understand that you have some concerns about his current condition and the situation that has happened today. Can we have a chat?'

Explain assessment	I'm sorry to learn of all that has happened to your husband today. I have seen him just now and done an assessment of his condition.	He denies that he has exposed himself intentionally. He denies any active psychiatric symptom currently.	However, I'd like to check with you more about his condition. Were you present when the incident took place? Can you tell me more about what happened? Have you noticed any recent changes in your husband? Has there been a change in his mood or his personality? How has his memory been?
Explore risks	Thanks for sharing with me. I understand that it has been a difficult time for you. Prior to the incident today, can I check whether your husband has been involved in similar incidents previously?	Can you tell me more? Do you remember how frequently these incidents happen?	Were the police involved? Did the police press charges against him?
Dealing with confidentiality	It seems to me that you have some information that you wish to share. The information that you share will be kept confidential and is important for us in helping your husband with his current condition.	I'm very concerned to hear that there was an episode in which your husband nearly exposed himself to your grandchildren. I'm sorry but this involves a risk to a third party, in this case, your grandchildren.	It is thus essential for me to break confidentiality given the nature of the information shared, as it would involve a risk to your grandchildren. We might need to inform the child protection services. I'm very sorry to be having to inform you about this.

(Continued)

Explain possible investigations, assessment and treatment	It sounds to me that your husband has been experiencing significant memory difficulties for the past year or so. One of my considerations for his current condition might be that of dementia.	I would need to speak to him again to gather more information. The information that you have provided me with regard to his memory difficulties is helpful as well.	We would also need to run some baseline blood investigations and probably also organize a baseline scan of his brain. This would help us in establishing the diagnosis. We might also recommend that he undergo further cognitive testing and maybe a neuropsychological battery of tests. If he does have dementia, there are a variety of options which we could recommend in terms of how best we could help him with his current condition.
Picking up on possible depressive symptoms in the carer	How have you been coping thus far? It seems to me that you are quite affected by all that has happened. How has your mood been for you?	Do you find yourself having interest in the things that you used to enjoy? How has your sleep been for you? What about your appetite?	Apart from this, are there other stressors in your life? Have you ever felt that life is hopeless and no longer worth living? I understand that you are in a difficult position currently in view of the ongoing issues involving your husband and the potential risks he poses to your grandchildren.

Common pitfalls

a. Failure to cover the range and depth of the information required for this station

Quick recall*

- Indecent exposure is an offence under the 1824 Vagrancy Act.
- Exhibitionism, the exposing of the genitals to the opposite sex, is characterized into the following two main groups:
  - Type I: inhibited young men of relatively normal personality and good character who struggle against the impulse but find it irresistible. They

---

* Adapted from B.K. Puri, A. Hall and R. Ho (2014). *Revision Notes in Psychiatry*. London, UK: CRC Press, p. 607.

expose with a flaccid penis and do not masturbate. They expose to individuals, not seeking a particular response. The frequency of exposure is often related to other sexual stresses and anxieties, such as marital conflict or pregnancy in the spouse.

- Type II: less inhibited, more sociopathic men. Individuals expose with erect penis in a state of excitement and may masturbate. Pleasure is obtained, and little guilt is shown. The person is more likely to expose to a group of women or girls and may return repeatedly to the same place. The person seeks a response from the victim, either shock or disgust. There are fewer attempts to resist the urge to expose. The behaviour is associated with other psychosexual disorders and other types of offences. These may lead to more serious mental illness.

- Eighty per cent do not reoffend if they are charged with a first offence. The chances of reconviction rise dramatically with the second offence. There is a small group of recidivists who persist, but these tend to reduce in number in their 40s. It is generally a harmless nonviolent offence, except in a minority who may progress to more violent offences.

- There is a good prognosis associated with being married, good social relationships and a good work record.

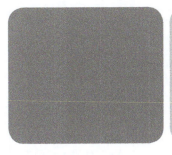

General Adult Psychiatry

STATION 137: SEASONAL AFFECTIVE DISORDER – HISTORY TAKING

Information to candidates

Name of patient: Victoria

You have been tasked to speak to Victoria. She has just returned from a holiday in Singapore a few weeks ago. She claims that the harsh weather in the United Kingdom has affected her mental health well-being.

Task

Please take a history of her symptoms to come to a diagnosis. You may wish to take notes as her husband wants to speak to you after you have assessed her.

CASC construct table

The CASC construct table is formatted such that candidates will be able to cover adequately both the range and the depth of the assessment required in this station.

Starting off: 'Hello, I am Dr Melvyn. Thanks for coming today. Can we have a brief chat to help me to understand you better?'			
Explore circumstances	I understand that you are here because you have been having some difficulties lately.	I'm sorry to be hearing that. Can you tell me more?	

(Continued)

---

* Stations 137 to 152 are entirely NEW stations which the authors have devised. These NEW stations are devised because very often during the original CASC examination, there might be variation from the original college station or the college might also introduce an entirely new station. The authors hope that these new stations will help candidates to prepare for the unexpected and not be taken aback during the examination when faced with an entirely new station.

Elicit core symptoms of depression	How has your mood been since the time you have been back to the United Kingdom? Have you found yourself losing interest in things which you used to enjoy previously?	How has your sleep been? Do you have any difficulties with sleep? Have you found yourself sleeping more than usual? What about your appetite? How has it been? Do you find your appetite better than usual? Do you tend to crave sugary/sweet food? What about your energy level? Do you find yourself having many difficulties in getting through a typical day?	How has your concentration been? Do you find yourself being able to concentrate on things which you used to enjoy? I'm sorry to hear that you find that your mood has been low. Sometimes when people are having low mood, it is not uncommon for them to have abnormal experiences as well. I wonder whether there are times in which you've been alone and have experienced any abnormal experiences. By that I mean hearing things which are not there or seeing things which are not there. Can I check whether you have felt this way before? Was there any association with the weather and seasonal changes? How often have you been feeling this way?
Risk assessment	I understand that it has been a difficult time for you. Do you feel guilty or responsible for anything? Do you feel as if you have committed a sin or done something very wrong?	What are your thoughts about the future? Have you had thoughts that your future is useless and no longer worth living?	Have you had thoughts that life is no longer worth living? When was the last time that you had such a thought? Do you still have those thoughts now? Have you made any plans to end your life?
Assessment of comorbid psychiatric disorders	Have there been times in which you feel that others around you are plotting against you?	Do you feel in control of your own thoughts? Do you feel in control of your own actions and emotions?	Have you used alcohol before? How often do you use? Do you use any other drugs?
Explore for significant personal history	Have you seen a psychiatrist before?	Is there anyone in the family who has any mental health conditions that I need to know of?	

Quick recall*

- Seasonal affective disorder (SAD) is a form of recurrent depressive disorder in which the sufferers consistently experience low mood in the winter months. Symptoms include increased appetite, craving for sugar or rice, low energy, increased sleep and weight gain.
- The prevalence of the disorder has been estimated to be 3% in Europe.
- Aetiology: melatonin and pineal gland abnormalities. Biologically vulnerable individuals are affected by the actual effect of the changes in the seasons and specific anniversary or environmental factors in winter.
- Clinical features: The clinical features of SAD are similar to that of atypical depression. These include hypersomnia, hyperphagia, tiredness and low mood in winter.
- *International Statistical Classification of Diseases and Related Health Problems (ICD) criteria:*
  1. Three or more episodes of mood disorder must occur with onset within the same 90-day period of the year for 3 or more consecutive days.
  2. Remission also occurs within a particular 90-day period of the year.
  3. Seasonal episodes substantially outnumber any non-seasonal episodes that may occur.

STATION 138: SEASONAL AFFECTIVE DISORDER – EXPLANATION AND MANAGEMENT

Information to candidates

Name of patient: Mr Brown

You have been tasked to speak to her husband, Mr Brown. You have assessed his wife in the previous station. He wants to know more about your assessment and the proposed treatment for his wife.

Task

Please speak to him about the diagnosis and the appropriate treatment. Please also address any concerns that he might have.

CASC construct table

The CASC construct table is formatted such that candidates will be able to cover adequately both the range and the depth of the assessment required in this station.

---

* Adapted from B.K. Puri, A. Hall and R. Ho (2014). *Revision Notes in Psychiatry.* London, UK: CRC Press, pp. 380, 381.

Starting off: 'Hello, I am Dr Melvyn. I understand that you have some concerns about your wife's condition. Can we have a chat?'			
Explain diagnosis	I have seen your wife previously, and she has granted me consent to speak to you about her condition. I understand that you are very concerned about her condition. Is there anything in particular that you wish to share about how she has been?	Thanks for sharing. I'm sorry to hear that it has definitely been a very difficult time for you and your family. It seemed to us that she might be having an episode of seasonal affective disorder (SAD). Have you heard of this before?	SAD is actually a form of depression. It comes and goes, and usually individuals experience low mood in the winter months. Their mood improves thereafter. Some of the symptoms of this disorder are like what you have shared with me.
Explain differences between SAD and depression	In depression, for most individuals, their mood is low, and they also experience a reduction in their interest.	Associated with the low mood, individuals might have difficulties with sleep and also experience a reduction in their appetite.	Unlike seasonal depressive disorder, individuals with SAD usually experience increased lethargy and have an increased need for sleep and tend to over eat.
Explain possible aetiological causes	No one knows the precise cause of the condition thus far.	There are some suggestions that there might be hormonal changes that are responsible for the mood symptoms.	
Discuss management	With regard to management, we could try medications and other approaches. There are some medications that we could consider to help her cope with her symptoms.	There are some of our patients who have benefited from an alternative therapy, which is light therapy. There has been a significant amount of evidence demonstrating the efficacy of light therapy.	At times, other forms of therapy might be indicated as well. These might include psychotherapy or talking therapy. Have you heard of these before? Very commonly, we do refer our patients to receive psychotherapy and, in particular, cognitive behavioural therapy (CBT).
Explore concerns	I know that I have provided you with quite a lot of information.	Do you have any questions for me?	

Quick recall*

- In SAD, there is a regular temporal relationship between the onset of depressive episodes and a particular time of the year.

---

* Adapted from B.K. Puri, A. Hall and R. Ho (2014). *Revision Notes in Psychiatry*. London, UK: CRC Press, p. 381

- Depressive episodes commence in autumn or winter months and end in spring or summer months as the hours of daylight increase.
- The onset of bipolar disorders may be seasonal as well.

STATION 139: DEPOT MEDICATIONS

Information to candidates

Name of patient: Mr Anderson

Mr Anderson suffers from chronic schizophrenia. However, he is poorly compliant with oral medication and has relapsed again, believing that 'agents' from the 'matrix' are out to get him. Your consultant has decided to start him on an intramuscular depot medication. His wife is here and is very concerned to be hearing this. She wants to know more from you.

Task

Please speak to the wife of Mr Anderson and address all her concerns and expectations.

CASC construct table

The CASC construct table is formatted such that candidates will be able to cover adequately both the range and the depth of the assessment required in this station.

Starting off: 'Hello, I am Dr Melvyn. I understand that you have some concerns about your husband's condition. Can we have a chat?'			
Explain medication and rationale for commencement	I understand that you have some concerns about your husband's condition. I hope that we can make use of this session to clarify your doubts about his condition. Do you know the reasons your husband has been admitted to the inpatient unit?	The team noted that your husband has not been compliant with the oral antipsychotic medications that we have prescribed to him as an outpatient. For his condition (psychosis), it is of utmost importance for patients to be compliant with their medications. There is a high chance of relapse if they are not compliant with their medications. To this end, we have noted that your husband has had a total of three admissions this year, and they were all due to him not being concordant with his medications.	Thus, we have made the recommendation that he be commenced on an intramuscular medication. This medication will be slowly released into his body over weeks, and hence, it will lessen the chances of him needing an admission if he is not going to be concordant with the oral medications that we have prescribed for him. We hope that with the introduction of this medication, his condition will be more stable, and our community psychiatric nurse can monitor him in the outpatient setting.

(Continued)

Explain administration methodology	As your husband will be starting out on the medication for the first time, what usually happens is that we would administer a test dose of the medication to him. This medication is usually given in the muscular areas of the body.	It could be given on the upper arms or in the buttock region. It would be administered by our nurses in a private room.	If there are not side effects from the test dose of the medication administered, we will proceed to administer the medication periodically. Typically, we will require our patients to receive the dose of the medication once every 4 weeks. The time for the next administration of the medication usually also depends on which particular antipsychotic your husband is given.
Explain potential benefits	The benefits of using an intramuscular depot for patients are that it would help to prevent relapse due to non-concordance with medications. As the depot medication is given usually once per month, it is easier for patients to receive it, compared with the need to remember to take their oral medications on a daily basis.	The depot medications would bring about the same benefits as that of the oral medications. It would help in the control of positive symptoms or the abnormal experiences that your husband used to be facing.	In the longer term, we hope that the depot medication could bring about better stability in your husband's condition. With better stability, we hope that he would then be better able to enjoy a better quality of life.
Explain potential adverse effects	The side effects associated with the depot medications are largely similar to that of the oral medications. They have the same tendency to cause extra-pyramidal side effects. Have you heard of those before? Can I take some time to explain to you if you have not heard of them before?	Other common adverse effects might include pain at the site of administration. Some patients do also complain of increasing anxiety.. Some patients do also complain of marked sedation after they receive their dose of depot medication.	

Quick recall*

- Between 5% and 25% of schizophrenics are unresponsive to conventional neuroleptics.
- Five to ten per cent are intolerant owing to adverse neurological side effects.
- Forty to sixty per cent of schizophrenics are noncompliant with oral medications. Possible reasons are as follows:
  - Limited insight into the disease
  - Limited beneficial effect
  - Unpleasant side effects
  - Pressure from family and friends
  - Poor communication with the medical team
- Depot neuroleptics increase compliance and reduce relapse rates.
- Continuous therapy is superior to intermittent treatment. It results in fewer relapses and a lower overall dose of neuroleptics.
- Of those who stop medication, 60%–70% relapse within a year, and 85% relapse within 2 years, compared with 10%–30% of those who continue on active medication.
- Schizophrenia patients are often non-adherent to antipsychotics. The National Institute for Health and Care Excellence (NICE) guidelines recommend the following interventions to enhance adherence:
  - Improve communication: Adapt the communication style to suit the patient's needs.
  - Increase the patient's involvement: The analysis of risks and benefits will help the patient to make the decision.
  - Understand the patient's perspective: Explore about general or specific concerns.
  - Determine the type of non-adherence: intentional or unintentional.
  - Provide information: Provide further information in the form of a leaflet.
  - Monitor adherence in a non-judgemental way: The psychiatrist should explain why he or she is interested in patient's adherence and let the patient understand his or her good intention.
  - There should be further intervention to increase adherence.

STATION 140: SECTIONING – ASSESSMENT

Information to candidates

Name of patient: Mr Templar

You have been tasked to speak to Mr Templar. He turned up at the hospital and demanded to see a nurse with whom he claimed to be in a relationship. When

* Adapted from B.K. Puri, A. Hall and R. Ho (2014). *Revision Notes in Psychiatry*. London, UK: CRC Press, p. 365.

his demand was refused, he waved a knife and was arrested by the police. He was admitted under the Mental Health Act, and you have been asked to assess whether he needs to continue to be detained under Section 2.

Task

Please speak to him and obtain a history with the view of deciding whether he needs to be continued to be detained under Section 2.

CASC construct table

The CASC construct table is formatted such that candidates will be able to cover adequately both the range and the depth of the assessment required in this station.

Starting off: 'Hello, I am Dr Melvyn. I understand that you have been to the hospital today to look for one of the nurses and the police have since arrested you. Can we have a chat?'			
Assess current behaviour	Can you tell me why you are under police custody at this moment? What is your relationship with the nurse? What have you done to her thus far? Do you know her name? How do you feel towards her?	How much do you know about her? Do you know her number? If you do, how often do you call upon her? Would you resort to leaving a voice message if she did not respond to your call? Do you mind telling the contents of your voice message? Do you happen to know where she lives? How did you get to know about it?	Why did you need to take the above actions? Do you want to be close to her? From your view, how does your behaviour affect her daily life?
Risk assessment	Are you planning to do anything to the nurse? If so, would you mind telling me the details? Do you plan to harm her? If yes, what will you do? Is this part of your fantasy?	Have you ever applied force on her? What was her reaction? Did she defend herself? Will you do it again in the future?	Have you thought of harming yourself? Or are you so stressed with the current situation that you have had thoughts of ending your life? Has anyone tried to stop you from following her? If yes, what did you do? Do you carry a weapon? Will you use it to harm others who try to stop you?

(Continued)

Differentiation between types of stalker	Incompetent stalker: Did you encounter any difficulty having a relationship in the past? Does the nurse remind you of the unpleasant past? Rejected stalker: When you are ignored or rejected by the nurse, how do you feel? Do you feel that both of you were in a relationship? Do you hope to reconcile by following her?	Intimacy seekers and erotomania: Are you in love with her? Do you think she is in love with you? Do you think she will love you? How certain are you that she is in love with you? Could it be a misunderstanding? Do you have sexual feelings towards her? Resentful stalkers: Have you tried to frighten her? Are you taking revenge on her?	You have done a lot of following her. Do you feel stressed? Do you want to continue this behaviour? Have you thought of changing yourself? Do you think you need treatment?
Forensic and psychiatric history	Did you have trouble with the police in the past? If yes, what was the reason? Were you charged subsequently? Did you break any court order in the past? Have you seen a psychiatrist in the past?	How often do you drink? What kind of alcohol do you drink? What would you do if you were drunk? Do you also use any recreational drugs?	
Sectioning	Thanks for sharing with me the information. I will need to discuss this with the rest of the team.	In the meantime, I'm sorry to inform you that you might need to be detained under Section 2 of the Mental Health Act.	I understand that your relative is here. Could I speak to her?

Quick recall*

- In this condition, the person holds the delusional belief that someone, usually of a higher social or professional status or a famous personality or in some other way 'unattainable', is in love with him or her. The patient may make repeated attempts to contact that other person.
- Eventually, rejections may lead to animosity and bitterness on the part of the patient towards the object of attention.

---

* Adapted from B.K. Puri, A. Hall and R. Ho (2014). *Revision Notes in Psychiatry*. London, UK: CRC Press, p. 370.

- In hospital and outpatient clinical psychiatry, patients are more likely to be female than male, whereas in forensic psychiatry, male patients are commoner.
- Overall, females outnumber males.

Overview of delusional disorder

- According to *ICD-10*, a delusional disorder is an ill-defined condition, manifesting as a single delusion or a set of related delusions, being persistent, sometimes lifelong and not having an identifiable organic basis.
- There are occasional or transitory auditory hallucinations, particularly in the elderly.
- Delusions are the most conspicuous or only symptoms and are present for at least 3 months. For the diagnosis, there must be no evidence of schizophrenic symptoms or brain disease.
- *ICD-10* includes the previously used term 'late paraphrenia', although there is some evidence that there are differences between persistent delusional disorder and late paraphrenia.
- Magnetic resonance imaging (MRI) scans in a group of late-onset schizophrenics and late-onset delusional disorders showed that the lateral ventricle volumes in the delusional disorder patients were much greater than those of schizophrenics and almost twice those of controls.
- Mono-delusional disorders feature a stable, encapsulated delusional system, which takes over much of a person's life. The personality is preserved.
- There is a point prevalence of 0.03% and a lifetime risk of 0.05%–0.1%.
- The mean age of onset is 35 years for males and 45 years for females.
- Onset is usually gradual and unremitting in 62%.
- There is an equal sex ratio of sufferers.
- Sufferers are often unmarried, with high marital breakdown and low reproductive rates.
- Introverted, long-standing interpersonal difficulties might predispose individuals towards delusional disorder.
- Family history of psychiatric disorder but not that of delusional disorder or schizophrenia is a predisposing factor.
- There is evidence of minimal brain disorder in 16% of the patients.

STATION 141: SECTIONING – EXPLANATION TO RELATIVE

Information to Candidates

Name of patient: Mrs Templar

You have been tasked to speak to the patient's partner. She has turned up and demands to speak to you. She is quite upset that her husband has been detained against his will, and she is demanding an explanation.

Task

Please explain to her about the usage of the Mental Health Act. Please address all her concerns and expectations.

CASC construct table

The CASC construct table is formatted such that candidates will be able to cover adequately both the range and the depth of the assessment required in this station.

Starting off: 'Hello, I am Dr Melvyn. I understand that you have some concerns about your husband's condition. Can we have a chat?'			
Acknowledge distress, try to calm relative down and use reflective listening	I understand that you have some concerns about your husband's condition. Thanks for meeting up today.	I hope I will be able to take this opportunity to help address any of your concerns, particularly with regard to the fact that your husband is currently on section.	
Explain sectioning	Sectioning refers to having an individual admitted to a hospital despite their disagreement. Usually this is done under the Mental Health Act.	An individual could be sectioned if he or she is deemed to have a mental health condition which requires further assessment and treatment. At times, a section may be applied if there are threats to one's own health or the safety of others.	The section that your husband is currently on is Section 2. Section 2 requires the individual to be in the hospital for 28 days.
Explore whether the relative could appeal against the decision	I hear your concerns about having your husband in the hospital and that your husband is on a section.	Should you wish to appeal against this, you could do so via the mental health tribunal.	Otherwise, you could also approach the hospital managers.
Address other concerns	Do you have any other questions for me?		

Candidates are recommended to refer to the Royal College of Psychiatrists Mental Health leaflets on sectioning for further information.

STATION 142: OPPOSITIONAL DEFIANT DISORDER (ODD)

Information to candidates

Name of patient: Charlie

You are a general practitioner, and the parents of Charlie are here to see you. They tell you that their 11-year-old son, Charlie, is exhibiting difficult behaviour such as being disrespectful, spiteful and argumentative at home and school. His behaviour has started to concern his parents and teachers.

Task

Please take a history from the parents to establish a diagnosis. Please also perform a risk assessment.

CASC construct table

The CASC construct table is formatted such that candidates will be able to cover adequately both the range and the depth of the assessment required in this station.

Starting off: 'Hello, I am Dr Melvyn. I understand that you have some concerns about your son's condition. Can we have a chat?'			
Introduction	Thanks for taking time off today. I hope that I can make use of the time that we have to gather more information about your son.	With this information, it would help us in the formulation of the right diagnosis with regard to his condition.	
Symptoms of oppositional defiant disorder	Can you tell me more about how long he has been having these behavioural difficulties? Have they been there for 1 year or more? Does he annoy or argue with other people? Can you tell me more?	Does he tend to blame others for his mistakes? Have there been problems with assigning him tasks to do? Does he comply with the instructions that you have provided him with?	Does he seem to be always spiteful and angry towards yourselves? Does he routinely throw temper tantrums?
Symptoms of conduct disorder	Can I enquire more about other symptoms? Has there been a time in which he has violated the rights of other people or even animals, such as bullying or fighting with others? Has there been an occasion in which he has tortured animals?	Has he been involved in any vandalism acts? Has he ever set fire to properties around? Does he break rules at home or at school?	Has he been involved with the police before? Has he ever shoplifted, or used any weapons before? Has he been involved in truancy or any prior substance abuse?

(Continued)

Assess for risk factors and impact of ODD	Have there been difficulties previously with disciplining your child?	Has his behaviour had any impact on his academic grades? Has his behaviour had any impact on his interpersonal functioning?	Has his behaviour had any impact on your relationship (parental relationship)?
Assess for other risk factors	Has he done anything to harm himself before this?	Has he done anything recently that might result in harm towards others?	
Other relevant information	Can I know whether he has been seen by a psychiatrist before? Does he have any other conditions? Does he have attention deficit hyperactivity disorder (ADHD)? Does he also have learning difficulties?	Is there anyone in the family who has any mental health history that I need to know of?	
Summarize	Thanks for sharing more about his condition.	Based on my assessment, it seems like he has a condition known as oppositional defiant disorder.	Have you heard about it? Is it alright that we arrange another time in which I can discuss more about the condition with you?

Quick recall*

- Oppositional defiant disorder is defined as recurrent patterns of negativistic, hostile and disobedient behaviour towards authority figures for 6 months. The child should have at least four symptoms: losing temper, arguing with adults, refusing to comply with adults' requests, annoying others, being angry, actively defiant, blaming others for personal mistakes and showing spiteful behaviour.

Management

- Behaviour therapy: Discourage oppositional defiant behaviour and encourage appropriate and adaptive behaviour. Parents can coach them to develop adaptive responses.
- Individual psychotherapy: Restoration of self-esteem may lead to positive responses to external control.
- Parental training eliminating harsh and punitive parenting; increasing positive parent–child interactions.

---

* Adapted from B.K. Puri, A. Hall and R. Ho (2014). *Revision Notes in Psychiatry*. London, UK: CRC Press, p. 636.

- Prognosis: Two-thirds of the children with oppositional defiant disorder no longer meet the diagnostic criteria after 3 years. One-third of the children will develop conduct disorder.
- Children with early-onset, more severe symptoms and comorbidity of ADHD are three times more likely to progress to a diagnosis of conduct disorder.
- Being argumentative, non-compliant, rule-breaking and demonstrating spiteful hurtful behaviour predicts aggressive conduct disorder.
- Children with oppositional defiant disorder have a higher chance of developing mood disorders, anxiety disorders and substance abuse disorders in adolescence and adulthood.

STATION 143: SUICIDE RISK ASSESSMENT

Information to candidates

Name of patient: Sandra

You are the core trainee working in the accident and emergency department. Sandra has been brought into the emergency services again as she attempted suicide by jumping from a high precipice. She has been admitted to the emergency services two times earlier this month for self-harm.

Task

Please speak to her and take a history to assess her suicide attempt and assess for her current risk. Please also assess for depressive symptoms and obtain further relevant information.

CASC construct table

The CASC construct table is formatted such that candidates will be able to cover adequately both the range and the depth of the assessment required in this station.

Starting off: 'Hello, I am Dr Melvyn. I understand that you have just been brought into the emergency services by the police. Can we have a chat?'			
Enquiries about suicide attempt	I'm sorry to hear that you have been arrested by the police and brought into the hospital. I understand that you attempted to jump from a high precipice today. Can you tell me more about it? What precipitated you to do that?	Did you make any plans before doing it? Did you make any efforts to avoid discovery? Did you leave any suicide message or last note?	How were you discovered? Can you tell me more?

(Continued)

Assess for symptoms of depression and other relevant history	How has your mood been for the past 2 weeks? Have you experienced a loss of interest?	Do you have any difficulties with your sleep? How has your appetite been for you? Are you able to concentrate on your tasks?	Sometimes, when their mood is low, people do have other symptoms. Have you experienced any strange experiences, such as hearing things that are not there or seeing things that are not there? Is there a family history of suicide or self-harm? Does anyone in the family have depression?
Assess current suicide risk in the emergency	What is your view towards the suicide attempt? Do you regret it? Do you feel remorseful about it given that you are now in the hospital?	Do you still feel that life is not worth living? Do you still have thoughts of ending your life?	We might be able to organize some form of treatment for you. Will you be keen for that?
Assess for the cause of current suicide attempt and ongoing stress	Is there any ongoing stress that you are experiencing?		

This station is a variation of the commonly assessed suicide risk assessment station.

Please refer to the previous notes about suicide risk assessment.

STATION 144: ABNORMAL GRIEF REACTION

Information to candidates

Name of patient: Mr Brown

You are the core trainee working in local mental health service. You are about to see a 50-year-old patient who came to the clinic with his son's death certificate. The patient's 12-year-old son, Peter, passed away 8 months ago.

Task

Please take a history from the patient and assess the cause of death of the patient's son. Please assess the patient and decide if the patient suffers from normal or abnormal grief reaction.

CASC construct table

The CASC construct table is formatted such that candidates will be able to cover adequately both the range and the depth of the assessment required in this station.

Starting off: 'Hello, I am Dr Melvyn. Can we have a chat about how you have been?'			
Empathetic opening/ introduction and identification of the cause of death of son and exploration of events leading to death	Thanks for coming today. I'm sorry to learn about what has happened. I understand that it has been a very difficult time for you. I hope I can help understand you better and help you deal with what you're going through.	I'm sorry but I would like to understand more about what has happened. Can you tell me more?	What happened prior to the death of Peter? *(Use patient's son's name to demonstrate that you are empathetic towards his concerns).*
Inquiry about symptoms of normal grief reactions after Peter's death	Can you tell me how you felt when you learnt about the passing of your son?	How long did those feelings of shock last? Were there times in which you tried to search for him? Did you bargain spiritually as to why it had to be your son?	Was there a phase in which you went into denial whilst you were negotiating the death of your son? How long did these symptoms last?
Inquiry of symptoms of abnormal grief	Aside from the feelings that you have shared, were there other feelings that bothered you?	Have there been times in which you have been feeling that life is no longer worth living, and that you might be better off dead? Have you made any plans to join your son (or the deceased)? Do you feel extremely guilty for what has happened?	Sometimes, when people are going through a difficult time, they do have abnormal experiences. Have you had any unusual experiences? Have you heard voices when there was no one around? What have you done to your son's belongings? Have you kept them the way they used to be?
Establish the duration of grief symptoms	Can I check how long you have been feeling this way?	Have these feelings been persistent for more than 8 months?	

(Continued)

Assess symptoms of depression	Aside from you having low mood ever since the death of your son, have you had other difficulties? Do you have any difficulties with enjoying the things you used to enjoy?	How has your sleep been? Do you have difficulties with initiation of sleep or difficulties with maintaining sleep? Do you find yourself waking up much earlier than usual? How has your appetite been? Do you feel that you have enough energy to get through the day? Have you had any difficulties concentrating on daily activities?	Was there a time in which you felt that life was no longer worth living? Have you made any plans to end your life? Can you please tell me more? When was the last time you had such suicidal ideations?
Obtaining other relevant information	I'm sorry to hear that it has indeed been a very difficult time for you. Can you tell me how you have been coping? Are there other family members who have been supportive towards you?	How has the passing of your son affected your life in general? How was your relationship with your son? How has your relationship with your wife changed after your son's demise?	Have you seen a psychiatrist before? Is there anyone in your family who has a mental health history? Have you experienced other losses before?

Remember to ascertain risk factors for abnormal grief: enmeshed or ambivalent relationship with the deceased; sudden, traumatic and unexpected death of the deceased; poor social support; multiple previous bereavements and presence of previous psychiatric disorder.

Quick recall*

- Bereavement reactions or grief usually has three phases. The stunned phase lasts from a few hours to a few weeks. This gives way to the mourning phase, with intense yearning and autonomic symptoms. After several weeks, the phase of acceptance and adjustment takes over. Grief typically lasts about 6 months.

---

* Adapted from B.K. Puri, A. Hall and R. Ho (2014). *Revision Notes in Psychiatry*. London, UK: CRC Press, p. 381.

Atypical grief is divided by Parkes into the following:

- Inhibited grief: absence of expected grief symptoms at any stage
- Delayed grief: avoidance of painful symptoms within 2 weeks of loss
- Chronic grief: continued significant grief-related symptoms for 6 months

It is important to understand the differences between depression and bereavement. The following features are common in depression but not in bereavement:

- Active suicidal ideations
- Depressive symptoms that are out of proportion with loss
- Feelings of guilt not related to the decreased
- Marked functional impairment for longer than 2 months
- Marked psychomotor changes lasting more than a few days
- Preoccupation with worthlessness

Management

- Grief is usually managed in the outpatient setting, but the inpatient setting is indicated for patients at high suicide risk.
- Psychiatrist needs to assess and distinguish normal grief from abnormal grief.
- Grief work is supportive psychotherapy that allows expression of loss and its meaning and works through the issues. It also provides a secure base, identifies factors that block natural grief and addresses social isolation and spiritual issues.
- Family involvement and psychoeducation.
- If a psychotropic drug is indicated, careful dosing is required to avoid side effects. Maintenance treatment is required for severe prolonged grief.
- Rehabilitative efforts emphasize stage-appropriate tasks such as developing vocational and social skills.

STATION 145: BORDERLINE PERSONALITY DISORDER AND SUBSTANCE ABUSE

Information to candidates

Name of patient: Sharon

You are the core trainee working in a local mental health service. Sharon, a 30-year-old woman, comes to see you as she has cut her thighs and has been disturbed by recurrent thoughts of harming herself. She also admits that she has been using amphetamines on a regular basis.

Task

Please take a history from the patient and assess for borderline personality disorder. Please also explore with the patient more about her substance usage history.

CASC construct table

The CASC construct table is formatted such that candidates will be able to cover adequately both the range and the depth of the assessment required in this station.

Starting off: 'Hello, I am Dr Melvyn. Can we have a chat?'			
Introduction and using open-ended questions to start the interview, building rapport	Thanks for coming today.	I understand that you have been going through a tough time. Can you tell me more?	I'm sorry to hear that you've been cutting. Is there a reason for you to do so? Can you share with me more with regard to the stressors that you have been experiencing in life?
Symptoms of borderline personality disorder: chronic feeling of emptiness, unstable emotions, impulsive behaviour	How would you describe your personality? How do you usually cope when your relationships do not turn out well? How do you feel when your relationships end? Do you feel or worry about being abandoned, especially so in between relationships? How many relationships have you had now? How long does each relationship last for you?	Can you tell me how you feel about yourself and about your future? Some people do tell me that they have this feeling of chronic emptiness. Have you had such feelings and experiences before? How would you describe yourself? Do you think you are someone who is very impulsive? • drugs, excessive spending, car speeding, promiscuous sexual behaviour. Do you worry about your identity and purpose in life?	How has your mood been? Do you find that there is much fluctuation in your mood, especially in reaction to things around you? What do others say about your mood? With all these stressors that you have been enduring, has there been a time when you have had unusual experiences? By that I mean hearing voices or seeing things that are not there?
Suicide risk assessment	Can you tell me whether something similar to this has happened before? Previously, have you also cut yourself? When did this first start?	Have you done anything more serious than this? Have you made any attempts to end your life? Have you been hospitalized before for a suicide attempt? Can you tell me more?	Do you have thoughts currently that life is no longer worth living? Have you made any plans to end your life? Can you share with me more about the plans that you have made? What do you think would prevent you from doing so?

(Continued)

Assessment of effect of stimulants	Thanks for sharing with me more about your drug usage. Can you tell me when you first started using these drugs? How often have you been using them? How much do you use, and how do you use them?	How do you feel after using those amphetamines? Do you feel high and good? Do you feel that you have increased energy? Do you become more agitated?	Are you able to sleep after taking the amphetamines? Have you experienced any strange symptoms, such as paranoia, after consumption of the amphetamines?
Assessment withdrawal symptoms of stimulants	Can you tell me more about what happens if you do not use the amphetamines?	Do you feel low and depressed in your mood? Do you tend to feel tired and lethargic?	Do you overeat or oversleep? How was your interest during those periods?

If the patient injects drugs, you should offer to look at the sites of injection to assess any infection/abscess.

Quick recall*

- The prevalence of borderline personality disorder is 1%–2%.
- The gender ratio is 1:2 (males:females).
- The age of onset is usually during adolescence or early adulthood.
- The suicide rate is 9%.
- The ICD-10 classifies emotionally unstable personality disorder into impulsive and borderline type. The *Diagnostic and Statistical Manual of Mental Disorders,* 5th edition (*DSM-5*) does not propose the concept of emotionally unstable personality disorder and only has borderline personality disorder. The patient meets the general criteria for personality disorder if he or she presents at least three of the following symptoms of impulsive type:
  - Affect: tendency to outbursts of anger or violence with inability to control the resulting behavioural explosions and unstable and capricious mood.
  - Behaviour: marked tendency to act unexpectedly and without consideration of consequences, marked tendency of quarrelsome behaviour and conflicts with others, especially when impulsive acts are thwarted or criticized, and difficulty in maintaining any course of action that offers no immediate reward.

Elicit borderline personality disorder (key questions to ask):

- Do you have problems with your anger control? How often do you get into quarrels?
- How often do you feel empty inside of yourself? What do you do when you feel empty?

---

* Adapted from B.K. Puri, A. Hall and R. Ho (2014). *Revision Notes in Psychiatry.* London, UK: CRC Press, p. 443.

- How is your relationship with other people?
- How would you feel if your friend or partner left you? Do you have a strong feeling of abandonment?
- Do you think that your friends would view you as a moody person?
- How often do you hurt yourself? Why do you cut yourself? Do you want to re-experience the pain of the past?
- Commonly associated conditions includes depression, post traumatic stress disorder (PTSD), substance misuse and bulimia nervosa.

Management:

Inpatient treatment and therapeutic communities	Indications for admission: a. Life-threatening suicide attempt b. Imminent danger to other people c. Psychosis d. Severe symptoms interfering with functioning that are unresponsive to outpatient treatment Risk of hospitalizations include the following: a. Stigma b. Disruption of social and occupational roles c. Loss of freedom d. Hospital-induced behavioural regression
Psychotherapy	• Long-term inpatient psychotherapy is recommended because patients can handle challenges in their daily life with support from psychotherapists. • Dialectical behaviour therapy and mentalization-based therapy are recommended treatments for people with borderline personality disorder. • The NICE guidelines recommend that therapists should use an explicit and integrated approach and share this with their clients. • The guidelines also recommend that the therapists should set therapy at twice per week and should not offer brief interventions. • Supportive psychotherapy helps to diminish the suicidal behaviours and impulsive acts whilst awaiting a remission, since the long-term prognosis of the disorder is good. • CBT focuses on maladaptive cognitions about oneself and other people. Behaviour therapy improves social and emotional functioning. • Transference-focused therapy aims at correcting distorted perceptions of significant others and decreasing symptoms and self-destructive behaviour. • Family therapy is frequently offered to borderline adolescent patients and is regarded by many as the treatment of choice for these patients. • Social skills training.
Pharmacotherapy	• The psychiatrist can prescribe a selective serotonin reuptake inhibitor (SSRI, such as fluoxetine) to treat mood, rejection sensitivity and anger. If the second SSRI is not effective, the psychiatrist could consider adding on a low-dose antipsychotic for anger control and an anxiolytic for anxiety control. • Mood stabilizers such as sodium valproate medications can be added if the above-mentioned are not effective.

Course and prognosis:

- Impulsivity improves significantly over time. Affective symptoms have the least improvement.
- Poor prognosis is associated with early childhood sexual abuse, early first psychiatric contact, chronicity of symptoms, high affective instability, aggression and substance use disorder.

Information about amphetamines:

Psychotic-like states result from acute or chronic ingestion. It leads to paranoia, hallucination and sometimes a delirium-like state. The effect usually lasts for 3–4 days. In contrast to paranoid schizophrenia, amphetamine-induced psychosis is associated with visual hallucinations, appropriate affect, hyperactivity, hyper-sexuality and confusion. Thought disorder and alogia are not found in amphetamine-induced psychosis. It usually resolves with abstinence but may continue for some months. In the withdrawal state (or crash), the person will develop fatigue, hypersomnia, hyperphagia, depression and nightmares. Following chronic use, profound depression and fatigue occur. Long-term use leads to central nervous system (CNS) serotonergic neuronal destruction.

Child Psychiatry

STATION 146: SELF-HARM IN YOUNG PEOPLE

Information to candidates

Name of patient: Mary Jane

Mary Jane is a 16-year-old girl who has presented to the emergency room with repeated episodes of self-cutting. The medical student, who is on attachment to the emergency room, has spoken to her and is currently very concerned about her condition. He wishes to discuss the history he has obtained with you, the on-call resident.

Task

Please speak to the medical student and answer any questions he has about the patient.

CASC construct table

The CASC construct table is formatted such that candidates will be able to cover adequately both the range and the depth of the assessment required in this station.

Starting off: 'Hello, I am Dr Melvyn. I understand that you have some concerns about Mary Jane's condition. Can we have a chat?'

Differences between self-harm and suicide attempt	I understand that you have just spoken to Mary and have obtained a history from her. Are you able to give me a summary of the history you have obtained? Thanks for providing me with the summary of her condition.	Do you have any questions for me about her condition? It seems to me that you are concerned about the differences between suicide and self-harm.	Self-harm refers to an episode in which an individual injures or harms him- or herself on purpose and not by means of an accident. Such form of self-harm might include cutting oneself or even overdosing on common medications.
Explain how to perform a suicide risk assessment	We need to assess each individual who presents with a self-harm episode and determine their suicide risk. Apart from a clinical interview, there are questionnaires that we could use to help us.	We need to assess whether the attempt was premeditated and whether the individual had prior planning for the attempt. Usually, someone who has a strong will to end their life might also make prior arrangements, such as leaving a last note or making some last financial arrangement.	In addition, we need to gather more information about the attempt. Signs of a suicide attempt might include attempts made to conceal the attempt. In addition, we need to ascertain whether there are any protective factors that would mitigate against subsequent self-harm attempts.
Explain possible reasons leading to self-harm	No one knows the actual aetiology resulting in self-harm.	For some individuals, they self-harm as an attempt to gain more control. Some of them self-harm as an attempt to relieve the tension that they are experiencing.	For some individuals, however, it might be a precursor to a more serious attempt – suicide – as they might have underlying psychiatric disorders that need treatment.
Discuss possible differential diagnosis	Some of the possible differential diagnoses currently include an underlying depression.	Further history would be required in order for us to determine whether an individual has depression. Collateral information is necessary as well.	Some personality disorders such as borderline personality disorder are associated with a greater rate of self-harm as well.
Explain possible management	For every patient, we need to determine the element of risk and determine whether an inpatient admission is indicated.	If the individual does have an underlying psychiatric disorder, at times, medication can be started.	Talking therapies such as psychotherapy and CBT might also be helpful.

(Continued)

Emphasize the importance of family support	It is also important to engage the family members and encourage them to provide more support for the individual.		

Quick recall*

- With regard to childhood-onset suicide and self-harm, suicide is considered to be very rare in prepubertal children. It may be caused by accident, or the child may exhibit stereotyped movements to the extent that either causes physical injury or marked interference with normal activities for at least 1 month.
- With regard to adolescent-onset suicide and self-harm: 20,000 young people in England and Wales are referred to hospital for assessment of self-harm each year. The rate of attempted suicide is 8%–9% in Western countries. The rate of suicidal ideation is 15%–20%. Suicide is common amongst young people at the age of between 14 and 16 years. The male-to-female ratio for suicide is 4:1. Suicide is the third commonest cause of death for young people after accident and homicide. Self-harm is the most common cause of admission to a general hospital.
- Aetiological factors include psychiatric disorders. For girls, self-harm is strongly predicted by depressive disorder. For boys, self-harm is strongly predicted by previous suicide attempt. Family issues such as loss of a parent in childhood, family dysfunction, abuse and neglect are all predisposing factors.

There has been an increase in adolescence suicide as a result of the following:

- Factors influencing reporting (copycat suicides resulting from media coverage; the fostering of illusions and ideals through Internet suicide groups and pop culture)
- Factors influencing the incidence of psychiatric problems
- Social factors

The common self-harm and suicide methods include the following:

- Self-harm: Cutting and scratching are common impulsive gestures. Cutting often has a dysphoric reducing effect.
- Suicide: Self-poisoning is a common method used by British adolescents. Using firearms is more common in the United States.
- Management of self-laceration: Offer physical treatment with adequate anaesthesia. Do not delay psychosocial assessment. Explain the care process. For those who repeatedly self-poison, do not offer minimization advice on self-poisoning because there is no safe limit. For those who self-injure repeatedly, teach self-management strategies on superficial injuries, harm minimization techniques and alternative coping strategies.

---

* Adapted from B.K. Puri, A. Hall and R. Ho (2014). *Revision Notes in Psychiatry.* London, UK: CRC Press, p. 650.

- Management of suicidal adolescents: Consider inpatient treatment after balancing the benefits against loss of family support. Involve the young person in the admission process. Electroconvulsive therapy (ECT) may be used in adolescents with very severe depression and suicidal behaviour not responding to other treatments.
- Prognosis for self-harm: 10% will repeat in 1 year. Higher risk of repetition in older male adolescents, history of suicide attempts, persistent suicide ideation, psychotic symptoms, substance misuse and use of methods other than overdose or self-laceration.

STATION 147: BULLYING – PAIRED STATION A

Information to candidates

Name of patient: Johnny

You have been tasked to speak to the mother of an 8-year-old boy, Johnny. His mother is extremely worried about her son as she feels that his behaviour has changed drastically ever since he got transferred over to a new school. He has been reluctant to go to school and will often make up excuses for not going. His teachers have feedback that he has not been paying attention in class, keeps fidgeting and, at times, appears to be on edge.

Task

Please speak to his mother and take a history to come to a diagnosis. You might want to take notes as his father is also waiting to speak to you.

CASC construct table

The CASC construct table is formatted such that candidates will be able to cover adequately both the range and the depth of the assessment required in this station.

Starting off: 'Hello, I am Dr Melvyn. I understand that you have some concerns about your son's recent changes in behaviour. Can we have a chat?'			
Acknowledge mother's distress and calm her down	Thanks for coming today. I understand that you have some concerns about your son's condition. I hope that I could find out more from you to decide how best to help your son with his current condition.	I know that it has been difficult for you, given the acute changes in his behaviour ever since he has been enrolled in the new school.	Please rest assured that we will try our best to help him with his condition.

(Continued)

History of presenting complaint	Can you tell me more about his condition? What abnormalities have you noticed?	Thanks for sharing. I understand that he has been refusing to go to school. Did he tell you the reasons why he has been refusing?	Can you tell me more with regard to the feedback you have obtained from his teachers? What have they told you? Of importance, can I know whether he has had such behaviours before? Is this the very first time he is presenting as such?
Elicit possible stressors – bullying	I understand that he has just been to the new school for a month. Did he share with you any stressors arising from school? Any other changes in his life?	Sometimes, children may avoid school as they find themselves being picked on whilst at school. Has he ever been bullied before? Any friends to talk to?	Bullying could be verbal, physical and even emotional. Bullying is common and does occur. There is no isolated reason as to why some individuals are being bullied. If there is such a possibility, you could help by listening to your child and taking their comments seriously and trying to work out ways with your child and the school to solve the problem.
Rule out other psychiatric symptoms	Have you noticed if his mood has been low for the past 2 weeks or so? Is he still able to enjoy things that he used to enjoy?	How is his concentration like in school and at home? Does he complain that it is tough to get through a single day? Any deliberate self-harm episodes? What is his personality like?	How has his sleep been for him? What about his appetite? Has he told you that he has had any abnormal experiences? Did he ever tell you that he finds his life meaningless and that he no longer wishes to live?

Quick recall*

- It is important to understand the difference between the concepts of school refusal as well as that of truancy.

---

* Adapted from B.K. Puri, A. Hall and R. Ho (2014). *Revision Notes in Psychiatry*. London, UK: CRC Press, pp. 644–645.

- School refusal is the refusal to attend or stay at school because of anxiety and in spite of parental or other pressure.
- Boys and girls are usually equally represented. There are three main incidence peak ages:
  - Separation anxiety at the age of 5 years
  - At the age of 11 years, which may be precipitated by the change from junior to secondary schooling
  - At the age of 14–16 years, which may be a symptom of a psychiatric disorder, such as that of depression and social phobia
- Truancy is an important differential diagnosis. Truancy is ego-syntonic and intended.
- There is usually an associated history of antisocial personality disorder.
- It is usually associated with large family size.
- There is usually inconsistent discipline.
- Truancy is more common in adolescents than in younger children.
- Truancy is not associated with psychiatric symptoms but wilful intention to skip classes.
- Truant students are usually outside home and usually engaging in alternative activities. They usually have poor academic performance.

STATION 148: AUTISM

Information to candidates

Name of patient: Mr and Mrs Brown

You are the core trainee working in the child and adolescent service department. Mr and Mrs Brown are here to see you. Their 9-year-old son suffers from autism, and they are very stressed about the child's behaviour.

Task

Please take a history from the parents to elicit symptoms of autism in their child. Assess relevant behaviour problems and comorbidity associated with autism that might have contributed to parental stress.

CASC construct table

The CASC construct table is formatted such that candidates will be able to cover adequately both the range and the depth of the assessment required in this station.

Starting off: 'Hello, I am Dr Melvyn. I understand that you have some concerns about your son. Can we have a chat about it?'			
Introduction and establishing age of first onset of symptoms	I received some information that your son has been previously diagnosed with autism. I understand that it has been a difficult time for you recently in view of his behavioural difficulties. I hope that we could have a chat to allow me to have a better understanding of his problems, so that I can help you.	Can I check when your child was diagnosed with autism? Was it before the age of 3 years old? How was his language development when he was much younger? Can you tell me more? What was his language development like when he was 12, 18 and 24 months, respectively?	How was his motor development when he was younger? Were there any delays with regard to his motor development? Was he seen by any doctor back then? Any assessment done?
Elicit symptoms of abnormal reciprocal social interactions	Can you tell me more about his other symptoms? Was he able to reciprocate normal social interactions? Did you notice that there was a paucity or failure of normal eye gaze?	Was he able to form normal friendships? Did he have trouble making friends?	Was he able to share toys with other children in school? Did he have any imaginary play? Did he tend to play alone? Can you tell me more?
Elicit symptoms of abnormal communication	How were his communication skills when he was much younger? Were there any difficulties?	Was there a lack of development of spoken language?	Did he fail to sustain a normal conversation? If he was unable to, can you tell me more about the problems he faced?
Check for restricted, stereotyped and repetitive behaviour	Did you notice any other abnormalities? Were there some restricted and stereotyped and repetitive behaviour that you notice?	Was he preoccupied with parts of objects or only certain objects? Was he able to shift from one activity to another easily? Did he tend to get upset when people disrupted his routine?	Was he able to play like how other children would do so?
Lack of creativity and fantasy	Did his teachers provide any feedback about his behaviour?	Have they commented that he has had difficulties with others?	Did they also comment that he tends to lack creativity and fantasy in play?

(Continued)

Behavioural problems	I understand that he has been having difficult behaviours. I'm sorry that you have been having a relatively difficult time dealing with his problematic behaviours. Can you share more about them?	Does he have any sleep disturbances? Is he able to eat normally?	Does he engage in any forms of self-harm? Is he very aggressive? Can you tell me more?
Check for comorbidity	Does he have any other problems? Does he also have associated learning difficulties?	Does he have any other medical problems that I need to know of?	In particular, does he have epilepsy? Is he on medications for that?
Obtain other relevant information	Can I check whether there is a family history of any psychiatric disorder? Is there a family history of autism as well?	Aside from the doctor's assessment, has he been for other assessment and therapy? Can you tell me more?	Were there any problems during the pregnancy of this child? Any post-delivery complications?

The parent in this station may be very frustrated and feeling guilty with regard to the child. The parent may also be in denial of the diagnosis. Remember to address these issues during the interview, instead of merely focusing on eliciting the symptoms of autism.

Quick recall*

ICD-10 diagnostic criteria and clinical characteristics:

1. The presence of abnormal development that is manifested before the age of 3 years, including abnormal receptive or expressive language, abnormal selective or reciprocal social interaction and abnormal functional or symbolic play. Children with autism are often attached to odd objects and have a relative lack of creativity and fantasy in thoughts.
2. Abnormal reciprocal social interactions include failure in eye gaze and body language, failure in development of peer relationships, lack of socio-emotional reciprocity and lack of spontaneous sharing with other people.
3. Abnormal communication includes lack of development of spoken language, lack of social imitative play, failure to initiate or sustain conversational interchange and stereotyped and repetitive use of language. Their language usages are frequently associated with pronoun reversals. A child with autism may say, 'You want the pencil' when he means he wants it. Echolalia and palialia are common.
4. Restricted, stereotyped and repetitive behaviours include preoccupation with stereotyped interest, compulsive adherence to rituals, motor mannerisms and preoccupation with part-objects or non-functional elements of play materials. Some children with autism enjoy vestibular stimulations such as spinning and swinging.

---

* Adapted from B.K. Puri, A. Hall and R. Ho (2014). *Revision Notes in Psychiatry.* London, UK: CRC Press, p. 624.

5. Other nonspecific problems include phobias, sleeping and eating disturbances, temper tantrums and self-directed aggression and self-injury.
6. There should be an absence of other causes of pervasive developmental disorders, socio-emotional problems and schizophrenia-like symptoms.

Women's Mental Health and Perinatal Psychiatry

STATION 149: BIPOLAR DISORDER AND PREGNANCY

Information to candidates

Name of patient: Sandra

You have been tasked to speak to Sandra, who is a 32-year-old female. She has been diagnosed with bipolar disorder since the age of 25 and has been tried on multiple medications. She has been stabilized more recently on sodium valproate. She has not needed an admission to the inpatient unit for the past 2 years. She has been married for the past 5 years and is planning to start a family. She noticed that she has missed her regular menstrual cycle for the past month and suspects that she might be pregnant. She is concerned about her medications and how they might affect her baby.

Task

Please speak to Sandra and address all her concerns and expectations. Please do not perform a mental state examination.

CASC construct table

The CASC construct table is formatted such that candidates will be able to cover adequately both the range and the depth of the assessment required in this station.

Starting off: 'Hello, I am Dr Melvyn. I understand that you have some concerns. Can we have a chat?'			
Explore possibility of pregnancy	I understand that you have some concerns that you like to discuss today. I hope that we could make use of this opportunity to clarify any doubts that you might have. I also hope to be able to provide you with the appropriate advice.	From my understanding, you have not had your routine menstrual cycle for the past month. Has this happened before? Are you currently on any other medication aside from the medications that we have started you on?	I wonder whether you have consulted your obstetrics doctor. Has he or she done any investigations for you to ascertain whether there is a chance that you might be pregnant? Thanks for sharing with me. Congratulations on your pregnancy!

(Continued)

Explore medication options and advise alternatives and explanation of rationale for switch	One of the concerns we have is that sodium valproate is not safe in pregnancy. There is a chance that it might result in neurological defects in the baby, and hence it should not be used during pregnancy.	The risk of this happening is 1 in 100. We could observe your mood for now after discontinuation of the mood stabilizer. If you do have a manic relapse, we could start you on antipsychotics such as olanzapine. If the antipsychotic does not work out well for you, we could recommend that you undergo a course of ECT.	Some patients do experience low mood or have symptoms suggestive of bipolar depression instead. For those with milder symptoms, we recommend a course of talking therapy, such as CBT. Have you heard about this before? If your mood remains persistently low, we could consider starting you on other medications. Fluoxetine, an antidepressant, has the most evidence base and would be the safest choice in pregnancy.
Explain side effects of new medications	The possible side effects of olanzapine might include sedation as well as weight gain. We need to monitor this to avoid longer-term issues such as high blood pressure, raised cholesterol and diabetes mellitus.	For haloperidol, we do need to monitor carefully to see whether you develop any adverse side effects such as tremors and rigidity. Please do let us know should you feel very restless after the commencement of these medications.	
Explain side effects associated with other mood stabilizers	I understand that you are concerned as to why you cannot be maintained on any of the other mood stabilizers.	The usage of lithium during pregnancy would result in heart abnormalities.	The usage of carbamazepine as well as lamotrigine would also result in other birth defects, and hence we need to be careful with regard to their usage. I understand that I have provided you with a lot of information. Please let me know if you have any other questions for me.

Quick recall*

The NICE and Maudsley's guidelines recommend the following:

- Treat with an antipsychotic if patient has an acute mania or if she is stable.
- Consider ECT or mood stabilizer if the patient does not respond to an antipsychotic.
- If lithium is used, the woman should undergo level 2 ultrasound of the foetus at 6 and 18 weeks of gestation.
- If carbamazepine is used, prophylactic vitamin K should be administered to the mother and neonate after delivery.
- The treatment of bipolar depression follows the recommendation of treatment for depression.

Drug choices for bipolar disorder in pregnancy:

- The risk of relapse is high if medication is stopped suddenly.
- Lithium: The incidence of Ebstein's anomaly is between 0.05% and 0.1% after maternal exposure to lithium in the first trimester.
- Valproate: Incidence of foetal birth defect (mainly neural tube defect) is 1 in 100.
- Carbamazepine: Incidence of foetal birth defect is 3 in 100.
- For mania: Haloperidol and olanzapine are indicated during pregnancy; ECT is indicated if antipsychotic fails.
- For bipolar depression: CBT is indicated for moderate bipolar depression. Fluoxetine has the most data on safety and is indicated for severe bipolar depression, especially for those patients with very few previous manic episodes.
- Valproate is the most teratogenic mood stabilizer and should not be combined with other mood stabilizers.
- Lamotrigine requires further evaluation because it is not routinely used in pregnancy. It could result in oral cleft (9 in 1000) and Stevens–Johnson syndrome in infants.

STATION 150: POSTNATAL DEPRESSION

Information to candidates

Name of patient: Amy

You are the core trainee working in the accident and emergency department. Amy gave birth 2 months ago. She needs to work and look after her baby daughter. She feels very stressed and exhausted. She has not gone to work for few days and cannot be contacted. Her supervisor called the police, and the police stopped her from hanging herself. She was sent to the emergency department.

---

* Adapted from B.K. Puri, A. Hall and R. Ho (2014). *Revision Notes in Psychiatry*. London, UK: CRC Press, p. 561.

Task

Please speak to her and take a history to establish the psychiatric diagnosis. Please also perform a relevant risk assessment.

CASC construct table

The CASC construct table is formatted such that candidates will be able to cover adequately both the range and the depth of the assessment required in this station.

Starting off: 'Hello, I am Dr Melvyn. I understand that you have just been brought into the emergency services by the police. Can we have a chat?'			
Introduction and checking for symptoms of postnatal depression and its impact on the care on the baby	I received some information about you. Can we have a chat so that I can understand you better and consider how best to help you? I know that it has been a very difficult time for you, but I hope that I can do my best to help. I understand that you have just recently given birth. Can you tell me more? What is the name of your baby? Was this your first pregnancy?	How has your mood been? How long have you been feeling this way? How has your energy been? Do you find yourself having enough energy to get through a day? How has your sleep been for you? What about your appetite? Is your sleep disturbed by your baby?	Can you concentrate on caring for your baby? Have you been feeling worthless and helpless? Do you feel that you are worthless as a mother?
Assess for symptoms for postpartum psychosis	Sometimes when one's mood is low, it is not uncommon for one to experience unusual experiences. Have you had those experiences before? By that I mean have you heard voices when no one is there or seen anything unusual?	Do you feel that there is something wrong with your baby? Do you feel that others are out there to harm you? Do you feel that others are plotting against you?	Has there been a time in which you find yourself being more irritable in your mood? When did this happen? What was your sleep like then? What about your energy levels?
Assess for risk factors of postnatal depression	Can you tell me more about your pregnancy? Was it a planned pregnancy or was it entirely unplanned?	Were there any problems during the pregnancy or the delivery? Were there problems during the confinement period?	Has your partner been supportive? Is he helping out in caring for your child? How do you feel towards your baby?

(Continued)

Assess for risk issues	Can you tell me more about what happened today that led to the police arresting you? Did you make any plans before this? Did you leave a suicide note? Did you take any actions to avoid discovery?	Have you had thoughts of doing anything to harm your child or baby? Can you tell me who has been helping you to care for your child? Have there been times when you neglect the care of your baby (feeding, etc.)? How about pinching/hitting the baby?	Do you still have thoughts that life is no longer worth living now that you are here in the emergency department? How have you coped with your stress so far? Have you been neglecting your own health and personal care too?
Other relevant information	Can I know whether you have seen a psychiatrist before? Is there anyone in the family who has a mental health history?	Have you used any alcohol or substances like drugs to help you cope with your mood symptoms?	Is there anyone else who is able to provide you with some support?

It is important to ascertain the number of children the patient has. Do not assume that this is her first child (especially when this is not specified in the stem of the question). Also check if she is planning for another baby now.

Remember to ask for the name of the baby early in the interview. This helps to personalize the interview and improves empathy.

Risk assessments towards the baby, others and to self must be fully explored.

Quick recall*

- Postnatal depression is a depressive illness not significantly different from non-psychotic depression in other settings.
- It is characterized by low mood, with reduced self-esteem, tearfulness, anxiety, particularly about the baby's health, and an inability to cope. Mothers may experience reduced affection for their baby and may have difficulty with breastfeeding.
- Common symptoms seen in the mother include irritability, tearfulness, poor sleep and tiredness, feeling inadequate as a mother and loss of confidence in mothering.
- Common symptoms related to the care and safety of the baby: anxieties about the baby's health and expressing concerns that the baby might be malformed and does not belong to her. There might also be reluctance to feed or handle the baby. 40% of patients do have thoughts of harming the baby.

Management

- The education of health visitors and midwives is necessary to identify cases early.
- The Edinburgh Postnatal Depression Scale is a 10-item self-report questionnaire, used by health visitors to identify postnatal depression during the course of their normal contacts with new mothers.

---

* Adapted from B.K. Puri, A. Hall and R. Ho (2014). *Revision Notes in Psychiatry*. London, UK: CRC Press, pp. 567–568.

- Nondirective counselling by health visitors individually or in groups is effective in one-third of the cases. Self-help groups and mother-and-baby groups are useful to combat isolation.
- In those with more severe symptoms or those unresponsive to counselling, antidepressant is indicated.
- If depression is severe, admission, preferably with the baby to a mother-and-baby unit, may be required.
- Suicidal mothers may have thoughts of taking their babies with them, so questions about the safety of the child would form part of the normal assessment of mothers of young children.
- ECT may be required, particularly if worthlessness, hopelessness and despair are present.
- Breastfeeding should not be routinely suspended.

Psychotherapies

STATION 151: PSYCHOTHERAPY – COGNITIVE ANALYTICAL THERAPY

Information to candidates

Name of patient: Mr Charlie Wayne

You have been tasked to speak to Mr Charlie Wayne, who is a 40-year-old male. He has been recently diagnosed with depression. He has previously responded to a course of antidepressants and interpersonal therapy. He is currently not keen to try medications again as it previously caused him some side effects such as sexual dysfunction. You have discussed his case with your consultant. In view of him having mild-to-moderate depression, the consultant has suggested that he could potentially be considered for cognitive analytical therapy.

Task

Please speak to Mr Wayne and explain to him what this form of therapy involves. Please address all his concerns and expectations.

CASC construct table

The CASC construct table is formatted such that candidates will be able to cover adequately both the range and the depth of the assessment required in this station.

Common pitfalls

a. Failure to cover the range and depth of the information required for this station

Starting off: 'Hello, I am Dr Melvyn. Can we have a chat with regard to the possible treatment options that we would like to recommend for you?'			
Clarification of the differences between interpersonal therapy and cognitive analytical therapy	I understand that you have previously been through both CBT and had a trial of antidepressant. Cognitive analytical therapy is different from the interpersonal therapy that you underwent before.	Cognitive analytical therapy focuses more on specific patterns of thinking and much less on interpersonal behaviour. It also does not focus on interpretations of transference as well.	
Explain common indications	Depression is just one of the conditions that are indicated.	Other conditions include neurotic disorder, personality disorders as well as individuals who have prior self-harm attempts.	
Provide an overview of the therapy process	The therapy involves the identification of traps and dilemmas as well as snags.	Traps refer to repetitive cycle of behaviour and their consequences that perpetuate on. Dilemma refers to false choices or unduly narrowed options.	Snag refers to extreme pessimism about the future, which typically stops a plan before it even starts.
Address any other concerns	Do you have any other questions for me?	Well, the duration of the therapy would usually last between 16 and 24 sessions.	

Quick recall*

- Cognitive analytical therapy (CAT) aims at changing maladaptive procedural sequences. CAT focuses on specific patterns of thinking and less on interpersonal behaviour. CAT focuses less on transference interpretation.
- The indications include neurotic disorders, personality disorder (such as borderline personality disorder), depression, deliberate self-harm and abnormal illness behaviour.
- Techniques include the following: Use open questioning and descriptive reframing during the assessment. Formulate a procedural sequence model. The model tries to understand the aim-directed action (e.g., formulate an aim, evaluate environmental plans, plan actions and evaluate results of actions).

Identify faulty procedures:

- Traps: Repetitive cycles of behaviour and their consequences become perpetuated.
- Dilemma: false choice or unduly narrowed options.
- Snag: extreme pessimism about the future and halting a plan before it even starts.

---

* Adapted from B.K. Puri, A. Hall and R. Ho (2014). *Revision Notes in Psychiatry*. London, UK: CRC Press, pp. 339–340.

- Write a re-formulation letter that begins with a narrative account of the client's life story and identifies repetitive maladaptive patterns. The letter also contains a diagram that illustrates the reciprocal roles between the client and procedural sequences model.
- Change maladaptive procedural sequences and predict the likely transference and countertransference feelings. Enactments become active during sessions.
- Towards termination, the therapist will issue a goodbye letter to the client that summarizes the progress and achievement of the therapy. The client also issues a goodbye letter to the therapist.
- Duration: 16–24 weeks.

Consultation Liaison Psychiatry

STATION 152: POST-CONCUSSION SYNDROME

Information to candidates

Name of patient: Mr Brown

You are the core trainee working in local mental health service. You are about to see a 45-year-old man, who comes to see you today because he has injured his head after he was assaulted by another man in a pub.

Task

Please take a brief history from the patient to assess post-concussion syndrome. Please also perform an appropriate risk assessment. Please also perform appropriate cognitive tasks.

CASC construct table

The CASC construct table is formatted such that candidates will be able to cover adequately both the range and the depth of the assessment required in this station.

Starting off: 'Hello, I am Dr Melvyn. Can we have a chat about how you have been?'			
Introduction and exploration of history relating to head injury	I'm sorry to learn that you have sustained a head injury recently. It must have been a very difficult time for you.	I'm sorry but can you tell me more about what happened that day? What injury did you sustain? Was there a period in which you actually blacked out? Was there a period of amnesia before or after the injury? Were you hospitalized? Any brain imaging done?	How were things after the injury?

(Continued)

Assessment of neurological symptoms	Recently, have you had any bodily symptoms after your head injury?	Have you ever had headache or giddiness?	Have you ever had tinnitus?
Assessment of psychiatric symptoms	How has your mood been since the head injury?	Do you find yourself being low in mood? Do you find yourself being anxious for no reason?	Have others commented that you appear to be more irritable than usual? Do you find yourself sensitive to noise/ lights around you?
Assessment of cognitive symptoms	How do you find your memory ever since the time you sustained the head injury?	Do you find yourself having difficulties with concentration? Do you find yourself having difficulties with your attention?	Are there difficulties with your short-term memory? Do you find yourself having problems recalling things in the past?
Risk assessment	As a result of your head injuries, have you had difficulties with walking? Have you sustained any falls recently?	Has there been a time in which you have forgotten to turn off the stove or left the fire on?	
Brief cognitive examination	I would like to spend the next few minutes assessing your memory. Would that be alright for you?	Candidates are to do the following tasks: Assess registration of three items: competency to perform serial 7 or WORLD backwards; verbal fluency and competency to assess recall of three items.	

Quick recall*

- Post concussion syndrome (PCS) occurs after minor head injury.
- PCS is associated with premorbid physical and social problems. It usually lasts from several weeks to 3 months and is more likely to be persistent in women.
- Common physical symptoms include headache, nausea and sensitivity to light and noise.
- Common psychological symptoms include cognitive impairment, poor concentration and irritability.

Acknowledgements

Some of these stations have been contributed jointly by Dr. Cheow Enquan (MBBS, MRCPsych), specialist registrar, Institute of Mental Health, Singapore.

---

* Adapted from B.K. Puri, A. Hall and R. Ho (2014). *Revision Notes in Psychiatry*. London, UK: CRC Press, p. 499.

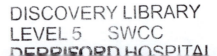

INDEX

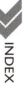